Plague and the End of Antiquity

Plague was a key factor in the waning of Antiquity and the beginning of the Middle Ages. Eight centuries before the Black Death, a pandemic of plague engulfed the lands surrounding the Mediterranean Sea and eventually extended as far east as Persia and as far north as the British Isles. It persisted sporadically from 541 to 750, the same period that witnessed the distinctive shaping of the Byzantine Empire, a new prominence of the Roman papacy and of monasticism, the beginnings of Islam and the meteoric expansion of the Arabic Empire, the ascent of the Carolingian dynasty in Frankish Gaul, and, not coincidentally, the beginnings of a positive work ethic in the Latin West.

In this volume, twelve scholars using history, archaeology, epidemiology, and molecular biology have produced a comprehensive account of the pandemic's origins, spread, and mortality, as well as its economic, social, political, and religious effects. The historians' sources are in Arabic, Syriac, Greek, Latin, and Old Irish. The archaeologists' sources include burial pits, abandoned villages, and aborted building projects. The epidemiologists use the written sources to track the disease's means and speed of transmission, the mix of vulnerability and resistance it encountered, and the patterns of reappearance over time. Finally, molecular biologists, newcomers to this kind of investigation, have become pioneers of paleopathology, seeking ways to identify pathogens in human remains from the remote past.

Lester K. Little is Dwight W. Morrow Professor Emeritus of History at Smith College and former Director of the American Academy in Rome. He is a past President of the Medieval Academy of America and also of the International Union of Institutes of Archaeology, Art History, and History in Rome. He is the author of *Benedictine Maledictions: Liturgical Cursing in Romanesque France* and *Religious Poverty and the Profit Economy in Medieval Europe*.

D1550830

Plague and the End of Antiquity

The Pandemic of 541–750

Edited by
LESTER K. LITTLE

Cambridge University Press in association with
The American Academy in Rome

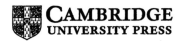

CAMBRIDGE
UNIVERSITY PRESS

CAMBRIDGE UNIVERSITY PRESS
Cambridge, New York, Melbourne, Madrid, Cape Town, Singapore, São Paulo, Delhi

Cambridge University Press
32 Avenue of the Americas, New York, NY 10013-2473, USA

www.cambridge.org
Information on this title: www.cambridge.org/9780521718974

First published 2007
Reprinted 2007 (twice), 2008
First paperback edition 2007
Reprinted 2009

Printed in the United States of America

A catalog record for this publication is available from the British Library.

Library of Congress Cataloging in Publication Data

Plague and the end of antiquity : the pandemic of 541–750 / edited by
Lester K. Little.
p. cm.
Includes bibliographical references and index.
ISBN-13: 978-0-521-84639-4 (hardback)
ISBN-10: 0-521-84639-0 (hardback)
1. Plague – Europe – History – To 1500. 2. Plague – Byzantine Empire – History –
To 1500. I. Little, Lester K.
[DNLM: 1. Plague – history – Byzantium. 2. Plague – history – Europe.
3. Disease Outbreaks – history – Byzantium. 4. Disease Outbreaks – history – Europe.
5. History, Medieval – Byzantium. 6. History, Medieval – Europe. WC 350 P6975 2007]
RA644.P7P39 2007
614.5'732–dc22 2006009895

ISBN 978-0-521-84639-4 hardback
ISBN 978-0-521-71897-4 paperback

Contents

IV THE LATIN WEST

V THE CHALLENGE OF EPIDEMIOLOGY
AND MOLECULAR BIOLOGY

Contributors

Ann Dooley is Professor of Celtic Studies at the University of Toronto. She received her Ph.D. from that university, co-founded the Celtic Studies Program there, and now teaches both there and at the Centre for Medieval Studies. She is the author of *Playing the Hero: Reading the Early Irish Saga Táin Bó Cuailnge* (2006).

Jo N. Hays is Professor of History at Loyola University of Chicago. His recent publications include: *The Burdens of Disease: Epidemics and Human Response in Western History* (1998); "Disease as Urban Disaster: Ambiguities and Continuities," in G. Massard-Guilbard et al., eds., *Cities and Catastrophes: Coping with Emergency in European History* (2002); and *Epidemics and Pandemics: Their Impacts on Human History* (2005).

Hugh N. Kennedy is Professor of Middle Eastern History at the University of Saint Andrews. His publications include *The Early Abbasid Caliphate: A Political History* (1981), *Muslim Spain and Portugal: A Political History of al-Andalus* (1996), *Armies of the Caliphs: Military and Society in the Early Islamic State* (2001), and *The Prophet and the Age of the Caliphates: The Islamic Near East from the Sixth to the Eleventh Century,* 2nd ed. (2004).

Michael Kulikowski is Associate Professor at the University of Tennessee, Knoxville. He is the author of *Late Roman Spain and Its Cities* (2004) and co-editor of *Hispania in Late Antiquity: Current Approaches* (2005). In 2005–6 he held the Solmsen Fellowship at the Institute for Research in the Humanities at the University of Wisconsin.

Lester K. Little is Dwight W. Morrow Professor Emeritus of History at Smith College, former Director of the American Academy in Rome, and a past

President of the Medieval Academy of America. His books include *Liberty, Charity, Fraternity: Lay Religious Confraternities at Bergamo in the Age of the Commune* (1988), *Benedictine Maledictions: Liturgical Cursing in Romanesque France* (1993), and, with Barbara H. Rosenwein, *Debating the Middle Ages: Issues and Readings* (1998).

John Maddicott is Fellow and Tutor in Medieval History at Exeter College, Oxford. A Fellow of the British Academy, he is the author of *Thomas of Lancaster, 1307–22* (1970), *Simon de Montfort* (1994), and numerous articles on Anglo-Saxon history and on English history of the thirteenth and fourteenth centuries.

Michael McCormick is the Goelet Professor of Medieval History at Harvard University. His most recent book, *Origins of the European Economy: Communication and Commerce, A.D. 300–900* (2001), won the Haskins Medal of the Medieval Academy of America. In 2002, he received a Distinguished Achievement Award from the Andrew W. Mellon Foundation, which he is applying to explore the intersection of the natural sciences and archaeology in the historical investigation of the later Roman Empire and the early Middle Ages.

Michael G. Morony is Professor of History at the University of California, Los Angeles. His publications include *Iraq After the Muslim Conquest* (1984) and *Between Civil Wars: The Caliphate of Mū'āwiyah* (1987), the latter being his translation of a ninth-century work on the period from 661 to 680.

Robert Sallares is a Research Fellow in the Institute of Science and Technology and Department of Biomolecular Sciences at the University of Manchester. He is the author of *The Ecology of the Ancient Greek World* (1991) and *Malaria and Rome: A History of Malaria in Ancient Italy* (2002).

Peter Sarris is University Lecturer in Early Medieval History at the University of Cambridge and a Fellow of Trinity College. He is also an external Fellow of All Souls College, Oxford. He has published *Economy and Society in the Age of Justinian* (2006).

Dionysios Stathakopoulos is a Research Fellow at King's College, London. He studied Byzantine and medieval history at the Westfälische Wilhelms-Universität in Münster and received his doctorate at the University of Vienna. He is the author of *Famine and Pestilence in the Late Roman and Early Byzantine Empire: A Systematic Survey of Subsistence Crises and Epidemics* (2004).

Alain J. Stoclet is Maître de Conférences at the University of Lyons II – Lumière and a Research Fellow of the National Center for Scientific Research, working with a group on the history and archaeology of the medieval Christian and Muslim worlds. He is the author of *Autour de Fulrad de Saint-Denis (v. 710–784)* (1993) and *Immunes ab omni teloneo. Études de diplomatique, de philologie et d'histoire sur l'exemption de tonlieux au Haut Moyen Age et spécialement sur la Praeceptio de navibus* (1999).

Preface

Plague helped carry out Antiquity and usher in the Middle Ages. Eight centuries before the Black Death did its part to carry out the Middle Ages and usher in the Renaissance, a similar pandemic of plague engulfed the lands surrounding the Mediterranean Sea and eventually extended as far east as Persia and as far north as the British Isles. Its sporadic appearances persisted from 541 to 750, the same period that witnessed the distinctive shaping of the Byzantine Empire, a new prominence of monasticism and of the Roman papacy, the gradual Christianizing of the Celtic and Germanic peoples, the beginnings of Islam, the rapid accumulation of the Arabic Empire, the ascent of the Carolingian dynasty in Frankish Gaul, and, not coincidentally, the beginnings of a positive work ethic in the Latin West.

Twelve specialists have here combined history, archaeology, epidemiology, and molecular biology to produce a comprehensive account of the pandemic's origins, spread, and mortality, as well as its economic, social, political, and religious effects. The historians' sources are written in Arabic, Syriac, Greek, Latin, and Old Irish. The archaeologists' finds include burial pits, abandoned villages, and aborted building projects. The epidemiologists use the written sources to track the disease's means and speed of transmission, the mix of vulnerability and resistance it encountered, and the patterns of its comings and goings. And molecular biologists, newcomers to this kind of investigation, have become pioneers of paleo- or archeopathology, seeking ways to identify the pathogens in human remains from the remote past.

Given the vast scope and interdisciplinary demands of the subject, the time is not yet ripe for a lone author to undertake a continuous and fully integrated narrative of this 210-year pandemic, yet it is far clearer today than it was back in 1999 when a small group of colleagues assembled at the American Academy in Rome to plan a conference that would bring together the top specialists in various aspects of the pandemic's history. These colleagues were Lawrence I. Conrad, at the time a professor at the Wellcome Institute for the History of Medicine in London, an expert on disease and medicine in early Islam; Evelyne Patlagean, professor of Byzantine social and economic history at the University of Paris X – Nanterre; Barbara H. Rosenwein, professor of history at Loyola University of Chicago, a specialist in early medieval European social and religious history; and David Whitehouse, the director of the Corning Museum of Glass, a Roman archaeologist and glass specialist whose work has focused on the late antique–early medieval period. Our conversations over three days gave us a broad view – available nowhere in print – of the pandemic of 541–750 and laid the groundwork for a conference eventually held at the American Academy in Rome in December 2001. The guidelines set down for the conference specified that the disciplines of history, archaeology, and epidemiology be represented, and that the major linguistic-cultural groups in which the historical documentation was written be represented.

Three holdovers from the planning group, Lawrence Conrad, David Whitehouse, and I took part in the conference. Among the others who participated was a specialist in the role of epidemics in human history, Jo N. Hays of Loyola University of Chicago. For the archaeology and history of Syria, Hugh Kennedy of St. Andrews and Michael Morony of UCLA joined us. Two Byzantinists, Dionysios Stathakopoulos, then at the University of Vienna, and Peter Sarris from Cambridge, the former placing greater emphasis on the written sources, the latter on material remains, also took part. For the Latin West, we had the participation of Alain Stoclet of the University of Lyons II on Frankish Gaul, Michael Kulikowski of the University of Tennessee on Visigothic Spain, and John Maddicott of Oxford on Anglo-Saxon England.

Also present was Michel Drancourt, the lead author of a study published in 1998 by a team of scholars at Marseilles who succeeded in identifying the plague pathogen in human remains from burial pits dating from two well-documented plague epidemics in Provence, those of 1720 and 1590. M. Drancourt gave a detailed explanation of the procedures followed in that pioneering study. In addition, another experienced practitioner of paleopathology, Robert Sallares of the University of Manchester, participated. A classicist who became a microbiologist with a vast knowledge of epidemiology, he analyzed some human remains found in a dig at Lugnano, about sixty kilometers north of Rome. The director of that dig, David Soren of the University of Arizona, dated those burials to the middle of the fifth century AD, and Dr. Sallares identified the cause of death as malaria, the first such positive identification of malaria in remains from Antiquity. Lastly, Michael McCormick of Harvard, a historian equally at home in the Greek East and the Latin West, one moreover, like Hugh Kennedy, Michael Kulikowski, and John Maddicott, particularly well versed in archaeology, and whose major concern at the time was the totality of the means of communication in the Mediterranean Basin, rounded out the conference by indicating the way to a molecular history of the pandemic.

Apart from the conclusions of substance reached at that gathering, it became clear, with regard to method, that future study of this subject should be conducted with a full awareness, in even the most minute of local studies, of the pandemic's vast temporal and geographic range, and that historians and archaeologists need to keep abreast of the latest developments in epidemiology and molecular biology, precisely the areas that have made the most significant advances in recent years.

Eleven of the papers presented in Rome became essays in this book; the twelfth essay, that by Ann Dooley of the University of Toronto on Ireland, is a later addition. Lawrence Conrad, Michel Drancourt, and David Whitehouse chose not to have their papers included, which is unfortunate given the valuable contributions they made to the conference. Works by all three, though, are cited herein and are listed in the bibliography. Moreover, a brief section on the Arabic sources, culled mainly from earlier publications by Prof. Conrad, appears in the first of the introductory essays. Just one essay in this book is a reprint of a previous publication, that of John Maddicott on England, which appeared in *Past and Present* in 1997. That article was at once so fresh and so thorough that the fact of its prior publication not only did not disqualify it for inclusion here but rendered Dr. Maddicott's involvement in both the conference and this publication imperative. It is thus a pleasure to acknowledge with gratitude the permission to reprint it granted by the Past and Present Society.

Thanks are also owed to Jessie and Charles Price and the Howard Gilman Foundation for generous grants in support of this project, the latter facilitated by the foundation's former Director, Dr. James A. Smith, and one of its trustees, the late Hon. Marcello Guidi, as well as the Vice President for Development of the American Academy in Rome, Elizabeth

Gray Kogen. The Academy's President, Adele Chatfield-Taylor, backed the project enthusiastically from start to finish. The conference benefited greatly from the organizing skills of Milena Sales, as did the notes and bibliography of this volume from the editorial skills of Maggie Hanson and Kristina Giannotta.

Lester K. Little

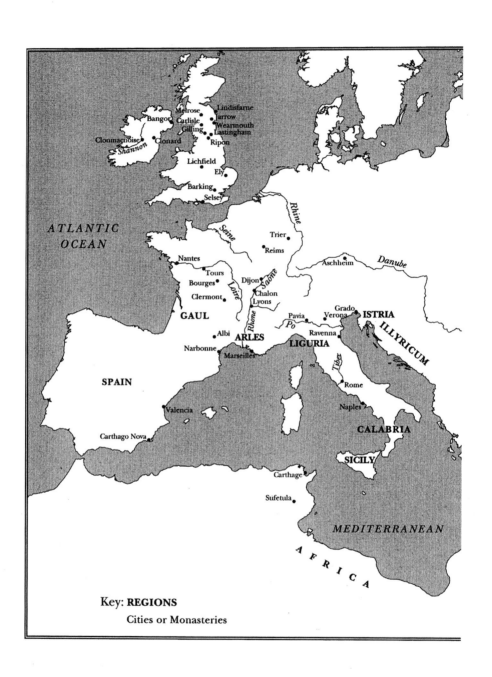

Melrose
Lindisfarne
Bangor
Carlisle
Jarrow
Gilling
Wearmouth
Lastingham
Clonmacnoise
Clonard
Ripon

Shannon

Lichfield
Ely

Barking
Selsey

ATLANTIC
OCEAN

Rhine

Seine

Trier
Reims

Nantes

Aschheim

Danube

Tours
Bourges

Dijon
Saône

Clermont

Loire

Chalon
Lyons

GAUL

Rhône

Pavia
Grado
Verona
ISTRIA

ILLYRICUM

Po

Ravenna

Albi
ARLES

LIGURIA

Narbonne

Marseilles

Tiber

SPAIN

Rome

Valencia

Naples

Carthago Nova

CALABRIA

SICILY

Carthage

Sufetula

MEDITERRANEAN

A F R I C A

Key: **REGIONS**

Cities or Monasteries

Presence of Plague between 541 and 750

This map shows only places specifically mentioned in the sources as having been struck by plague at least once during the pandemic, although many of them were, of course, struck several times. Overall, it bears the imprint of the Roman Empire, with two exceptions: one being Ireland, which was brought into frequent contact with Britain and the Continent by missionaries starting in the fifth century; and the other being Persia, which lay beyond a border that was frequently traversed in the sixth, seventh, and eighth centuries by Byzantine, Persian, and eventually Arab armies. The place names on the map refer either to regions (whether areas, provinces, whole countries, or the like) or to cities, except for those in the British Isles, where only monasteries are specifically cited as being hit by plague, and where the inclusion of Carlisle is meant to refer not to the city but to an unnamed monastery near it.

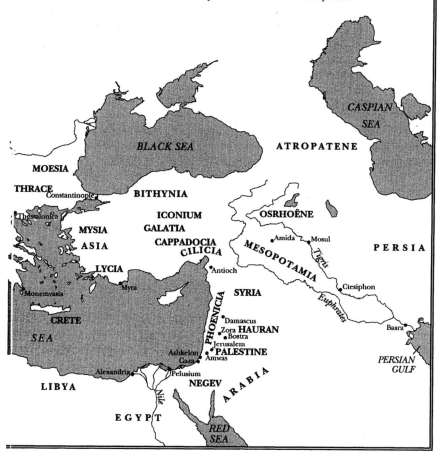

Plague and the End of Antiquity

I

INTRODUCTION

1

Life and Afterlife of the First Plague Pandemic

Lester K. Little

In the summer of 541 AD a deadly infectious disease broke out in the
Egyptian port city of Pelusium, located on the eastern edge of the Nile
delta. It quickly spread eastward along the coast to Gaza and westward to
Alexandria. By the following spring it had found its way to Constantinople, capital of the Roman Empire. Syria, Anatolia, Greece, Italy, Gaul,
Iberia, and North Africa: none of the lands bordering the Mediterranean
escaped it. Here and there, it followed river valleys or overland routes and
thus penetrated far into the interior, reaching, for example, as far east as
Persia or as far north, after another sea-crossing, as the British Isles.[1]

The disease remained virulent in these lands for slighty more than
two centuries, although it never settled anywhere for long. Instead, it
came and went, and as is frequently the case with unwelcome visitors, its
appearances were unannounced. Overall, there was not a decade in the
course of those two centuries when it was not inflicting death somewhere
in the Mediterranean region. In those places where it appeared several
times, the intervals between recurrences ranged from about six to twenty
years. And then, in the middle of the eighth century, it vanished with as
little ceremony as when it first arrived.[2]

Thus did bubonic plague make its first appearance on the world historical scene. Diagnosis of historical illnesses on the basis of descriptions
in ancient texts can rarely be made with compelling certainty because
all infectious diseases involve fever and the other symptoms tend not to
be exclusive to particular diseases. Plague, however, is a major exception

---

[1] Scarborough and Kazhdan, "Plague."
[2] Biraben, *Les Hommes et la peste*, 1:27–32.

because of the unmistakable appearance of buboes on most of its victims, those painful swellings of the lymph nodes that appear in the groin, in the armpit, or on the neck just below the ear. Taken together, the dozens of epidemics of this disease that broke out throughout the Mediterranean basin and its hinterlands between the mid-sixth and mid-eighth centuries constitute the first historically documented pandemic of plague, the first of three.[3]

THE THREE PANDEMICS

What came before were lethal epidemics to be sure, but of diseases that still lack generally agreed-upon diagnoses. The most notable of these were the 'plague' at Athens in 430 BC described by Thucydides, in which Pericles died, the Antonine Plague in Galen's time that stretched over much of the Roman Empire between 169 and 194, in which Marcus Aurelius died, and that of a century later, between 250 and 270, in which another emperor, Claudius Gothicus, died. Smallpox, typhus, and measles were most likely the diseases involved in those epidemics.[4] Meanwhile Greek and Roman medical writers, who commented on and anthologized the works of Hippocrates, apparently knew of plague, if only as an endemic disease. In the works compiled by such writers as Aretaeus of Cappadocia (mid-first century AD), Rufus of Ephesus (late first century AD), and Oribasius (late fourth century AD), plague appears not as a disease experienced or observed, but as one heard about from the far side of the Mediterranean.[5] They made frequent reference to cases in Egypt and Libya, less often in Syria, in which the sick and deceased had malignant buboes. Thus the presence of endemic plague in the ancient Near East centuries before the outbreak at Pelusium appears reasonably well attested. Then, when the disease did appear in full view of literate observers beginning in 541, some of these individuals gave convincingly precise descriptions of plague symptoms. And as this debut took place during the reign of the Emperor Justinian, Byzantinists especially refer to this outbreak as the "Plague of Justinian" or the "Justinianic Plague."[6]

[3] Brothwell and Sandison, *Diseases in Antiquity*, 238–46; Cockburn, "Infectious Diseases."

[4] Thucydides, *Peloponnesian War* 2.47–54, vol. 1:340–57; Gilliam, "Plague under Marcus Aurelius"; Duncan-Jones, "Impact of the Antonine Plague"; Zosimus, *New History* 1:26, 37, 46, pp. 8, 12, 14. On epidemics in the Roman Empire: Rijkels, *Agnosis en Diagnosis*.

[5] Conrad, "Plague in the Early Medieval Near East," 73.

[6] Allen, "'Justinianic' Plague." Michael McCormick suggests "Justinianic Pandemic" in the title of his essay in this volume.

The second pandemic, well known to all readers of history as the "Black Death," erupted in Central Asia in the 1330s, reached the Crimea by 1346, and then moved on the following year to Constantinople and thence to ports all around the Mediterranean. It spread more widely and moved further inland than it had eight hundred years before, for example, by reaching Scandinavia and also far into the Arabian peninsula for the first time. For more than a century and a half it continued to recur with notable regularity, but then became sporadic, though still deadly, vanishing from Europe in 1772, but lingering in the Near East until the 1830s.[7]

The third pandemic broke out in China in the second half of the nineteenth century. It reached massive proportions and gained world attention in 1894 when it struck Canton and Hong Kong. While Europe, which so suffered from the Black Death, has barely ever been touched by this third, nameless pandemic, the disease has found its way to much of the rest of the world, excluding the polar regions but including the United States. Where sailing ships of the Age of Exploration, which fell within the time period of the second pandemic, failed to export plague to the New World, the speedier steamship succeeded. Plague crossed the Pacific to Honolulu and from there to San Francisco in 1899, and a gigantic disease pool has since developed among the wild rodent and small ground-mammal populations of the western, especially the southwestern, states. Modern medicine has for the most part successfully isolated the occasional outbreaks of plague, and yet the disease shows no signs of going away.[8]

Besides reaching the Western Hemisphere, the third pandemic gave occasion for the identification of the pathogen. In the years preceding its outbreak, the new science of microbiology had taken hold, most famously in the rival French and German schools of Louis Pasteur in Paris and of Robert Koch in Berlin. When word of the outbreak of plague in 1894 at Hong Kong spread, Shibasaburo Kitasato of Tokyo, a student of Koch, rushed to the scene, as did Alexandre Yersin, a Pasteur student who was then working in French Indochina. An intensely competitive race ensued. Although Kitasato was the first to claim victory, the scientific community eventually awarded that claim to Yersin. The bacillus he isolated and described was duly named *Yersinia pestis*. Between 1894 and 1897 Yersin developed the first anti-plague serum for vaccinations, and

---

[7] Horrox, *Black Death*; Biraben, *Les Hommes et la peste*; Dols, *Black Death in the Middle East*.

[8] Benedict, *Bubonic Plague in Nineteenth-Century China*; Link, *History of Plague in the United States*.

by 1898 his colleague Paul-Louis Simond had unraveled the nexus of
bacilli, fleas, and rats while doing research in Bombay.[9] He found the
chief vector of *Yersinia* to be a flea, *Xenopsylla cheopis*, whose preferred
hosts in turn were rats, either *Rattus rattus*, the common stay-at-home
black rat, or *Rattus norvegicus*, the sea-going brown wharf rat. Contrary to
the long-held assumption that plague is a contagious disease, it is most
commonly by the bite of a rat flea that the highly toxic substance gets
injected into a human being and drains into a lymph node. Multiplying
rapidly, it there forms the painful swelling known as a bubo. Once fatal
to slightly more than half the people who contracted it, plague in recent
decades has become routinely curable, if timely diagnosis and medical
supplies permit, preferably by streptomycin, gentamycin, clorampheni-
col, or tetracycline.[10]

Can we be certain that the same disease was at play in all three pandemics? Or, to be more precise, can we be certain that *Y. pestis* was the
causal agent of either or both of the first two, pre-microbiology pandemics? This question rarely came up at all during most of the twentieth
century. Medical experts in the years around 1900, starting with Yersin
himself in the very paper of 1894 in which he announced his discovery, declared that both the Black Death and the earlier pandemic were
caused by the same plague bacillus as the one they could see under their
microscopes. To make such historical assertions, they had not scrambled
to become historians overnight. Instead, they were merely drawing on
their secondary-school learning in ancient and medieval history, which
had included some of the major descriptions of those earlier pandemics.
Thus the authority they gained from using the new science to identify the
pathogen during the third pandemic carried over sufficiently to validate
as well their readings of historical texts concerning the first two. Only in
recent years have some historians criticized those judgments and their
unquestioning perpetuation by other historians throughout the intervening century.[11] Yet also very recently, a completely new approach to these
issues has been developing. It is the work not of historians but, as in 1894,
of microbiologists, the heirs of Yersin and Kitasato, who now, redefined
as molecular biologists, are extending their use of DNA analysis from the
present and immediate past to the very remote past. Paleopathology is

[9] Brocke, *Robert Koch*; Debré, *Louis Pasteur*; Mollaret and Brossollet, *Alexandre Yersin*.
[10] Dennis et al., *Plague Manual*, 11–41.
[11] Twigg, *Black Death: A Biological Reappraisal*; Herlihy, *Black Death and the Transformation of
the West*; and Cohn, *Black Death Transformed*; for the historical judgments made by both
Yersin and Kitasato, ibid., 8.

becoming an increasingly viable tool of research, a point to which we shall return.[12]

THE EVIDENCE

Notwithstanding these promising laboratory developments, written sources remain the preeminent tool of historians. The principal sources available for studying the Plague of Justinian are written in four languages: Syriac, Arabic, Greek, and Latin. The lengthiest account in any language, found in the *Ecclesiastical History* of John of Ephesus, was written in Syriac. By an astonishing set of circumstances, he was completing a mission from Constantinople to Alexandria at the time the plague arrived in Egypt. Upon his return trip overland through Palestine, Syria, and Asia Minor, he found himself keeping abreast of the parallel movement of the disease as he traveled. In Palestine he saw entire town populations wiped out. "During the tumult and intensity of the pestilence," he wrote, "we journeyed from Syria to the capital. Day after day we, too, used to knock at the door of the grave along with everyone else. We used to think that if there would be evening, death would come upon us suddenly in the night. Although the next morning would come, we used to face the grave during the whole day as we looked at the devastated and moaning villages in these regions, and at corpses lying on the ground with no one to gather them." According to John, some people carried corpses all day, while others spent the day digging graves. Houses and farms were abandoned. Animals forgot their domestication. "Crops of wheat in fertile fields located in all the regions through which we passed from Syria up through Thrace, were white and standing but there was no one to reap them and store the wheat. Vineyards, whose picking season came and went, shed their leaves, since winter was severe, but kept their fruits hanging on their vines, and there was no one to pick them or press them." In his *Lives of the Eastern Saints,* John reported on one monastery that buried eighty-four of its members who had died of the plague. Other Syriac writings contain details of later outbreaks in Iraq, Egypt, Syria, and Palestine, including the *Chronicle of Zuqnīn,* whose monastic author, in recounting the epidemic of 743–745, specified that the victims had swellings in the groin, the armpit, or the neck.[13]

[12] Drancourt et al., "Detection of 400-year-old *Yersinia pestis.*"
[13] John of Ephesus, *Lives of the Eastern Saints* 17.1, p. 261; *CZ,* pp. 95, 174. Most of John's *Ecclesiastical History* is incorporated in the *CZ.*

The situation with Arabic sources is altogether different. To begin with, written Arabic was still very rare in the sixth century. Moreover, the Arabian Peninsula itself seems to have escaped this plague pandemic. But already in the sixth year of the Islamic era, corresponding to 627–628 AD, Arabic sources do contain a number of references to an outbreak of plague that devastated Sasanian Iraq; they call it the Plague of Sharawaygh for the Sasanian ruler it killed along with many inhabitants of Ctesiphon, the capital city. Then, after the death of Mohammed in 632 and the consolidation of power within Arabia under the first caliph, the Arabs went on the offensive in Syria, Palestine, and Iraq. With the conquest of Syria virtually complete by 638, the Arabs were beset for the first time with a major epidemic, this one named the Plague of Anwas (for a village where they first encountered it).

These earliest Arabic testimonies concerning plague have not come to us directly from the seventh century. Later scholars, especially some located in Basra, refashioned them and incorporated them into larger, more systematic works, including plague chronologies and consolation treatises. The first of these included al-Asmai (died 862), a lexicographer who compiled a list of plague epidemics with their dates and their assigned names. Another was the historian al-Madaini (died 840), who worked independently of al-Asmai, although probably with common sources, and who provided considerable detail on the effects of the epidemics that struck Basra. And to mention just one more Basran scholar, al-Mubarrad (died in 899 or 900) wrote one of the earliest books of consolation, a type of work that told of the terrible encounters of Muslims with past epidemics, whether victims or survivors, to bolster the courage of present-day and future believers in confronting this dreadful scourge. But in the case of this writer and his book, we encounter another level of the complexity in untangling the Arabic sources dealing with the first plague pandemic, for this work is mainly known from those portions of it incorporated into the plague treatises that began to appear in the 1360s in the wake of the Black Death. Thus the earliest extant writings on the plague in Arabic, whether lists of epidemics or treatises, date from the ninth and later centuries, while of course referring back to works – now lost – of the seventh and eighth centuries.[14]

The principal Greek source is the work of the historian Procopius of Caesarea, who was present at the court of Justinian in Constantinople in the early 540s. In his *Persian War*, Procopius says with reference to this time, "there was a pestilence by which the whole human race came

---

[14] Conrad, "Arabic Plague Chronologies and Treatises," 52–70.

near to being annihilated.... It started among the Egyptians. Then it moved to Palestine and from there spread over the whole world.... In the second year it reached Byzantium in the middle of the spring." He says that for the majority of those stricken the onset of fever was the first sign, and then there developed after a few days a bubonic swelling, either in the groin, in the armpit, or beside the ears. He reports that the mortality rose alarmingly, eventually reaching more than ten thousand each day. Procopius also mentions that the emperor himself was taken ill, but only in his *Secret History* did he go on to reveal that there were rumors at court that Justinian had died and that speculation about the succession flourished. Justinian, however, recovered and reigned for two more decades.[15]

The lawyer Agathias undertook to continue the history of Procopius. He says that after 544 when plague ceased in Constantinople, it had never really stopped but simply moved on from place to place, until it returned to the city almost as though it had been cheated on the first occasion into a needlessly hasty departure. This was the spring of 558, when "a second outbreak of plague swept the capital, destroying a vast number of people." The form the epidemic took was not unlike that of the earlier outbreak. A swelling in the glands in the groin was accompanied by a high fever that raged night and day with unabated intensity and never left its victim until the moment of death.[16]

Another testimony in Greek came from the Antiochene lawyer Evagrius "Scholasticus." Plague broke out in 594 while he was at work on his *Ecclesiastical History*, and in a passage of that book he notes that this was the fourth episode of the plague in his experience, going back to 542 when the disease first arrived in Antioch and he himself, then six years old, suffered from its fevers and swellings. In each of the later outbreaks he lost servants and family members, including most recently a daughter and a grandson.[17] We need emphasize that all three of these leading Greek sources, Procopius, Agathias, and Evagrius, were knowledgeable about earlier epidemics, yet clearly stressed the dreadful newness of the epidemics that started in 542.[18]

Of the Latin writers on this pandemic, Gregory of Tours (539–594) had the most to say. A native of Clermont and descendant of a Gallo-Roman family proud of its senatorial rank, he served as bishop of

[15] Procopius, *PW* 2.22–23, pp. 451–73; *SH* 4.1, 18.44, pp. 42–43, 226–27.
[16] Agathias, *The Histories* 5.3, 10, pp. 37–41, 145–46.
[17] Evagrius, "Evagre, *Histoire ecclésiastique*" 4.29, pp. 389–92; Allen, *Evagrius Scholasticus*, 190–94.
[18] Patlagean, *Pauvreté économique*, 87.

Tours from 573 to 594. In his *History of the Franks* and also in his *Lives of the Fathers*, he gives testimony to the first appearance of the plague in Gaul, which took place in the Rhone Valley in 543. The context was his telling of the saintly life of his uncle, Bishop Gallus of Clermont, in whose time, he says, "that illness called inguinal raged in many regions and most notably it depopulated the province of Arles." Gallus prayed that his diocese be spared and the Angel of the Lord came to him in a vision to assure him that his prayers would protect his people. Thus assured, Gallus led his people in various forms of devotion and indeed not a single one of them at Clermont died of the plague.[19]

Things went differently at Clermont in 571 under Bishop Cautinus, who scurried from one place to another to avoid the plague. "So many people were killed off in the whole region and the dead bodies were so numerous that it was not even possible to count them. There was such a shortage of coffins and tombstones that ten or more bodies were buried in the same grave. In St. Peter's church alone on a single Sunday three hundred dead bodies were counted." Gregory describes the sore "like a snake's bite" that appeared in a victim's groin or armpit, leading to death a few days later. He finishes off the paragraph by saying that Bishop Cautinus came back to Clermont, got the infection, and died on Good Friday, "on the same day and at the same hour as his cousin Tetradus. Lyons, Bourges, Chalon-sur-Saône, and Dijon were decimated by this plague."[20]

Gregory's references to plague in northern Gaul extend to Reims, which was protected miraculously by a relic of St. Rémi, and Trier, which was protected by the saintliness of Bishop Nicetius, but no further, while in the South these extend to Narbonne and Albi. His reference to the bishop of Nantes contracting plague suggests that the disease reached westward to the mouth of the Loire where it flows into the Atlantic. This in turn suggests that the probable route for the plague between Gaul and both Cornwall and Ireland was through Nantes, the port used in some instances by Irish monks in their travels to and from the Continent in the years around 600.[21]

---

[19] Gregory of Tours, *Historia Francorum* 4.5, pp. 144–45 and *History of the Franks*, 199–200; idem, *Liber vitae patrum* 6.6, pp. 684–85 and *Life of the Fathers*, 39–40.

[20] Gregory of Tours, *Historia Francorum* 4.31, pp. 166–68 and *History of the Franks*, 224–27.

[21] Gregory of Tours, *Liber in Gloria confessorum* 78, pp. 795–96 and *Glory of the Confessors*, 82–83; idem, *Liber vitae patrum* 17.4, p. 731 and *Life of the Fathers*, 110–11; idem, *Historia Francorum* 6.33, 6.15, pp. 274, 258–59 and *History of the Franks*, 364, 346–47. For the connection between Gaul and Ireland, see Wooding, *Communication and Commerce*, 64–68, 93–104. My thanks to Prof. Lisa Bitel for this reference.

The port of entry for the disease into Gaul in the first place, we can assume, was Marseilles, since the earliest report we have of it in Gaul was in the Rhone Valley. While Gregory did not mention Marseilles in his passage on the outbreak of 543, he has an astonishing tale to tell of the one there in 588, astonishing for the bits of etiological insights it contains. "A ship from Spain put into port with the usual kind of cargo, unfortunately also with it the source of this infection. Quite a few of the townsfolk purchased objects from the cargo and in less than no time a house in which eight people lived was completely deserted, all the inhabitants having caught the disease. The infection did not spread through the residential quarter immediately. Some time passed and then, like a wheat field set on fire, the entire town was suddenly ablaze with the pestilence...At the end of two months the plague burned itself out. The population returned to Marseilles, thinking to be safe. Then the disease started again and all who had come back died. On several occasions later on Marseilles suffered from an epidemic of this sort."[22]

The final epidemic written up by Gregory was that of the year 590 in Rome, as reported to him by a cleric named Agiulf whom he had sent to Rome to get saints' relics for the church of Tours. In the closing months of 589, continuous rains caused the Tiber to flood much of the city, destroying many churches and, notably, the papal granaries. Agiulf told of countless serpents that came down the river, especially a giant dragon, and of how they all drowned. "As a result there followed an epidemic, which caused swellings in the groin. This started in January." One of the first victims was Pope Pelagius II, and many others followed. The people of Rome turned to a deacon from one of the great senatorial families, who took the name of Gregory, the first pope to do so, and thus was born one of the most influential reigns in papal history, that of Gregory I, saint, Father of the Church, and surnamed "the Great" (590–604). Agiulf's report contains what purports to be the text of a sermon given by the new pope about the plague, which he saw, not surprisingly, as divine punishment. Pope Gregory stressed the need for all to reflect upon and repent of their own sins because the deaths they were seeing about them every day were so sudden that they left no time for victims to put their lives in order. The Romans were being carried off not one by one but in droves. "Homes are left empty, parents are forced to attend the funerals of their children, their heirs march before them to the grave." The sermon concludes with a plan for acts of penance and litanies and processions of supplication.

---

[22] Gregory of Tours, *Historia Francorum* 9.22, p. 380 and *History of the Franks*, 510–11.

The passage itself concludes with an account of how these devotions were carried out, the account made dramatic by Agiulf's testimony that on one day as he saw the solemn procession passing through the streets, eighty people fell dead on the ground.[23]

The major indigenous Latin source on the plague for Italy is Paul the Deacon, a Lombard scholar who lived and wrote two full centuries later than Gregory of Tours. His *History of the Lombards* includes mention of four separate outbreaks. The first of these occurred in Liguria in 565, when there began to appear "in the groins of men and in other delicate places a swelling of the glands accompanied by intense fever." The victim either died on the third day or, once having survived beyond that day, had some hope of recovering. Paul does not tell us anything more specific about this particular outbreak, but he follows with a dramatic description of its effects upon individuals, families, and whole communities. "The dwellings were left deserted by their inhabitants, and the dogs only kept house. The flocks remained alone in the pastures with no shepherd at hand. You might see villas or fortified places lately filled with crowds of men, and on the next day, all had departed and everything was in utter silence. Sons fled, leaving the corpses of their parents unburied; parents forgetful of their duty abandoned their children in raging fever. If by chance long-standing affection constrained anyone to bury his near relative, he remained himself unburied, and while he was performing the funeral rites he perished; while he offered obsequies to the dead, his own corpse remained without obsequies." The common perception that plague has little impact on the countryside is contradicted by his comments: "You might see the world brought back to its ancient silence: no voice in the field; no whistling of shepherds; no lying in wait of wild beasts among the cattle; no harm to domestic fowls. The crops, outliving the time of the harvest, awaited the reaper untouched; the vineyard with its fallen leaves and its shining grapes remained undisturbed while winter came on; . . . pastoral places had been turned into sepulchers for men, and human habitations had become places of refuge for wild beasts."[24]

Paul gives a report many times shorter than that by Gregory of Tours of the outbreak in Rome in 590. He begins it as Gregory did with the flooding of the Tiber, the huge dragon heading downstream, and the connection between this flooding and the inguinal pestilence that followed right away, "wasting the people with such destruction that out of a

[23] Gregory of Tours, *Historia Francorum* 10.1, pp. 406–9 and *History of the Franks*, 543–47.
[24] Paul the Deacon, *Historia Longobardorum* 2.4, p. 74 and *History of the Lombards*, 56–58.

countless multitude, barely a few remained." There followed the death of Pope Pelagius and the advent of Gregory the Great. Of the third outbreak of inguinal plague, he merely says that it took place in 593 in Ravenna, Grado, and Istria.[25]

The fourth and final outbreak reported by Paul was that of 680, a very severe pestilence that raged through July, August, and September. In Rome, so many people were dying that bodies were placed two by two on biers for transport to the tombs outside the city. To this point, his account follows almost identically the entry under Pope Agatone (678–681) in the *Liber pontificalis*. But then Paul added information about Pavia, the Lombard capital, where the combination of people either dying or fleeing left the city so empty that grass and bushes grew in the streets and marketplaces.[26]

The sixth century had begun with high promise for Italy. Following upon a century that had brought population decline, de-urbanization, widespread destruction, and gravely weakened institutions, the Gothic king of Italy Theodoric set out on a course of revival. The long career of his secretary Cassiodorus reflects the changing fortunes of the peninsula. The letters that this wealthy, well-educated Roman aristocrat prepared for the king tell us, in refined classical Latin, of plans to restore order, reform institutions, and repair such damaged parts of the infrastructure as aqueducts, roads, and bridges. He wrote a history of the Goths that justifies to Roman readers the passing of dominance to a people whom the Romans had thought of and treated as barbarians. But all this came to naught in the reigns of Theodoric's successors when in 533 the Emperor Justinian, who never for a moment accepted that the original heartland of the Roman Empire remain forever in Germanic hands, sent an army westward to reconquer North Africa from the Vandals and then Italy from the Goths. In this latter war, recounted to us by Procopius and thus known from the Byzantine point of view as the "Gothic War," Italy suffered far greater damage than at any earlier time in imperial history. The war dragged on for nearly two decades and some parts of Italian territory passed back and forth from one side to the other several times. Cassiodorus withdrew from public life to set up a monastery on his estate overlooking the Ionian Sea. He gave his monks the charge of copying

[25] Paul the Deacon, *Historia Longobardorum* 3.24, 4.4, pp. 104–5, 117 and *History of the Lombards*, 127–28, 152–53.

[26] Paul the Deacon, *Historia Longobardorum* 6.5, p. 166 and *History of the Lombards*, 254–55. *Liber pontificalis*, 193–94.

down the great writings of Christian and pagan antiquity alike, lest these be lost. A Gothic writer named Jordanes rewrote Cassiodorus' *History of the Goths* so as to justify to a Gothic audience the Roman, that is, Byzantine, reconquest. And it was in the 530s and 540s that Benedict of Nursia, after fleeing from the disorders of Rome, founded his monasteries at Subiaco and at Montecassino.

These are just some of the indications that fundamental change was underway throughout Italy when, in 543, the first epidemic of plague struck. The next one that we know about, from Paul the Deacon, hit in 565, and it was in 568 that the Lombards began their migration into the Italian peninsula. Two centuries later, in the final years of the Lombard kingdom, it was in Italy that the pandemic struck for the last time, in Naples and Sicily in 749–750.[27]

For North Africa, we have the testimony of the Latin poet Corippus. In 549 he recited at Carthage his epic poem, the *Johannis*, on the recently concluded war between the Byzantine army (under a general named John Troglita) and Berber tribes. In the midst of the war a terrible pestilence arrived by sea. Death was so widespread that people became desensitized to it, no longer shedding tears even for their loved ones or observing those rites traditionally due the deceased. Social breakdown was further evident in the scramble among survivors to take possession of the properties and belongings of the victims. Wealthy widows were more sought after than young maidens. References to a later plague epidemic in North Africa, in 599 and 600, are found in the correspondence of Pope Gregory the Great.[28]

The writings under discussion here have in common that for the most part they are artfully contrived historical narratives, in which the choices and style and point of view of the author are present in every paragraph. They differ markedly from archival material, which is supposed to contain data entered on a regular basis over a long period of time. Such archival material abounds from the time of the second pandemic, not to mention the third, and yet is nearly completely absent from that of the first, rendering these narratives all the more precious.

To fold into the historical narratives of the first plague pandemic, we need to search out evidence of the material remains produced by

---

[27] For the dates of this final round, see the essay in this volume of Michael McCormick.

[28] Corippus, *Iohannidos* 3.343–89, pp. 60–62. Gregory the Great, *Letters* 9.32, 10.20, pp. 706, 729.

archaeological investigation. These include such constructions as domestic and public buildings, markets and transport infrastructures, and systems of water supply and waste disposal. For the archaeology of pandemics, however, one is often confronted with little more than negative evidence – not the best sort for establishing proof – evidence such as the abandonment of structures and indeed of entire communities, or a marked break in a long-range pattern of building and expansion.[29] Still, such investigations often yield our best evidence of depopulation. Thus while the sources, of whatever sort, are not nearly so numerous for the first pandemic as they are for the second, evidence there is nonetheless, even if not easy to come by or to interpret.

MODERN SCHOLARSHIP

What, then, of modern scholarship? Its beginning is found in two bibliographical studies, one on the Greek and Latin sources by Valentin Seibel, a German, in 1857, and the other on Arabic sources by Alfred von Kremer, an Austrian, in 1880.[30] Unfortunately, this promising start did not lead to productive results. There has never been a book on the subject and only a very few articles.[31] Although some historical subjects can boast of traditions of scholarship that have been both innovative and stimulating, this one instead has been not just sparse but notably unimaginative.

Not only is there no comprehensive study of the entire first pandemic, there are no comprehensive studies of this plague in the major geopolitical and cultural–linguistic subdivisions of the Mediterranean world, such as the Latin West or the Near East.[32] Given such a record, it is not astonishing that this first plague pandemic, which lasted for more than two hundred years, has not entered the historical canon. Yet, these same two hundred years witnessed among other significant things the Lombard takeover in Italy, the breaching of the Balkan frontier by the Slavs, the transformation of the eastern Roman Empire into the Byzantine Empire, the Christian missions from Rome to England and thence to Germany as

---

[29] Hodges and Whitehouse, *Mohammed, Charlemagne and the Origins of Europe*, 52–53. See also the essay in this volume by Hugh Kennedy.

[30] Seibel, *Die grosse Pest*; von Kremer, "Über die grossen Seuchen."

[31] Several of the articles are discussed in Stathakopoulos, "Justinianic Plague Revisited."

[32] Several of the essays in this volume are intended to remedy this problem. See as well the dissertation of Conrad, "Plague in the Early Medieval Near East" and Stathakopoulos, *Famine and Pestilence*.

well as those from Ireland to Scotland and Frankish Gaul, and, perhaps
most significantly, the beginnings of Islam and the Arab conquests.[33]

What is utterly astonishing is the lack of attention shown to the first
pandemic by the numerous experts on the second one. The Black Death,
as solid a part of the historical canon, or master narrative, as the Norman
Conquest or the Protestant Reformation, has long continued to attract
historical investigators, and yet those most interested in it have shown
little curiosity about whether it had any precedent. For them, its history
begins in the fourteenth century. The exception is a medical historian,
Jean-Noel Biraben, who teamed up with the medieval cultural historian
Jacques Le Goff to produce an article on the Justinianic Plague in 1969.
This article in turn became the first chapter of Biraben's substantial history of the Black Death, but Biraben made no attempt to link the two
pandemics, as if no memory of the first still lingered at the time of the
second. Textbooks, too, which presumably define or at least enshrine
what is canonical, routinely devote space to the Black Death, often indeed
including a map, but leave out mention of the earlier pandemic.[34]

In a remarkable study of how six major epidemics affected different parts of the modern world, Sheldon Watts begins with the human
response to plague in western Europe and the Middle East between 1347
and 1844. At one point he interrupts his narrative to refer to the account
of the epidemic at Athens by Thucydides and then resumes his narrative by saying, "When plague re-emerged in 1347 (an earlier, all but
forgotten, pandemic had raged from 541 to 755 CE),...." In a book
that is both learned in its details and rich in thoughtful interpretations,
Watts is not unusual in giving nothing more than this passing nod to the
Justinianic Plague. Scholars have for the most part left the first plague

---

[33] The point was made many years ago by Peter Brown when he suggested "that the hushed
generations following the great visitation of the plague after 543, which saw the saddened
old age of Justinian, the maturity of Pope Gregory I, and the youth of Mohammed,
might repay more close consideration as a possible turning point in the history of the
Mediterranean." Brown, *Society and the Holy*, 67.

[34] Biraben and Le Goff, "La Peste dans le Haut Moyen Age," and Biraben, *Les Hommes
et la peste*, 1:25–48. The lack of attention to the earlier pandemic in a textbook, while
common, is particularly puzzling in the case of one very distinguished historian of the
Black Death who was also a very influential textbook author. In the course of his general
account, he rightfully asserted the prerogative of such authors to give special weight to
his particular interest; thus the Black Death, as he told it, had major social, economic,
and political consequences. But he devoted just one sentence to the outbreak of plague
during the reign of Emperor Justinian. See Chambers, *Western Experience*, 259, 421–26,
465–66.

pandemic unacknowledged, or where they have mentioned it, they have treated it as forgotten or, as in this case, worthy at most of a parenthetical interjection.[35]

We need to ask why this scholarship has been so unsatisfactory. Part of the answer has to do with academic and cultural divides, and part with adherence to the canons of positivist rules of evidence. The area over which the pandemic spread was phenomenally rich in cultural and linguistic diversity, a condition that remains undiminished in our time. Thus, few scholars in the world have the necessary skills for reading sources from all the areas covered. Moreover, the academic divisions among disciplines, areas, and chronological eras maintain both their unity and their identity largely by rewarding only achievement within their conventionally fixed boundaries.

In 1989 the French Byzantinist Jean Durliat issued a challenge to fellow scholars to study the plague. Best known as a protagonist of the school that stresses continuity instead of decline and fall from Roman imperial to Carolingian times, Durliat seemed to have made up his mind from the start. He surveyed separately each discipline and subdiscipline to see what evidence it had supplied concerning the plague pandemic: art history, archaeology, epigraphy, numismatics, paleography, and so on. Both individually and even all together, he concluded, these had supplied very little. Narrative sources, on the other hand, Durliat granted were relatively abundant, but he hastened to minimize the significance of these for their derivative quality (for example, by asking whether Procopius did not borrow heavily from Thucydides) and for their rhetorical exaggerations (for example, by asking whether there really were ten thousand deaths per day at Constantinople). His answer was to send his colleagues, the art historians, the archaeologists, the epigraphers, and so on, back to their respective sources to try to squeeze more evidence from them. There is nothing inherently wrong with asking specialists to try to glean more from their sources, but it is clearly not enough.[36]

What is called for is scientific cooperation. This subject requires the expertise of specialists with different disciplinary approaches, minimally those of history, archaeology, and molecular biology. In addition, it requires the expertise of specialists on all of the geographical areas where

---

[35] Watts, *Epidemics and History*, 4.

[36] Durliat, "La peste du VIe siècle," 1:107–19. See also the response by Biraben, ibid., 121–25.

the pandemic is known to have penetrated. Not only is there a need for comparative studies of different plague outbreaks within the vast geographical and chronological parameters of this pandemic, but also a need for comparative studies of different pandemics.[37]

THE FIRST TWO PANDEMICS COMPARED

The second plague pandemic, which is so much more thoroughly documented than its Justinianic predecessor, can perhaps for that very reason shed light on our subject. Historical comparisons should not be expected to establish rules for what ought to have or must have happened; instead they serve the more modest role of raising questions that can in turn become hypotheses. We have extensive material on the pattern of the disease's returns or recurrences in the fourteenth and fifteenth centuries. If one could overlay this pattern upon the much more sketchy information on recurrences in the earlier pandemic, useful hypotheses about some of the latter's "missing" information could perhaps follow.

The unresolved issue of the nature of the immunity conferred upon plague survivors, for example how strong and how long lasting it is, if it exists at all, is insistently raised by some of the descriptions of fourteenth-century recurrences. To cite just the first four English instances: "In 1361 a general mortality oppressed the people. It was called the second pestilence and both rich and poor died, but especially young people and children." "In 1369 there was a third pestilence in England and in several other countries. It was great beyond measure, lasted a long time, and was particularly fatal to children." "The fourth pestilence arrived in York and was particularly fatal to children." And finally, "In 1390 a great plague ravaged the country. It especially attacked adolescents and boys." Had the plague become a children's disease, meaning that it found victims mostly among those born since its previous visitation? It is enough to make us consider carefully Agathias' observation that in the epidemic of 558 "people of all ages were struck down indiscriminately, but the heaviest toll was among the young and vigorous," or the meaning of the name given an outbreak at Basra in 706 as the "Plague of the Maidens." The value of

---

[37] There is a developing body of work by paleoecologists interested in establishing connections among major natural phenomena such as volcanos, asteroids, climate change, and pandemics. While very promising, such work to date has failed to establish convincing instances of causal connections having to do with the Justinianic Pandemic. For references and summaries, see Keys, *Catastrophe,* and Antoniou and Anastasios, "Sixth-Century Plague."

such comparisons can only increase to the extent that the biomedical community can offer more convincing evidence that the pathogens in the different pandemics were the same.[38]

A major step in this direction, alluded to briefly above, was taken in 1998 with the publication of a study claiming that human remains of the early modern period yielded evidence of *Y. pestis*. A team of molecular biologists at Marseilles led by Michel Drancourt, Olivier Dutour, and Didier Raoult, working together with archaeologists and historians, obtained human remains that could be reasonably supposed to come from epidemics that struck the Marseilles region in 1590 and 1720, since burials from quarantine hospitals are well documented in those years. They "hypothesized that the dental pulp of unerupted teeth would be a lasting refuge of *Y. pestis* and would be a suitable material on which to base molecular detection of the bacterium for reasons including durability, good taphonomic [fossilizing] conservation, and encapsulation." The skulls were x-rayed and then the teeth were extracted and fractured longitudinally. "Powdery remnants [of blood] were scraped from the dental pulp cavities into sterile tubes for further DNA extraction" and the final result of this investigation was a positive identification of *Y. pestis*. The same group published in 2000 similar results from research they conducted on remains from the middle of the fourteenth century, thus pushing their discovery right back to the very beginning of the Black Death.[39]

While it is ironic that Yersin and Kitasato, who were the first to exploit a new scientific understanding to expose the causative agent of plague in their time, based their diagnoses of past epidemics purely upon their reading of historical texts, it is now for the first time becoming possible for some of our contemporaries to make diagnoses of past epidemics as scientifically precise as those that Yersin and the others made of the epidemic they observed in 1894. To be sure, the Marseilles scholars have had both detractors and competitors.[40] Among these, some have published negative results, but in 2005 scholars at Munich following the methods used by the Marseilles group reported the presence of *Y. pestis* DNA in skeletal remains from Aschheim in Upper Bavaria, remains we need note

---

[38] Horrox, *Black Death*, pp. 85, 88, 91; Agathias, *The Histories* 5.10, p. 145; Conrad, "Arabic Plague Chronicles and Treatises," 55.

[39] Drancourt et al., "Detection of 400-Year-Old *Yersinia pestis* DNA"; Raoult et al., "Molecular Identification."

[40] Cooper and Polnar, "Ancient DNA"; Cohn, *Black Death Transformed*, 248; Gilbert et al., "Absence of *Yersinia pestis*-Specific DNA."

found at a site whose date archaeologists place in the second half of the sixth century. Thus, rapid progress on the biomedical front is lending crucial support to the work of historians and archaeologists. Moreover, the Munich group accomplished something quite other than confirm what historians knew or suspected all along. Because there are no known extant texts indicating that the Justinianic Plague reached Bavaria, this collaboration of archaeologists and molecular biologists produced the first such indication. And because plague is attested more than once in late sixth-century northern Italy, including Verona in particular, it is not unreasonable to imagine the disease reaching southern Bavaria from Verona via the Brenner Pass.[41]

Such collaboration may eventually prove valuable for the history of plague in East Asia. There surely were epidemics in that vast area of the world, including some that fall within the dates of the first plague pandemic, such as the series of epidemics reported in the first half of the seventh century in China, or the epidemic that ravaged Japan between 735 and 737, but the lack of specificity about symptoms in the written sources there make scholars wary of being able to identify the particular diseases involved.[42] This question is relevant to the history of the first plague pandemic. To date, the original outbreak of the second pandemic is believed to have taken place in the Central Asian steppes, and it was the unification of much of the Eurasian landmass by the Mongols that facilitated not just the eastward travels of Marco Polo to China but also the westward progress of plague to the Black Sea and from there to the Mediterranean. But no such certainty pertains to the route taken by plague prior to its arrival at Pelusium in 541.[43] The problem with waiting for DNA analysis of human remains is that in most places researchers would be at the mercy of luck. While the scholars at Marseilles knew a great deal about the history of plague in their region and thus had every reason to think they could locate remains of plague victims, the archaeologists at Munich had good reason for choosing the site of their dig, but finding plague victims was not their main purpose. They found human

[41] Gutsmiedl, "Die justinianische Pest nördlich der Alpen?"; Wiechmann and Grupe, "Detection of *Yersinia pestis* DNA"; Reimann et al., "Vereint in den Tod." Paul the Deacon, *Historia Longobardorum* 3.23, p. 104 and *History of the Lombards*, 126–27.

[42] Twitchett, "Population and Pestilence in T'ang China," 42–47; Farris, *Population, Disease, and Land*, 53–73. I am very grateful for helpful advice from two experts on the history of disease and medicine in China, Prof. Nathan Siven of the University of Pennsylvania and Prof. Carol Benedict of Georgetown University.

[43] But see the argument on this point in the essay in this volume by Peter Sarris.

remains and submitted some of them (many more await study) to the latest developments in paleopathology. Thus, in China and elsewhere where there is no expectation of finding remains with traces of *Y. pestis* from the first pandemic, archaeologists will have to wait for those occasions when they encounter human remains from the appropriate era, especially if these are found in mass graves that are suggestive of epidemics, to call upon their colleagues in the paleopathology lab.

EFFECTS

Less directly dependent upon the identity of the disease but in no way less important is the study of its effects: economic, social, military, political, and religious. Massive mortality in traditional societies, even if it reaches all social levels, usually leads to an increase in the value of labor. The standard response of survivors from among the controlling classes is to complain about the difficulties of finding servants and laborers, and then to complain about what they see as the exorbitant demands for higher wages by those survivors whom they do find to work for them. Once again, the evidence from the time of the Black Death is abundant and thus helpful in understanding the significance of the bits and pieces of evidence remaining from seven and eight centuries earlier. In what is probably the most widely read description of the Black Death, namely the preface to the *Decameron*, Boccaccio reports sadly that, "the countless numbers of people who fell ill, both male and female, were entirely dependent either upon the charity of friends (who were few and far between) or the greed of servants, who remained in short supply despite the attraction of high wages out of all proportion to the services they performed."[44] But listen also to the archbishop of Canterbury, Simon Sudbury, sounding off in 1378 about the survivors within the severely depleted ranks of his clergy, describing them as "so infected with the sin of greed that, not satisfied with reasonable wages, they hire themselves out for vastly inflated salaries."[45] It is in the light of such complaints that we can see the significance of the lament of John of Ephesus concerning the "scandalous profits" being taken by those who carried away the dead and the greatly increased cost of getting laundry done in Constantinople in 544. Indeed, court dress there became much simplified at that time as a result.[46]

---

[44] Horrox, *Black Death*, 30.
[45] Ibid., 311.
[46] Patlagean, *Pauvreté économique*, 172.

Governments typically reacted by attempting to roll back the changes wrought by market forces. The Ordinance of Laborers, promulgated in England in 1349, captures the problem in a single sentence: "Since a great part of the population, and especially workers and servants, has now died in this pestilence, many people, observing the needs of masters and the shortage of employees, are refusing to work unless they are paid an excessive salary." A related but separate problem was that some workers preferred "to beg in idleness rather than to work for their living." As for what the ordinance has to say about wages, landlords were admonished not to pay workers any more than the rates that prevailed back in 1346, that is, before the plague's arrival. As for the lack of workers, all able-bodied workers who were offered employment had to accept, while lords were admonished to retain the service of only as many of their tenants as they really needed.[47] To this ordinance we can compare an edict issued by Justinian in 544 in which he announced the end of the pestilence and ordered that current prices and wages be set back to their pre-plague levels.[48]

The relationship between the wealthy and those who served them was based upon far more than mere wages, above all familiarity. This familiarity had great advantages for both sides of the relationship, but it also allowed for the possibility of intimidation. Thus, an accompaniment of the increased value of work is the new mobility of workers. Apparently it was better for workers to wander and ask for higher wages from strangers with whom they had no ties or memories or obligations. Furthermore, at the time of the Black Death, many peasants still had servile obligations (roughly half of all European peasants in 1348 were still serfs), so mobility was necessarily tied to their quest for better remuneration. The English Statute of Laborers of 1351 goes beyond the earlier ordinance by spelling out in great detail the maximum allowable wages for a ploughman, a shepherd, a dairymaid, a swineherd, and so on, and then turns to the issue of mobility by ordering sheriffs to arrest laborers, craftsmen, and servants who have fled from one county to another and to restore them to their home territories.[49] In like fashion, slavery persisted in many areas well into Late Antiquity. Slaves obviously did not have the option of asking their owners for higher compensation, so they had to escape in

---

[47] Horrox, *Black Death*, 287.

[48] Novella 122 in *CIC*, 3.592–93.

[49] Horrox, *Black Death*, 316; see the works of Hatcher on this and related points: *Plague, Population and the English Economy* and "Aftermath of the Black Death."

order to make their way as wage earners. The law codes of the Germanic kingdoms that succeeded the western provinces of the Roman Empire provided punishments for runaway slaves and all those who assisted them. In the latter half of the sixth century and through the seventh, there took place in both Visigothic Spain and Lombard Italy an escalation of repressive measures (a nearly certain sign of a failed policy) having to do with runaways. According to one leading Iberian historian, the population of the Visigothic kingdom had by 700 come to constitute one vast social police force for hunting down slaves; punishments were now provided for any who failed to cooperate with this operation. Thus, to material remuneration we must add the legal and social status of workers to appreciate the economic and social impact of a plague pandemic, whether that of the fourteenth and fifteenth centuries, in which serfdom virtually disappeared from western Europe, or that of the sixth and seventh centuries, which saw the end of ancient slavery, at least in Italy and Spain.[50]

The very concept of work also underwent a significant change at this time, even though attitudes do not change in the same way or, especially, at the same speed that law codes or battles or political fortunes do. In Roman culture there was a fundamental opposition between leisure (*otium*) and work (*negotium*). The first referred not to laziness or aimlessness but to an honorable and agreeable search for wisdom through intellectual or artistic pursuits; the second meant literally the negation of leisure (neatly captured in the English word *busi-ness*). Work could also be expressed by the word *labor*, which was considered to be painful and sad. One way of expressing the change that came about in the Latin West in the sixth century was the simultaneous rise of work to respectability and the descent of leisure to its connotation of aimless passing of time. The key text is the *Rule for Monks* composed by Benedict of Nursia in the middle years of the sixth century, wherein spiritual reading is work, not leisure, and the younger monks need supervision so that they will not fall into laziness but will read. Much of what Benedict set down is a distillation of a much longer rule, the so-called *Rule of the Master*, dating from a few decades earlier, but what he had to say about work flatly contradicted this forerunner, and can therefore be considered new. In his chapter on manual labor, Benedict used the word *labor* instead of *negotium* and he gave it a positive value. Benedict's influence might never have reached beyond his community at Montecassino, but Pope Gregory the Great rescued his reputation and his rule from obscurity by writing a life of Benedict; by the early ninth

[50] Blum, "Rise of Serfdom," 810–12; Bonnassie, *From Slavery to Feudalism*, 48–49, 94–96.

century, Benedict's rule became the exclusive rule for monks in the Latin church.[51]

The mortality resulting from the plague had military and political effects that are difficult to measure but no less important because of that. Study of the countryside, for example, including some of the empire's most productive regions, has shown that plague was quite as active there as in the cities. And as peasants formed the backbone of the Byzantine army, it comes as no surprise to learn that the army faced severe manpower shortages in the later sixth and seventh centuries. The ever-greater induction of barbarians into the army indicates a policy of resorting to searches beyond the usual sources for fresh recruits. Moreover, this was an army that had to be paid, and as fewer workers on the soil had to produce larger shares of tax revenue, the imperial government was perennially on the verge of fiscal collapse and unpaid soldiers had frequent resort to mutiny. One major question concerning military matters is how to evaluate the role of plague mortality among the various factors that contributed to the weakness of the Byzantine army in the face of the Arab advances.[52]

The decimation of rural populations did not go unnoticed by the living. The Byzantine imperial government resettled peasants in Thrace to regain some of the resources and revenues lost there from depopulation; it had also to transfer people to Constantinople. The extensive demographic losses in the Balkans, caused by barbarian raids as well as plague, left much of the region open to settlement by Slavs.[53] In the view of Paul the Deacon, the relative emptiness of Italy from the combined effects of the Byzantine reconquest and the plague made the advent of the Lombards into the peninsula, which started in 568, practically unopposed.[54] A large migration of Arabs into Syria was similarly facilitated by the high plague mortality in that land.[55] In all these matters, most of the evidence is circumstantial and thus wide open to interpretation, which in some cases was spun into political propaganda. After a lengthy and all-out war against Umayyad rule resulted in a complete Abbasid victory in 750,

---

[51] Rouche, "Une révolution mentale"; Ovitt, "Manual Labor"; Freedman, *Images of the Medieval Peasant*, 15–39; I am grateful to Paul Freedman for allowing me to read the first chapter of his book prior to its publication.

[52] Kaplan, *Les hommes et la terre*, 459–60; Treadgold, *History of the Byzantine State*, 236–41, 246–48; Evans, *Age of Justinian*, 164; Whitby, "Recruitment in Roman Armies," 63.

[53] Patlagean, *Pauvreté économique*, 302; Conrad, "Plague in the Early Medieval Near East," 485–86; Duby, *Early Growth*, 71: "The voids created by the disasters of the sixth century invited reconquest."

[54] Paul the Deacon, *Historia Longobardorum* 2.26, pp. 86–87; *History of the Lombards*, 80.

[55] Conrad, "Plague in the Early Medieval Near East," pp. 239–40.

and then it appeared that plague was not coming back after that date, the new regime's leaders claimed that God put an end to the plague pandemic because of their overthrow of the Umayyads.[56] And in what seems an echo of a similar claim, namely that the Carolingian overthrow of the Merovingians in 751 (when a new Christian rite of anointment replaced descent from the Germanic gods as the source of legitimacy) explains why God ended the pandemic, a twelfth-century writer linked ecclesiastical anointment with the royal capacity to cure victims of the "inguinal plague."[57]

The first plague pandemic was hardly the first natural disaster to confront Christians. One particularly apt precedent is the pestilence that raged in the Roman Empire between 250 and 270. Christians suffered not only sickness and death from it, but accusations as well that that they had caused it by their unwillingness to participate in the state religion. Bishop Cyprian of Carthage wrote a vigorous refutation of these accusations but then also wrote a tract, *On Mortality,* to rally the faithful to be steadfast in their Christian commitment. He taught them that death is to be welcomed rather than feared; that reluctance to die shows too great an attachment to worldly joys; and that suffering and dying from the disease would free them from the world and move them along earlier than anticipated to eternal glory. Besides encouraging those who were wavering, Cyprian had to console those who felt deprived of the martyrdom they longed for. He assures the servants of God "among whom confession is contemplated and martyrdom is conceived in the mind, the intention dedicated to good is crowned, with God as judge. It is one thing for the intention to be lacking for martyrdom; it is another thing for martyrdom to have been lacking for the intention."[58]

Earthquakes in the Rhone Valley in the 470s led the bishop of Vienne to institute a series of pious actions called rogations, for which the faithful prepared by fasting for three days and then which involved processions, Psalm-singing, and prayers for deliverance from the natural calamity.[59] Also in the Greek East, earthquake in the fifth century called for a response, which was expressed by the parading of icons in what Peter

---

[56] Dols, "Plague in Early Islamic History," p. 380.

[57] Bloch, *Les Rois thaumaturges,* 41–42 and the preface by Jacques Le Goff, xiii–xiv; see in this volume the essay by Alain Stoclet, who first called my attention to this matter.

[58] Cyprian, *De mortalitate* 1–17, pp. 20–37.

[59] Leclercq, "Rogations"; Cabrol, "Litanies"; Gregory of Tours, *Historia Francorum* 2.34, pp. 97–98 and *History of the Franks,* 149–50.

Brown has referred to as "great intercessory processions and solemn junkets."[60]

Thus when the plague arrived, prelates were not entirely lacking in tried and tested responses. During an epidemic in Mesopotamia in 573, the Nestorian patriarchs confronted plague with a complex of devotions very similar to rogations. Gregory of Tours tells us that his uncle, Bishop Gallus, saved Clermont by instituting rogations and by leading many from his flock on a forty-mile walk to the shrine of Saint-Julien of Brioude. They sang Psalms as they went and he prayed fervently that his city and its people be saved. We have already seen Gregory's cautionary tale contrasting the behavior of Bishop Cautinus, who tried unsuccessfully to escape from the plague, with that of his conscientious uncle.[61]

The Frankish King Guntran was a figure whom Gregory of Tours knew very well and who appears frequently in the pages of his history. When plague had been reported at Marseilles in 588, the king was staying in a village further up the Rhone Valley. He ordered the people to eat only barley bread and drink only water, and then he had them assemble for rogations. "He seemed so anxious about all his people that he might well have been taken for one of our Lord's bishops rather than a king." And so it was that at Rome in 590, the new pope, Gregory I, called for three days of fasting and prayer, and processions from seven major churches all directed towards Santa Maria Maggiore, "that there we may at great length make our supplication to the Lord with tears and groans, and thus be held worthy to win pardon for our sins."[62]

The frequent retellings of how saintly bishops, a good king, and a great pope dealt with plague meant that their humble successors had authoritative models to follow when disaster struck. These same models were immediately re-activated in the fourteenth century when the Black Death appeared, although of course they were often put to use in the interim.[63] During the two-century span of the first pandemic there were other indications of intensified piety, particularly characterized by humility, contrition, and supplication. The spectacular growth of monasticism is one such indication. A second is the continuation of church construction

[60] Brown, *Society and the Holy*, p. 277; Dagron, "Quand la terre tremble."
[61] Ebied and Young, "Treatise in Arabic," 96; *De patriarchis nestorianorum*, 2:25–26; Gregory of Tours, *Historia Francorum* 4.5 and 4.31, pp. 144–45, 167–68 and *History of the Franks*, 199–200, 226–27.
[62] Gregory of Tours, *Historia Francorum* 9.21, 10.1, pp. 379–80, 408–9 and *History of the Franks*, 509–10, 546.
[63] Horrox, *Black Death*, 111–57.

even in those places where the archaeological evidence, such as the lack of new buildings, abandonment of existing ones, and the shrinking of communities, suggests population decline. Churches built in such an environment were not responding to a need to serve a larger number of worshippers but to the spiritual needs of patrons. Still another indication is the rise of the votive mass, a variant form of the mass for use on a particular occasion, such as war, plague, or bad weather, that had its origin in the sixth century. By the middle of the eighth century there were about sixty such variants on the liturgical books.[64]

The intensification of devotion had its obverse in backsliding or what the orthodox could only see as reversions to "paganism." Gregory of Tours mixes up his stories about good models with others about colorful eccentrics such as the bogus Christ of Bourges, who misled simple folk into erroneous belief and meaningless acts of devotion. Scripture had prepared Gregory for such imposters, for he introduced his account of the one at Bourges by citing the Gospels where Jesus said that famine and pestilence and earthquakes would take place and that false Christs and false prophets would accordingly appear. Bede makes a similar connection in his account of the plague epidemic in England in 664, when St. Cuthbert was still preaching to the uninitiated but then in addition had to deal with setbacks among people converted quite recently. "For many of them profaned the faith they held by wicked deeds, and some of them also at the time of the plague, forgetting the sacred mystery of the faith into which they had been initiated, took to the illusive cures of idolatry, as though by incantations or amulets or any other mysteries of devilish art, they could ward off a plague sent by God the Creator."[65]

The loss of faith was but a part of the unraveling of community and the abandonment of social norms that apparently accompanied the plague wherever it went. The challenge for leaders everywhere was to keep communities together. St. Boniface, the Anglo-Saxon monk who headed the mission to evangelize the Germans, asked Pope Gregory II about this matter in 726 and received the following answer: "You ask whether, in the case of a contagious disease or plague in a church or monastery, those who are not yet attacked may escape danger by flight. We declare this to be the height of folly, for no one can escape from the hand of God."[66] For

---

[64] Hughes and Hamlin, *Celtic Monasticism*, 5. Reference is again made to the chapter in this volume by Hugh Kennedy; Amiet, "Votive Masses."

[65] Matthew 24.7 and Mark 13:22; Gregory of Tours, *Historia Francorum* 10.25, pp. 437–38 and *History of the Franks*, 584–86; *Two Lives of Saint Cuthbert*, 180–87.

[66] Boniface, *Letters of Saint Boniface*, 55.

the Arabs, the same problem engendered much discussion. Because they encountered it only outside of their homeland, this was at least at first mainly a problem for their armies. The main response to emerge was that when plague struck a place where they happened to be, a phenomenon to be explained only as a willful act of Allah, they should not flee for fear of violating their obligation to accept Allah's will. But because at the very time in 638 when Arab troops first encountered plague, the caliph was on his way from Medina to Syria with a large retinue, and news of the epidemic came to him, he chose to follow Bedouin tradition and avoid the danger by turning back to Medina. This act became the model for what Muslims should do if they approached an area that was disease-ridden.[67]

Practice was of course another matter, as in the case of the commanders of the army in Syria as well as, later on, the califs, who had their mountain retreats for quick escapes, even though the troops were ordered to stay put, at least in the early years of the conquests, in the garrison towns.[68] Perhaps they had a slight advantage because these towns were segregated from the communities of the conquered peoples. Still, the problem of flight cannot have been easily dispensed with, for death by plague came to be accepted as one of the ways to gain martyrdom.[69] This solution seems at first glance the very antithesis of the view of Cyprian of Carthage, who had to console those Christians who lamented that dying of a disease was robbing them of the opportunity to become martyrs. And yet Cyprian's argument that God's sending of the epidemic offered the faithful an opportunity to die and go sooner than expected to heaven was perhaps not so essentially different from the Islamic consolation of martyrdom.[70]

EXPIATION AND MEMORY

No study of the impact of the plague pandemic on religion, in particular western Christianity, would be complete without reference to the creation of a new saintly cult specifically intended to deal with plague, namely that of St. Sebastian. The most familiar of all plague saints thanks to the paintings by virtually every Renaissance artist of note, Sebastian was

[67] Dols, "Comparative Communal Responses," 276; Conrad, "Plague in the Early Medieval Near East," 199.

[68] Conrad, "Plague in the Early Medieval Near East," 170–75, 449–65; idem, "Historical Evidence," 269–74.

[69] Lewinstein, "Revaluation of Martyrdom," 82, 89; Dols, "Plague in Early Islamic History," 377; Sublet, "La peste prise aux rêts de la jurisprudence," 144–45.

[70] Cyprian, *De mortalitate* 17, pp. 36–37.

the Justinianic Plague's gift to the Black Death. The connection between Sebastian and plague was made, at the latest, in the year 680. Following his report of the plague outbreaks of that year in Rome and in Pavia, Paul the Deacon goes on to say that a certain man at Pavia had a revelation in which he was informed that the epidemic would not cease there until an altar of St. Sebastian the Martyr was set up in the church of St. Peter in Chains. Accordingly the Pavesi had relics brought from Rome and an appropriate altar set up just as the miraculous voice had instructed; sure enough, the pestilence ended. At about the same time a mosaic depicting Sebastian in Roman court dress and carrying a martyr's crown was placed on a wall of the more famous church of St. Peter in Chains, the one in Rome.[71] We need to inquire how the connection of this saint with this epidemic came about.

According to the pious legend that serves as the earliest extant account of his life, Sebastian was a closet Christian who served in the imperial guard of Diocletian, a risky position to occupy given the intensity of the persecution of Christians just then. Of course Sebastian's faith was eventually discovered, and the emperor reacted by ordering that he be shot and killed with arrows. His would-be executioners so filled his body with arrows that he "looked like a porcupine"; thinking him dead, they threw out his body. Some Christians who were hoping to give him a proper burial found him, and what is more, found him alive, so the pious widow Irene nursed him back to health. Once he was strong again, instead of hiding or fleeing Sebastian boldly reappeared before the emperor, who ordered his men to beat him until they were really sure he was dead. They completed their task this time and threw the remains into the great sewer (*cloaca maxima*). Even so, Sebastian appeared to the pious matron Lucina in a vision and directed her to recover his remains and have them put to rest in the catacombs on the Via Appia.[72]

Because the common practice for depicting a martyr in Christian iconography is to show the saint either undergoing fatal torture or else posing with the instruments of his or her torture, viewers of those many paintings of St. Sebastian could understandably deduce that he died of multiple arrow wounds. Yet for all that follows, at least from the year 680 on, the main point of the story is that Sebastian suffered that terrible, first attempt on his life – and recovered. To be sure, shortly after he regained

[71] Paul the Deacon, *Historia Longobardorum* 6.5, p. 166 and *History of the Lombards*, 255; *Liber pontificalis*, 193–94.
[72] *Acta S. Sebastiani* 23, cols. 1148–50.

his health he gained martyrdom by being beaten to death, but still, he had triumphed over the arrow wounds inflicted by the emperor's henchmen.

What do the arrows signify? Both the Judeo-Christian and the Greco-Roman traditions had something to say on this question. In Psalm 7:13 arrows are instruments of divine punishment: "If one does not repent, God will sharpen his sword; he has bent and strung his bow; he has prepared his deadly weapon, making his arrows fiery shafts." And in the very first lines of the *Iliad*, because of the terrible wrongs committed by Agamemnon and the entreaties of those whom he wronged, Apollo, son of Zeus, "distant, deadly archer," and "god of plague," "came down like night" and let fly his pestilence-laden arrows from his silver bow. "He cut them down in droves and the corpse fires burned on, night and day, no end in sight. Nine days the arrows of the god swept through the army."[73] We are not left to guess whether Roman aristocrats of later times had read their Homer. With reference to the epidemic at Rome in 590, Gregory the Great mentioned the pestilence "that depopulated this city" (*quae hanc urbem depopulavit*) and in which "one could see with one's physical eyes the arrows pouring out of the sky striking down individuals."[74] And thus by a remarkable inversion, the Greek god who sent down pestilence upon people by shooting arrows at them re-emerged in the seventh century as a Christian hero who, having suffered numerous arrow wounds and survived, now took upon himself in Christ-like fashion the arrow wounds (read: plague infections) of those who petitioned him for relief from the plague. Over the next few centuries the cult of Sebastian grew in Rome and spread elsewhere in Europe. The few surviving images of Sebastian from these times show him in the traditional manner with his martyr's crown or else as a soldier with a spear, whereas the familiar scene of his body penetrated by arrows did not come into fashion until the fourteenth century.[75]

The first plague pandemic left little in the way of visual representation, but the principal exception, composed of various elements that coalesced only over a long stretch of time, is a unique and dramatic monument. The initial elements were the theme of divine punishment preached by Pope Gregory the Great in 590 – "I see my entire flock being struck down by the sword of God's wrath" – and the penitential processions he

---

[73] Homer, *The Iliad* 1.10–68, pp. 77–79.
[74] Gregory the Great, *Dialogues* 4.37.7, in vol. 3:128–31.
[75] Marshall, "Manipulating the Sacred."

then organized.[76] The second element is the mausoleum of the Emperor Hadrian, a massive drum-shaped cylinder poised on the right bank of the Tiber, roughly opposite its predecessor and model, the mausoleum of Augustus. Thanks to the Gothic War, it had been incorporated into the city's defensive walls by the middle of the sixth century.[77] The third element is the cult of St. Michael the Archangel, which began with his miraculous appearance in the late fifth century atop Mount Gargano, located on a peninsula in Apulia that juts out into the Adriatic Sea. In most places where the cult spread subsequently, its propagators sought sites at high elevations, appropriate for a messenger from heaven. The cult was active in Rome perhaps as early as the seventh century, but in any case in 852, after a destructive raid by Saracens, Pope Leo IV topped off his rebuilding of the walls by dedicating a chapel to St. Michael on top of Hadrian's Tomb. By that time at the latest, the building was known as the Castle of the Holy Angel (*castellum sancti angeli*).[78]

The key element that then wove together all these others was the account of the events of the year 590 as related by James of Voragine in his *Golden Legend*, which was completed in the 1260s. James' version adds an important detail to the oft-repeated story of the pope's organizing of penitential processions and supplications, namely, a miraculous sign of divine approval. One day the air began to clear, and, as James tells it, Gregory looked up and "saw, above the castle that in the past was called the Tomb of Hadrian, the angel of the Lord wiping a bloody sword and sheathing it. He understood thereby that his prayers had been answered and that the plague was over."[79] This triumphant conclusion to the story about Gregory brought the added authority of the Hebrew Bible, for it was a recasting of the story of God's displeasure with David, when God sent the angel to inflict a pestilence that killed 70,000 Israelites. Still not satisfied, God then sent the angel to destroy Jerusalem, but David made an altar and made offerings and supplications that persuaded God to relent and order the angel to stay his hand. Here we arrive at the relevant moment: David looked up and saw the angel of the Lord standing between heaven and earth, at first with his sword drawn and stretched over Jerusalem, but then at the Lord's command, the angel sheathed his

---

[76] Gregory of Tours, *Historia Francorum* 10.1, p. 407 and *History of the Franks*, p. 545.
[77] *Castel Sant'Angelo*, 20–33.
[78] *Culte et pèlerinages à saint Michel*; Krautheimer, *Rome*, 75, 117–20.
[79] James of Voragine, *Golden Legend*, 2:202.

sword.[80] This Old Testament prototype for the story of Pope Gregory is now largely forgotten, but the huge eighteenth-century bronze statue of an angel sheathing his sword that now stands atop the castle, visible from vantage points all over Rome, serves as a reminder of divine mercy and of Gregory's crucial role in securing it at the close of the sixth century.[81] This dramatic figure is also a reminder that the pandemic of 541 to 750 is a chapter of human history that deserves far better than a parenthetical phrase.

[80] 1 Chronicles 21:14–27. I am very grateful to Prof. Malcolm Bell III of the University of Virginia for bringing this biblical text to my attention.

[81] *Castel Sant'Angelo,* 91–97, 146–52. The present statue, made in 1752 by the Flemish sculptor P. A. von Verschaffelt, replaced a marble statue made in 1554 by Raffaele da Montelupo. There are indications of still earlier versions dating back to the thirteenth century. See D'Onofrio, *Castel S. Angelo,* 162–72.

2

Historians and Epidemics

Simple Questions, Complex Answers

Jo N. Hays

In this essay, I pose some questions that historians ask when they examine particular past epidemics or groups of epidemics, and I review some of the answers found in response to those questions. At some points, I even suggest their possible application to the Plague of Justinian. Most of the questions have been simple and obvious ones, but the answers, in some cases, have been complex and ambiguous; some of the complexities stem from historical uncertainty about whether disease should be constructed biologically or socially, a dilemma that the historiography of epidemics reflects. Different civilizations have reached different understandings of the general nature of disease. Modern historical writing, however, has reflected two relatively recent such understandings: the biological, reductionist view that rose to dominance in the late nineteenth century, and the more recent conviction that diseases are social constructs. Those two (at times conflicting) understandings now set the questions that historians of disease attempt to answer. Because disease is, in part, a "biological process," as Henry Sigerist defined it in 1943, questions about past epidemics have included "what *was* the disease" (in a biological, ontological sense), what were its physical effects, how did it spread, how many died or were sickened by it.[1] Convictions that diseases are social constructs have led to other questions: "What did the society make of it?" and "How did the society confront it or perhaps even *use* it?"

[1] Sigerist, *Civilization and Disease*, 1.

33

IN WHAT WAYS HAVE SOCIETIES PERCEIVED EPIDEMICS, AND HOW HAVE SOCIETIES RESPONDED TO EPIDEMICS?

These questions are intimately related, for societies have responded to epidemics in ways dictated by how they perceive them, and especially by how they perceive their causes. Epidemics, as Charles Rosenberg has pointed out, require a collective explanation of their cause and so have long posed porblems for societies that generally explained an individual's disease as a deviation (with an individual cause) from some norm of health.[2] Epidemic diseases have been variously ascribed to divine will, environmental corruption, contagion, malign spirits, individuals or groups (sometimes stigmatized as scapegoats), organisms external to the body, and spontaneous internal malfunctions. Each of these etiological positions has suggested different responses, but actual historical experience has most often reflected etiological uncertainty and disagreement. Etiological ambiguities have been the rule, not the exception, and those ambiguities have been reflected in the diverse and apparently contradictory responses of societies faced by epidemics. Attempts (such as Rosenberg's) to impose a clear chronological evolution on such different etiologies and responses, while stimulating, have faced a multitude of exceptions and complications.[3]

Do those "exceptions and complications" characterize responses to the Justinianic Plague? Did Hippocratic environmental traditions ("airs and places") intersect or conflict with the thoughts about contagion that Lawrence Conrad and others have explored?[4] How completely was the Christian notion of possession by demons domesticated in the sixth century? Or was the Justinianic Plague on too large a scale for such an "individual" interpretation? Alain Stoclet's essay confirms that (even in the Latin West) Asclepian and Hippocratic traditions persisted among pious Christian and ecclesiastical officials, and that fact suggests that either conflicting or compromised responses were commonplace over the Mediterranean Basin.

And – to take questions of response further – the essays in this volume concern a series of epidemics, called perhaps for convenience "*the* Plague of Justinian," which occurred in waves (numbered seventeen by Dionysius Stathokouplos in this volume, and fifteen in an earlier article

---

[2] Rosenberg, *Explaining Epidemics*, 294–95.
[3] E.g., ibid., 293–304; Kearns, "Zivilis or Hygaeia."
[4] E.g., Conrad and Wujastyk, *Contagion*, esp. 99–177.

by Biraben and Le Goff) between 541 and 750.[5] These phenomena are more akin to the plague epidemics between 1347 and the eighteenth century than they are to the single great 1347–1350 pandemic (the Black Death) properly speaking, and so some chronological evolution in etiologies and responses might be expected. Did such responses change over the two-century span of these epidemics? Did the pious Muslim response of resignation to God's will emerge only in the Abbasid period, while Muslims in the Umayyad period more often simply took flight?

Recent historiography has also clearly demonstrated that political, economic, or social conceptions intersect with more formal "etiology," whether that etiology is (for example) biomedical or theological. Thus, the cholera epidemic of 1832 in Paris inspired particular fear among a still-insecure bourgeois elite because the memory of political upheaval, both in 1830 and in 1792, drove that elite to associate the disease with threats from the lower orders. The cholera epidemic of 1848, in fact more serious (in terms of mortality and morbidity) than that of 1832, was regarded more calmly by a now-more-confident middle class.[6] How to explain the fact that the appearance of plague in Los Angeles in 1924 was denied by newspapers, which called it "malignant pneumonia," while poliomyelitis, ten years later, resulted in a panic (to which the authorities contributed) in the same city?[7]

Modern historians have attempted answers to questions about responses to, and perceptions of, epidemics by making use of a wide variety of sources: the records of governments and churches documenting their actions, the testimonies of witnesses of those actions, the writings of a wide range of "authorities" whose explanations of etiology carried contemporary weight, whether they spoke for religion, morality, "medicine," or folk-belief. In some cases we have been able to recover the experiences of the sufferers themselves, and so tell the story of an epidemic from "below." Part of the question "how was the epidemic perceived?" must surely be the further question, "perceived by *whom*?" Cholera in the 1830s baffled medical and political elites, but some poor city dwellers were convinced that governments, driven by Malthusian fears of overpopulation, were poisoning them.[8] British government attempts to compel smallpox vaccinations led some Norfolk villagers to believe "that the

---

[5] Biraben and Le Goff, "Plague in the Early Middle Ages."
[6] Kudlick, *Cholera in Post-Revolutionary Paris*, 29–30 and 41–42.
[7] Gregg, *Plague: An Ancient Disease*, 43; Paul, *History of Poliomyelitis*, 221.
[8] Morris, *Cholera*, 99–100.

state's encouragement of vaccination formed a plot to kill children under five, and Queen Victoria was a modern Herod."[9] Do sources exist from late antiquity and the early medieval period that would allow historians to interpret such views from below? How widespread were the talismans found by Stoclet in Gaul? And on another level of demotic response, what are we to make of the deliberate breaking of pottery noticed in Syria by Michael Morony? Do such actions illustrate a population in a traumatic shock? In the Philadelphia yellow fever epidemic of 1793, the citizenry fired guns into the air, perhaps in panic, but justified as environmental intervention to dispel a dangerous miasma.[10] Did a rationale underlie the Syrian pot-smashing?

WHAT CAN BE LEARNED ABOUT THE MORTALITY AND MORBIDITY INFLICTED BY EPIDEMICS? HOW MANY, AND WHO, DIED, WHERE AND WHEN?

Studies of modern epidemics also have a demographic component, which asks for some quantification of mortality (death rate) and morbidity (case rate) of the epidemic. Precise answers to demographic questions obviously depend on both accurate census data (for the total population), and diagnostic evidences of causes of death and illness. Finding either before the middle nineteenth century is rare, but that does not mean that the task hasn't been attempted. In addition to the elaborate estimates of the mortality of the so-called Black Death of 1347–1350,[11] information has also been shaken out of societies that seemingly have left little in the written record. Gunnar Karlsson, for example, has used a few chronicles, annals, and records of farm occupancy to reconstruct plague mortality in fifteenth-century Iceland, although "the fifteenth century is the only century in the history of Iceland about which we have no extensive written narratives."[12]

Other questions accompany a search for mortality and morbidity rates. If the search ultimately depends on "diagnosis" of causes of death or illness, then it also involves "but what *was* the disease, in modern (i.e. 'correct') biomedical terms"? We may not be able to decide that an epidemic

---

9 Digby, *Pauper Palaces*, 176.
10 Powell, *Bring Out Your Dead*, 51, 54, 71.
11 E.g., the most recent estimates by Benedictow, *Black Death*; compare with Biraben, *Les Hommes et la peste*, 1:156–84. A pioneering earlier discussion: Renouard, "Conséquences et intérêt démographiques," 459–66.
12 Karlsson, "Plague Without Rats."

killed 10% of a population (or, alternately, was responsible for a 10% increase in ordinary mortality rates) unless we can sort out different causes of death. "But what was the disease" has been a frequently asked question in disease historiography, one to which I will return, in part to discuss whether the question does or does not matter.

WHAT EFFECTS HAVE BEEN TRACED TO EPIDEMICS?

Historians have studied the effects of diseases on ideas, beliefs, and value systems; on the economy, either in the short run, the long run, or both; on the affected community's social structure; and on the positions and activities of political and other authorities. The experience of epidemics has contributed to changing etiological beliefs themselves; the apparent safety of medical personnel dealing with cholera cases in India combined with the failure of quarantine to stop the same disease's advance into Russia seemed to say to early nineteenth-century observers that that malady could not be contagious.[13] Did early medieval societies learn from their experiences with the Justinianic Plague? Michael Dols argued, in the 1970s, that Muslim experiences with the seventh-century plagues conditioned their responses to the fourteenth-century Black Death; there existed, Dols argued, a body of authoritative Islamic teaching that restrained panic and guilt in Muslim populations, while Christian communities, lacking such traditions, reacted differently.[14] Is it really true that Christian traditions from the Justinianic Plague inspired only fear, flight, and guilt?

In what different ways did Christian ideas change with the pandemic? Stoclet notices an increased emphasis on devotion to the Virgin Mary, perhaps introduced to succor a stricken population. And Michael Kulikowski proposes another possible shift in beliefs, both very important and very difficult to document: old burial habits in Visigothic Spain seem to have shifted rapidly under the pressure of epidemics; did those changes illustrate shifting relationships between the quick and the dead?

Epidemics have at times confirmed (and even promoted) existing social preconceptions. Modern social historians have documented a number of cases in which epidemics gave grounds for the further stigmatization of an already-marginalized group: the poor in Renaissance Italy (thought to harbor plague), Irish immigrants in nineteenth-century

---

[13] Ackerknecht, "Anticontagionism."
[14] Dols, *Black Death in the Middle East*, 291–97.

New York (associated with cholera), the poor all over the nineteenth-century western world (increasingly conflated with tuberculosis suffering), African Americans in the early twentieth century (a "syphilis-soaked" race), and the "4-H" (homosexuals, Haitians, hemophiliacs, and heroin addicts) group that seemed the focus of what was eventually called AIDS in the 1980s.[15] Those examples from modern history suggest the relevance of similar questions about the Plague of Justinian. What marginal populations existed in the sixth-, seventh-, and eighth-century Mediterranean and Europe? On what bases (religious belief, economic status, legal position, language, "barbarians") were they marginalized, and did epidemic disease confirm or strengthen that marginalization? In at least one curious case, documented by Kulikowski, pogroms against the Jews of Spain actually ceased during epidemics, apparently because the authorities needed population numbers more than they needed the psychosocial benefits of persecuting outsiders.

Such examples illustrate the social-construction side of disease. But diseases also have had more concrete economic or social effects, illustrating a disease's physical pathology as well as its social construction. Some social groups may actually have been at greater risk or have suffered higher mortality and morbidity rates than others during particular epidemics, and our findings about those facts may relate to our "modern" judgment of "but what was the disease?" And especially in those epidemics of unusually high mortality (that for instance associated with the fourteenth-century Black Death), high enough to make a real demographic impact (if only in the short run), economic changes might be expected. As is well known, much historical speculation has centered on the economic effects of the dramatically lowered population of Europe (and the Mediterranean Basin) in the wake of the Black Death,[16] and some of the same questions might be raised about the Justinianic Plague as well. Did Europe and the Near East move quickly from overpopulation, low wages, and high rents (and demands for labor services as part of tenancy), to underpopulation, high wages, and low rents (and freedom from "conditions")? Was productivity affected, and if so, how and where? Did greater disposable income for the survivors translate to more relative emphasis on luxury goods rather than staples? Was land occupied differently, with less attention to arable and more to pasture? Did high labor

---

[15] Carmichael, *Plague and the Poor*; Pullan, "Plague and Perceptions"; Rosenberg, *Cholera Years*, 59, 137–38; Smith, *Retreat of Tuberculosis*; Brandt, *No Magic Bullet*, 157–58.

[16] E.g., Miskimin, *Economy of Early Renaissance Europe*.

costs encourage the development of capital-intensive technology (analogous to the later wind and water power, printing presses, and cannon)? And of great importance: What sources might answer such questions?

It now seems likely that some such phenomena did appear in the wake of the Justinianic Plague. The volume of trade and of production declined generally in the mid-sixth century; in some places (Syria, at least, according to Hugh Kennedy), new housing ceased. The transmission of the epidemic, apparently by sea, meant that coastal cities (the greatest centers of wealth) were hit first and hardest, and perhaps their weaknesses rippled through the Mediterranean lands. Both Kulikowski (in Visigothic Spain) and Peter Sarris (in Byzantine lands) have detected attempts to tie increasingly scarce labor to land, attempts especially notable (in Sarris' view) in a time of legal and economic turmoil. But many interesting other possibilities remain.

Does a massive epidemic lead to a rapid demographic response, as the human population, perhaps seizing on newly favorable wage–price relations or newly available lands and opportunities, responds with earlier marriages and a birth boom? Robert Sallares has cautioned against exaggerating the long-term demographic significance of disease, given the reproductive recovery powers of human populations.[17] The case of India in the wake of the 1918–1919 influenza epidemic, however, suggests that such a recovery may be delayed, at least in the short run; I. D. Mills has argued that high morbidity in 1918 led to decreasing coital frequency, while mortality removed too many women of childbearing age and too many households were broken apart by the death of a partner.[18] (Mills' argument is strengthened by a known peculiarity of the 1918–1919 influenza pandemic: its particular severity for young adults, those from whom a rapid demographic recovery might have been expected.) A period of demographic stagnation ensued. The current AIDS epidemic in sub-Saharan Africa will be another test case for such demographic responses.

Still another category of effects, well-explored by historians, is the challenge to authority that epidemics (and the measures taken against them by authorities) have inspired. Different types of authority have been at stake: political, religious, intellectual, and professional. The perceived bungling by the governments of Naples, in particular, and Italy, in general, in response to the cholera epidemic of 1884 led to what Frank Snowden

[17] Sallares, *Ecology of the Ancient Greek World*, 222–24.
[18] Mills, "1918–1919 Influenza Pandemic," 17–23.

has called a challenge to the legitimacy of the liberal state, a challenge taken so seriously that when cholera next appeared, in 1911, the local and national governments attempted to deny that an epidemic crisis existed.[19] The resistance to authorities manifested in Italian cities in seventeenth-century plague years has been intensively studied.[20] Urban populations reacted to the decrees of city boards of health by pelting health officers with stones; and more generally (and perhaps suggestively) Giulia Calvi has uncovered a dense network of popular resistance to rules of quarantine, isolation in pest houses, sanitary cordons, health passes and inspections, resistance that might, alternately, be called "corruption" or "mediation between authority and popular culture." Surgeons could be bribed to certify deaths as not plague, allowing loved ones to be buried in churchyards; inspectors could overlook plague and allow families to remain in their homes, perhaps extracting material or sexual favors in return.[21] Clearly, gaps have existed between what authority decrees and what actually happens.

In some instances, authorities have used the crisis of an epidemic to strengthen their power. Quarantines certainly spurred popular resistance, but they also represented a considerable extension of the hand of government into daily lives. The Renaissance cities that located plague in their poorer quarters used that "fact" as an instrument of social control. Did the Justinianic Plague provide similar opportunities? Stoclet wonders whether epidemics in some way legitimized new dynasties such as the Abbasid and the Capetian. But the Justinianic epidemics may also have crippled state power, in ways that later and better-known plagues would illustrate. Sarris notes a suspicious coincidence of epidemics and periods of crisis in Byzantine state finance, crises likely produced by the declining tax base that followed on rural depopulation.

The seventeenth-century Italian experiences have also illustrated that epidemics can set one authority against another. Tensions between the authority of the church, which mandated pious processions and religious ceremonies in response to plague, and that of increasingly contagionist city–state authorities, who looked on such gatherings of the infected with horror, led at times to physical conflict. Seventeenth-century England experienced something similar, when Anglican theologians (especially

---

[19] Snowden, *Naples in the Time of Cholera.*

[20] E.g., works of Cipolla, *Christofano and the Plague; Public Health and the Medical Profession; Faith, Reason, and the Plague; Fighting the Plague.*

[21] Calvi, *Histories of a Plague Year,* esp. 155–96.

of the Puritan wing) emphasized the power of divine providence, the basic powerlessness of human action, and the necessity of prayer and divine services; those same theologians served a state committed to more active measures of isolation of the sick.[22] In the Moscow plague epidemic of 1771, many clergymen so violently disagreed with government policies (which proscribed traditional religious practices and services) that they contributed to a serious riot in the course of which an archbishop (seen as an agent of government) was murdered.[23] Another variation on the theme of authorities at odds has appeared in conflict between different levels of government. English local governments ignored the orders of the central Board of Health in the cholera epidemic of 1848–1849.[24] During the 1918 influenza epidemic, London's local borough councils went their own way in defiance of the Board of Health; Pittsburgh's mayor denounced the State Board of Health's closure of saloons, and in San Francisco, the city government ordered the population to wear gauze masks, which the State Board of Health ridiculed as unnecessary.[25]

The period of the Plague of Justinian seems rife with possible conflicts of authority, for it appears (to an outsider, at least) as an age of shifting religious domination and contested grounds: between Islam, Zoroastrianism, and Christianity, between differing versions of Christianity, and between differing local and more central polities, the seventh-century analogues of American federal–state confusion. Especially in zones of recent conquest or reconquest, were responses to epidemics complicated by such divided loyalties? In the Latin West, did responses to epidemic bring into focus tensions between secular and religious authority, or between greater and lesser patrons? Between new rulers and an old senatorial aristocracy, if such a term still had meaning?

As medicine came to claim greater authority in the nineteenth century, so doctors and hospitals became the targets of resistance. The cholera epidemic of the early 1830s saw violently dramatic attacks on doctors and hospitals in Paris, Manchester, Glasgow, and Edinburgh; the same were repeated in Marseilles and Naples in 1884, and in the Russian town of Khvalynsk, in 1892, a physician was battered to death by an angry crowd: "Ruffians jeered at the corpse and peasant women spit in the face of the deceased and railed at his imagined crimes, rejoicing that the

---

[22] Slack, *Impact of Plague*, 228–44.
[23] Alexander, *Bubonic Plague in Early Modern Russia*, 186–95.
[24] Durey, *Return of the Plague*, 207.
[25] Tomkins, "Failure of Expertise"; White, "Pittsburgh in the Great Epidemic," 227; Crosby, *America's Forgotten Pandemic*, 105.

poisoner had received proper retribution."[26] How strong was the hold of the hospital in the early Byzantine period? How relevant were hospitals to responses to an overwhelming and rapid epidemic?

It seems clear that challenges to authority are more likely when "authority" does not speak with a unified voice. Civic or religious authority responding to plague faced greater opposition in the seventeenth century than in the fourteenth. In the earlier case, etiologies and responses overlapped in important ways, with widespread agreement about different levels of cause that left different authorities free to respond to different levels without contradicting each other. In the later period, both churches and city-states had lost confidence in each other's answers, and each decided that they knew how to respond. The police corporal of Monte Lupo (1630), a man of little education, defended what we might call the "scientific" response against the arguments of the more-learned priest who spoke for "religion"; the countering authority of the state lay behind the corporal.[27] It is hard to imagine a western European, or North American, population in the twentieth century reacting against doctors in the way that the people of Khvalynsk did in 1892, or – for that matter – the way that the citizens of Paris and Manchester did in 1832; medical "authority," what is sometimes called "medicalization," had become too strong. (But remember that the word "medicalization" may imply that the claims of medicine are advanced, as the *New Shorter Oxford English Dictionary* puts it, "unwarrantedly"; those claims therefore, being socially constructed, may be conditional and transient.)

IN TERMS OF MODERN BIOMEDICAL UNDERSTANDING, WHAT "WAS" THE EPIDEMIC? AND DOES THAT QUESTION MATTER FOR HISTORICAL DISCUSSION?

Modern biomedical scientists will ask of past epidemics, "but what was the disease"?[28] The prospect of identifying the agent responsible for the Plague of Justinian seems bright. Literary evidence has long supported a diagnosis of bubonic plague, and now techniques of molecular biology, when allied with a determined and coordinated effort to identify plague burial sites, may settle the question. (See the accompanying essays of

[26] Kudlick, *Cholera in Post-Revolutionary Paris*, 186–87; Morris, *Cholera*, 108–14; Snowden, *Naples in the Time of Cholera*, 77–78 and 145–47; Frieden, "Russian Cholera Epidemic," 545.
[27] Cipolla, *Faith, Reason, and the Plague*, 75–76.
[28] The phrase comes from a title: Prins, "But What Was the Disease?"

Robert Sallares, who argues the possibility of *Yersinia pestis,* and that of Michael McCormick.)

I would like to ask here, "why does that matter"? Simply, knowing what disease caused an epidemic matters because it enables us to relate the incidence and spread of an epidemic to the social and physical environment that existed prior to its appearance, because it enables us to make better sense of some of the epidemic's social, political, and economic effects, and because estimates of mortality may be informed by such knowledge. But in historical writing the question of the identity of a disease has been complicated first by the historicist's desire to accept the testimony of the past on its own, and then by our now-well-established conviction that diseases are social constructions, or at least contain within them an important element of social construction.

In the late fifteenth century an apparently new disease began a dramatic sweep through Europe, and indeed through Asia as well. Europeans came to call this disease the "Great Pox." Only in the eighteenth century did the name "syphilis" begin to be widely used for "it," although the word did enter the discussion in the sixteenth-century poem of Fracastoro relating the disease to the blasphemy of the pagan shepherd Syphilis. But does a different word carry with it a large (and different) freight of meaning? If we say that "syphilis first appeared in Europe in the 1490s," are we committing ourselves to saying that "Europeans began to be infected by a specific microorganism called '*Treponema pallidum*' that resulted in thus-and-so symptoms"? Fifteenth-century Europeans did not think of the matter in those terms. "Poxes" existed along a continuum of pestilence; the "Great Pox" was not nearly as specific as associating it with a single parasite made it out.[29] Similarly, "phthisis" and "consumption" describe a wasting disease of the lungs; are those terms synonymous with "tuberculosis," when in fact what they describe may also have been lung cancer or silicosis, while "tuberculosis" includes what was once called "scrofula" and never called "consumption"? What we now call "AIDS" was for a time (thankfully brief) called "GRID," Gay-Related Immune Deficiency, and if the "meaning" of a disease encompasses its etiology, or its pattern of incidence, "GRID" seems a different disease than "AIDS." Should historians simply take the past on its own terms, and speak of Europeans suffering the "Great Pox" in the sixteenth century?

The subject, as it happens, has been especially explored with respect to "plague," particularly its great epidemic of the mid-fourteenth century. Was the "Black Death" a product of the microorganism now called *Y.*

[29] Arrizabalaga, *Great Pox;* Quétel, *History of Syphilis.*

pestis? That organism was first identified in the 1890s; shortly thereafter a convincing epidemiology, one that involved rodent hosts and insect vectors, was worked out. Most historians, I believe, have accepted the idea that the Black Death was caused by the spread of that organism through human populations, resulting in one of two (or three) different clinical manifestations of disease called bubonic plague, pneumonic plague, and septicaemic plague. Modern clinical descriptions of those diseases accord well with fourteenth-century evidence. On those bases, modern historians of the Black Death have constructed their arguments about its spread and (especially) about the environmental conditions that favored it.

But not all biological scientists are convinced. How could a disease most at home in rodent populations that move very little and not very far, conveyed by insects (especially the flea *Xenopsylla cheopis*) that only alight on humans accidentally and not by choice, have spread with such devastating rapidity through Europe and western Asia? How could the disease persist through winter months when the temperature range within which fleas flourish is so narrow? Could the victims of pneumonic plague diffuse the epidemic very easily or very far, given that disease's rapid onset of debility and death? In the light of these objections, could the Black Death really have been bubonic and/or pneumonic plague? Such arguments started to be made even before the identification of *Y. pestis*, for Charles Creighton suspected in 1894 that a relation existed between what he called the "plague virus" and typhus. J. F. D. Shrewsbury, in 1970, bothered by the biological improbabilities of *Y. pestis* as an agent for the Black Death, argued first that the assumptions of high mortality were overstated, and second that other diseases, especially typhus, helped account for the mortality that occurred; he did not, however, propose to banish *Y. pestis* entirely. Some later authors have been more ruthless. Graham Twigg, in 1984, made a case for anthrax as the culprit, and most recently Susan Scott and Christopher Duncan have urged the actual biological impossibility that *Y. pestis* could have accounted for the Black Death. Instead, they argue, that epidemic should be called a "haemorraghic plague," for which an unknown virus akin to the modern Ebola virus was responsible. Historical argument persists, as the writings of Samuel Cohn (dubious about "plague") and Ole Benedictow (vigorously reasserting plague's identity and importance) illustrate.[30]

---

[30] Creighton, *Epidemics in Britain*; Shrewsbury, *History of Bubonic Plague*; Twigg, *Black Death: A Biological Reappraisal*; Scott and Duncan, *Biology of Plagues*; Cohn, "The Black Death." Shrewsbury and Twigg were both heavily criticized by historians: e.g., C. Morris on Shrewsbury in *Historical Journal* and Gottfried on Twigg in *Speculum*. For rebuttals of Cohn, and of Scott and Duncan, see Sallares in this volume and Benedictow, *Black Death*.

To the historian, does it matter? I argued above that it does, but we should be aware of the difficulties when we impose modern constructs, two of which the Black Death illustrate: first, as Scott and Duncan et al. argue, the modern constructs may be the wrong ones; and second, even if those constructs are "right," does our modern "naming" of the epidemic interfere with our understanding of it and especially of contemporary responses to it? Jon Arrizabalaga, in his study of the reactions to the Black Death of contemporary university medical practitioners, puts the case clearly: "I am deliberately renouncing any attempt at retrospective diagnosis by the criteria of what current Western medicine understands by plague today. For in exploring disease perceptions and reactions by past human societies, we must not forget that the identity of the disease nowadays known as plague, just like the identity of other infectious diseases, relies on an intellectual construction we have inherited from a precise historical and cultural context – that of late nineteenth- and early twentieth-century laboratory medicine and, specifically, the germ theory. It would therefore be wrong to assume that when we talk about late medieval and early modern plague, we are dealing with the same disease that we recognize as plague today."[31] In a particularly persuasive argument along these lines, Andrew Cunningham maintains that "the dominance of the laboratory concept of disease has had a significant effect on our understanding of many *pre*-laboratory diseases – leading us to read them as if they were laboratory diseases; hence the coming of the laboratory has led to the *past* of medicine being rewritten to accord with the laboratory model of disease, and it has thereby been misunderstood." "The laboratory construction of plague," Cunningham concludes, "means that there is an unbridgeable gap between past 'plague' and our plague. The identities of pre-1894 plague and post-1894 plague have become incommensurable. We are simply unable to say whether they were the same, since the criteria of 'sameness' have been changed."[32]

But we should remember (as Cunningham recognizes) that diseases are only "culturally constructed" in certain ways. They also have a pathological reality. Beyond the perhaps-distorting power that "renaming" confers on us, coming to a "modern" understanding of a past epidemic does help historians with some other questions that they properly raise: questions relating to the human and physical environment that might allow a disease to spread, and that account for its decline or disappearance. What

[31] Arrizabalaga, "Facing the Black Death," 239.
[32] Cunningham, "Transforming Plague," 209–12.

factors about a given society made the epidemic possible, or more likely? Knowing something of the life cycles of the microbial or viral agents, their hosts, and the vectors that carry them relates disease to a society more clearly.

HOW DID THE LARGER ENVIRONMENTS, PHYSICAL AND SOCIAL, AFFECT THE ORIGIN AND SPREAD OF EPIDEMICS?

Several further questions may be subsumed under that heading. (a) What do we know about human settlements and movements? (b) What do we know about human nutrition? (c) What political or economic pressures did humans put on their environments?

Human Settlements and Movements

Density of human settlement has special importance for the spread of many diseases, especially airborne ones, whether bacterial (such as tuberculosis) or viral (such as smallpox). It is not simply a matter of keeping a chain of infection going easily, although that clearly is important in epidemics. In addition, some acute diseases need a reservoir of previously uninfected humans if an epidemic is to be sustained. Thus, measles and smallpox, both dependent on finding virgin soil, need a minimum population, a critical mass, to become epidemic.[33] Dense urban populations may also favor the easy movement of vectors from one person to another: fleas (especially relevant if human fleas, *Pulex irritans,* carry *Y. pestis*), lice (carrying typhus), mosquitoes (carrying malaria or yellow fever). And the density of a settlement may also affect its water supplies and the proximity of its people to quantities of human wastes; therefore waterborne diseases such as cholera, typhoid fever, and dysentery may also be density-determined. Density may, in recent times at least, have meant number of rooms per family, or the relation between number of rooms and population; tuberculosis among women may have declined in the late nineteenth century, in part, because housebound women gained a little more space in their dwellings.[34] Relevant housing conditions may also include building materials and styles; were medieval town dwellings companionable for rodents? Would a thatched roof house rodents and insects that a tile roof would repel?

[33] Summarized in Cliff and Haggett, "Epidemic Control."
[34] Cronje, "Tuberculosis and Mortality Decline."

How populous and densely settled were the lands of late antiquity and early medieval times? In some cases – sixth-century Spain, for instance, as Kulikowski argues – population density may not have been great enough to sustain prolonged epidemics. Were cities becoming larger or smaller, more or less dense, over the sixth, seventh, and eighth centuries? In seventh-century England, town populations had become significant for the first time since the end of Roman rule, and the coastal location of towns in England meant that they could provide diffusing links with the hinterland, as John Maddicott suggests. Constantinople's role as a plague diffuser may have been especially significant. Residential patterns have affected epidemiology. That the *poor* population of Syrian cities died first may be significant (according to Morony), both about the quarters of town in which those poor lived, and about the density of their settlements. And how crowded was Rome itself in the sixth century? Did its people still live in tall blocks of flats?

Another population variable that may affect an epidemic's history is age distribution. The young have been the traditional virgin target of such acute infections as measles and smallpox, and so (obviously) an unusually young population might be at a proportionally higher risk from such diseases. The same population might also be especially vulnerable to waterborne epidemics such as dysentery. Influenza usually affects the very young and the very old, although the 1918–1919 influenza pandemic was a notable anomaly, one whose severity to young adults may have had important later demographic effects. Do we know anything about age distribution in Late Antiquity, especially about any possible contrasts between different peoples? Was the Arabian eruption of the seventh and eighth centuries fueled by a bulging youth population?

Climate further affects a population's relationship to epidemic disease. Lower latitudes (and altitudes) (other things being equal) may harbor more hosts, vectors, and pathogens, so that a people who move to warmer climates may be more susceptible. Clothing may provide homes for insects, so warmer climates may in that way be healthier; but warmer climates also make bare feet more likely, which leads to the spread of various parasites through the feet. The colder climates of high latitudes also mean indoor crowding and a greater likelihood of person-to-person infection. And climate also affects yet another variable for disease (or resistance to it), nutrition; the links between weather disasters and famine have been real. "Conventional wisdom" about the climate of the sixth, seventh, and eighth centuries posits a prolonged drought and high temperatures in central Eurasia and the southern Mediterranean, and a cold, wet, and disturbed climate in northern and central Europe as well as Italy and the northern Mediterranean.[35] What effects did such conditions – and contrasts – have on human movement and patterns of settlement? On the lives of rodents, insect vectors, and microorganisms?

Human movement also plays a crucial role in disease propagation. A nomadic people may carry pathogens, hosts, and vectors with them. Human movements have had many causes: conquerors move into new territory, conscript or slave labor is driven into new territory, refugees are driven out of old territory, some populations live nomadic lives, others move seasonally from highland to lowland; others seek new opportunity in the next valley or across an ocean, still others are driven from home by famine. Some of those moving may carry pathogens with them; others may encounter a new disease environment when they arrive. In either case, the result may be what is now called a "virgin soil" epidemic. The classic such example is, of course, the horrific depopulation of the Americas in the wake of the appearance of Europeans and Africans in the sixteenth century, but other, more recent cases have also been studied, notably involving isolated island populations in the eighteenth and nineteenth centuries.[36] Europeans moving into sub-Saharan Africa faced new diseases for which their systems were ill prepared.[37] And on which side of the disease gradient were the Frankish Crusaders of the eleventh and twelfth centuries?[38]

The speed of movement presents another variable. A slow crossing of the Atlantic might mean that a chain of smallpox infection (for example) would exhaust itself before the ship reached America; that is, by the conclusion of the voyage everyone on the ship would have either died, recovered, or had demonstrated immunity probably because of an earlier, pre-voyage, case of the disease. Steamship travel made movement of pathogens more likely; jumbo jetliners make such movement more likely yet, and of course add the further hazard of crowding a large number

[35] Lamb, *Climate, History, and the Modern World*, 152–60. Sudden climatic change plays a central role in Keys, *Catastrophe*.
[36] E.g., McArthur, *Island Populations*; Stannard, *Before the Horror*; Cliff and Haggett, *Spread of Measles in Fiji*; Crosby, "Hawaiian Depopulation," 175–201.
[37] E.g., Curtin, *Death by Migration*.
[38] Compare Crosby, *Ecological Imperialism*, 63–67, with the implication in a review (of another book) by S. Watts in the *Bulletin of the History of Medicine*.

of people in a confined space, as did the earlier railways that moved vast crowds of often-unwashed pilgrims across the Indian subcontinent.[39]

What roles did human movement play in the repeated epidemics that make up the "Plague of Justinian"? Several sorts of movement seem likely, above all trade between the eastern Mediterranean, Africa, and Asia. The richness and extent of such trade in the age of the Justinianic Plague is becoming clearer, especially thanks to the work of Michael McCormick, and that trade surely played an important role in epidemiology.[40] As McCormick suggests, our knowledge of trade and our knowledge of infection patterns will reinforce and inform one another. The seas and oceans were highways, not barriers, in the sixth century.

Of course other people were on the move in the sixth and later centuries, especially soldiers, pilgrims, and those in flight from either soldiers or the disease itself. Did the military campaigns of Justinian, whether against Persians or Ostrogoths, relate to plague's diffusion? The sweeping conquests of the Arabs? Did Arab (or Byzantine) conquests promote a free trade area that encouraged commerce? Certainly such questions have been posed about the later Black Death: the Mongol Empire's movements across the vast Eurasian landscape may have dislodged bubonic plague from an ancestral home in central Asia.[41] Did that experience have a sixth- or seventh-century analogue?

Human Nutrition

Human nutrition may often be an important variable in a population's health, but its role in *epidemics* is less clear, especially if "epidemics" mean sudden surges in infections rather than persistent grave health problems, such as tuberculosis in the nineteenth century or lung cancer in the mid-twentieth. Population movement driven by famine is one evident cause of epidemic diffusion. Clearly, nutritional problems directly cause some diseases: scurvy and ergotism have received particular historical attention. Chronic diseases (tuberculosis, leprosy, or AIDS) are probably harder on the poorly nourished. But the cells and tissues of the starving may not provide adequate nutrition for parasitic microorganisms either, and in any case we have clear evidence that mortality from some acute

---

[39] Or so at least the International Sanitary Conference of 1866 believed: Arnold, *Colonizing the Body*, 186–87.

[40] McCormick, *Origins of the European Economy* and "Bateaux de vie, bateaux de mort."

[41] A central point of McNeill, *Plagues and Peoples*, 159–63.

epidemics either had little to do with the nutritional state of the victims (as seems true of bubonic and pneumonic plague) or was actually most severe among the apparently most healthy, a feature of the 1918–1919 influenza pandemic. But even in those cases, Ann Carmichael suggests, someone weakened by poor nutrition may be more vulnerable to "secondary" infections that appear in the wake of plague or influenza.[42] The Black Death of the fourteenth century, however, simply killed too many of its victims too quickly for their nutritional state to have mattered much.

Human Pressures on the Physical Environment

Humans have affected the environment for disease in many ways, apart from their movements. Plantation agriculture in nineteenth-century Egypt created an ideal environment for bilharzia.[43] John Ford's study of African trypanosomes provides some vivid examples of the relations between social and political change, environmental alteration, and disease incidence. According to Ford, pre-colonial African states had developed traditional frontier zones, whereas uncleared areas had been left for game, which thus isolated tsetse flies from the cultivated fields. European colonial political power disrupted those land arrangements and created conditions encouraging serious epidemics of trypanosomiasis, as game (no longer barred by the traditional guards) moved into areas of human settlement, bringing the tsetse flies with them. Criticizing what he called "*Pax Britannica* epidemiology," Ford called the result "not *pax* but *bellum*, an outbreak of biological warfare on a vast scale none the less terrible to its sufferers because they only vaguely perceived its cause while most colonial civil servants were quite unaware of the events that accompanied their advent."[44]

Those examples come from relatively recent history, and I cannot say whether modern human manipulative powers differ from those of late antiquity simply in degree or in absolute and more dramatic kind. But surely changing agricultural patterns, introducing new systems of irrigation, digging canals, constructing roads, all occurred in late antiquity and the early medieval period, and may have modified the relations between humans and parasites. For example, did the social and political settlement of the Anatolian peasantry in the reign of Heraclius have any such effects?

---

[42] Carmichael, "Infection, Hidden Hunger, and History."
[43] Farley, *Bilharzia*, 45–51.
[44] Ford, *Role of Trypanosomiases in African Ecology*, 489.

Answers to a previous question – "what was the disease?" – have contributed to approaches to possibly relevant environmental factors in an epidemic's spread. Consider how the assumption that *Y. pestis* was the causative organism in the Black Death has led to certain emphases about the human and physical environment. The disease spread as a result of contacts between people and infected rodents, with fleas the vector connecting the two populations. At some point, human-to-human transmission became involved, either through the medium of the human flea, or as the disease assumed pneumonic form and spread directly from one person to another through the respiratory system. Obviously, relevant environmental issues therefore include the movement of infected rat populations from one place to another (almost certainly mediated by humans, perhaps on ships, perhaps accompanying caravans); rodents companionable with humans, living in close proximity to them; human dwellings attractive to rats; a high level of human density, increasing the chances of human-to-human transmission; rodent burrows, human homes, clothing and bedding, all of which may be necessary to keep a flea population alive through the winter. The crowded towns of fourteenth-century Europe, filled with structures made of wood, wattle-and-daub, and thatch, represented such an environment; the extensive trade networks that connected northern Europe with the Mediterranean, and Europe with Asia, combined with intensive, more local, trade in grain, may have moved people, rodents, and fleas efficiently; the black rat, *Rattus rattus*, especially at home in crowded urban quarters, had established itself in Europe.

The disease of the Black Death appeared repeatedly in Europe from 1347–1350 until the late seventeenth or early eighteenth centuries, when it disappeared from at least western Europe. Why did it disappear?[45] Considerable historical discussion illustrates still another way in which "but what was the disease?" matters. One possibility is that the disease disappeared for "exogenous" reasons, in which human action played no role. Did a mutation occur in the causative organism? As Robert Sallares has argued, the periodicity of the great plague pandemics, as well as recent research on *Y. pestis*, makes such a possibility attractive.[46] Did humans acquire – if only by natural selection – greater resistance to its ravages? (A

[45] E.g., Appleby, "Disappearance of Plague"; Slack, "Disappearance of Plague: An Alternative View"; Cipolla, *Public Health and the Medical Profession*, 53–66; Sallares, *Ecology of the Ancient Greek World*, 268–71.

[46] Sallares, *Ecology of the Ancient Greek World*, 270. On the mutability of *Y. pestis*: Lenski, "Evolution of Plague Virulence," and Rosqvist et al., "Increased Virulence of *Yersinia pseudotuberculosis*."

possible shift in rat ecology, once advocated as another exogenous event, now seems less likely.[47]) Historians, perhaps uncomfortable with such vast impersonal forces, have concentrated more on human actions (certainly more familiar ground for us) as cause for plague's disappearance. Did humans deliberately or inadvertently interfere with the connections between themselves, rats, and fleas? Were cities constructed more spaciously, of different materials? Did quarantines eventually have an effect, stopping human traffic at least and perhaps with it the movement of fleas and infected rodents?

But notice how many of these speculations hinge on two beliefs, both possibly mistaken: (1) in *Y. pestis* as the prime causative agent, and (2) in the immutable character of *Y. pestis*. Take either of those away, and different historical discussions of an environment relevant to the spread of an epidemic result. Rats, fleas, and the human settlement and traffic that relate to them may cease to matter. Disappearance of plague can no longer be assigned to certain human acts, such as changing domestic architecture. If the Black Death was really an airborne virus, human density mattered more than ever; quarantine may have played an even more important role, since halting the traffic in people might have had a more certain effect than the indirect interference with the movement of rats and fleas that accompanied shipping and caravans.

If therefore a careful survey of "plague" gravesites from the Justinianic Plague can provide enough evidence to allow molecular biologists to establish the causative agent of the epidemics, historians will better know what features of the human, social, and physical environment properly form parts of the epidemic's story.

HAVE EPIDEMICS AFFECTED CONTEMPORARY
OR LATER IMAGINATIONS? HAVE EPIDEMICS THEIR
OWN HISTORIOGRAPHIES?

David Steel has suggested that plague epidemics have an "inherent structure" that mirrors literary conventions: an onset builds up to a climax, followed by a decline and a quiet fading away.[48] In a later and better-known version of the same point, Charles Rosenberg claimed that epidemics follow a "dramaturgic form": they "start in a moment in time, proceed on a stage limited in space and duration, following a plot line

[47] The rat theory was given currency by Helleiner, "Population of Europe," 4:84–85.
[48] Steel, "Plague Writing."

of increasing and revelatory tensions, move to a crisis of individual and collective character, then drift toward closure."[49]

Diseases, especially serious epidemics, have generated their own metaphors. As Susan Sontag memorably noticed, many of our modern metaphors of disease are political and military, speaking of invasions, defenses, conquests, subversions, aggressive therapies.[50] In Chicago in 1922, the commissioner of the Board of Health likened syphilis to a snake, and he proposed to drag it out of the bushes and "beat its head off in public." By 1937, the disease had become a fire that the public had "allowed to smoulder."[51] Within a decade, AIDS went from an overwhelming new plague meaning certain death for social deviants, to a chronic disease with an uncertain outcome that required less sense of crisis and more awareness of the costs of long-term care, but its metaphors changed more slowly.[52] Did the Plague of Justinian acquire contemporary metaphorical standing in the worlds of Islam and Christianity? What different effects flow from "God's anger" or "God's mercy"? It is certainly not for me to judge metaphors on the basis of an English translation published in 1914, but according to that rendering Procopius refers to the Plague of Justinian as a "scourge," which "attacked," "divided," "always moving forward and travelling at times favorable to it.... as if fearing some corner of the earth might escape it."[53]

Some such metaphors have taken more elaborate form, as authors have used plagues as frameworks for their literary constructions. Steel's article traced a long evolution of literary responses, both contemporary and later, to the Black Death and subsequent plague visitations.[54] Boccaccio used plague as a "powerful and inevitable background against which the masquerade of life with all its pleasures" could be more effectively portrayed; the blackness of the background made more vivid the color of the tales. Daniel Defoe's *Journal of the Plague Year* showed the value of sober piety and sense of duty; Alesssandro Manzoni's *I Promessi Sposi* used plague to explore social psychology, Harrison Ainsworth's *Old Saint Paul's* as an excuse for melodrama, and Albert Camus' *La Peste* as an illustration of the power of bureaucratic routine, as well as a reprise

---

[49] Rosenberg, *Explaining Epidemics*, 279.
[50] Sontag, *AIDS and its Metaphors*, 9.
[51] Poirier, *Chicago's War on Syphilis*, 1.
[52] Contrast the titles of two volumes, both edited by Fee and Fox: *AIDS: The Burdens of History* and *AIDS: The Making of a Chronic Disease*.
[53] Procopius, *PW* 2.22.1–11, pp. 451–55.
[54] Steel, "Plague writing," 90.

of Defoe's sober responsibility, transposed from a Protestant to a secular key.

Evolving metaphors may also relate to evolving historiography. Consumption appealed to the nineteenth-century Romantic imagination with its resultant languor, pallor, and the early deaths of such creative luminaries as Keats, Chopin, Weber, and Novalis;[55] when at the century's end it became pulmonary tuberculosis it gradually lost its social cachet and became a stigmatizing mark of poverty and bad habits. In the first sixty years of the twentieth century the incidence of tuberculosis fell (for a variety of reasons), and historians lost interest in it. Its revival in recent years has been mirrored by renewed historical attention, partly owing to its revived presence, but partly also because of its declassé character; social historians have found it a useful subject for a "bottom-up" approach.[56]

Faye Getz, in a persuasive article that appeared in 1991, illustrated the evolution of metaphorical and historical perceptions of the Black Death in the nineteenth and twentieth centuries.[57] These "modern" historiographies began with the rise of epidemiology as a research field the importance of which needed validation by its practitioners, led by Justus Hecker, whose *Der schwartze Tod in vierzehnten Jahrhundert* appeared in 1832. The longest chapter of Hecker's book, titled "Moral Effects," began with these words: "The mental shock sustained by all nations during the prevalence of the Black Plague, is without parallel and beyond description."[58] Hecker, and many later writers, saw the Black Death as an overwhelming natural event, one that excited humans to extremes of behavior and served as a decisive turning point in history, the transition between the Middle Ages and the Renaissance or even the "modern world." James Westfall Thompson (1921) likened the Black Death to the just-concluded Great War; Hans Zinsser (1934) treated epidemic diseases biographically, giving them their own terrible personae. Getz styled certain approaches to the plague "Gothic epidemiology," and the melodramas of nineteenth-century plague literature by Ainsworth, Mary Shelley (*The Last Man*), and Guilbert de Pixérécourt (*La Peste de Marseilles: Mélodrame historique*) illustrate her point. Echoes of "Gothic epidemiology" have continued to influence historical writing down to the recent past, at least: the focus on the extreme behavior of Flagellants and anti-Jewish massacres; views of the

55 Dubos and Dubos, *White Plague*, 44.
56 E.g., Smith, *Retreat of Tuberculosis*; Bryder, *Below the Magic Mountain*; Barnes, *Making of a Social Disease*; Feldberg, *Disease and Class*.
57 Getz, "Black Death and the Silver Lining."
58 Hecker, *Black Death*, 32.

sudden collapse of manorialism in the face of a changed supply–demand labor situation; the relation between high labor costs and late medieval technological innovation; the fine arts abruptly obsessed with images of death. Such emphases have manifested themselves in sources as varied as Barbara Tuchman's immensely popular *A Distant Mirror* (1978) and the studies of demographic catastrophe undertaken during the Cold War by the thermonuclear war-obsessed RAND Corporation.[59]

"Gothic epidemiology" therefore contributed to the more general historiographic view that sharply contrasted the Middle Ages with the Renaissance, generally to the discredit of the former. More recent Black Death historiography has revised some of these approaches, in large part, Getz believes, because of the more general re-evaluation of the Middle Ages and its relation to later periods. Had not medieval populations already begun to decline before 1347? Were medieval institutions and societies really so fragile that the epidemic could destroy them? The population declined rapidly, to be sure, but its continuation at a lower level had more to do with persistent epidemics in the next century or century and a half. Did a crisis really occur in art? Were the extreme social pathologies of the Flagellants typical, or did communities quickly re-establish their routines? Were economic changes underway well before 1347? Were the responses of medieval Christianity so eschatological, or did (as Robert Lerner argued) medieval Christianity provide help for ordinary people in their times of trouble?[60] This general historiographic context, in which gradual and partial transformations replace the abrupt and dramatic transitions encouraged by "Gothic epidemiology," may relate as well to attempts to downplay the importance of *Y. pestis*. Shrewsbury's revision of high mortality has not been widely accepted, but his and subsequent other questions about the role of a single great killer persist. Ann Carmichael asks: "Are plagues of this period dominated by the lethal action of *Yersinia pestis* in a human population, or do the economic disruption, the chaos, and poor personal and public hygiene push the death rates far higher than a killer microbe could unaided?"[61]

And while Carmichael emphasizes some dramatic responses to plague, and resultant harsh measures against the poor undertaken by cities convinced of a "politically privileged contagion theory," those responses were

[59] Tuchman, *Distant Mirror*; Hershleifer, *Disaster and Recovery*.
[60] Lerner, "Black Death and Western Eschatological Mentalities."
[61] Carmichael, "Contagion Theory and Contagion Practice," 254. Benedictow, *Black Death*, strongly reasserts the centrality of *Y. pestis*, at least in the mid-fourteenth century.

hardly those of hysterical panic. The leaders of Italian Renaissance cities, in Carlo Cipolla's phrase, acted as "Pre-Malthus Malthusians,"[62] in full knowledge of what they were doing. And in the Black Death itself, in the place of a Gothic horror, we now talk of the notaries of Perpignan drawing up wills and the people of Siena quickly resuming their political lives with little interruption. In that light, the novel by Camus, in which the ordinary people of twentieth-century Oran quietly go about their jobs, stands as a fictional treatment that (with great foresight) anticipated the historiographic re-evaluations of the Black Death and the late Middle Ages.

What motivates our re-evaluation of the Justinianic Plague? Is this re-evaluation part of a larger revision of the early Middle Ages, East and West? Will *Mohammed and Charlemagne* be revisited? Do we seek a better understanding of the relations of Europe with a region of intense contemporary – early twenty-first century – interest and importance? In asserting the importance of this series of epidemics ("removing them from the parentheses"), do we assume the mantle of Justus Hecker, building a case for dramatic and sweeping effects following in their wake? Is the Plague of Justinian responsible (even only partly) for the End of Antiquity? And if so, should we expect (or be resigned to) the appearance of a revisionist interpretation, perhaps sometime in the twenty-second century, which will put the Plague of Justinian back within parentheses?

[62] Cipolla, "Plague and Pre-Malthus Malthusians."

II

THE NEAR EAST

3

'For Whom Does the Writer Write?'

The First Bubonic Plague Pandemic According to Syriac Sources

Michael G. Morony

Syriac literature has a good deal to say about the first pandemic of bubonic plague from 541 to 749 CE. This includes information about the geographical spread and extent of the initial outbreak in the time of Justinian (541–543), the chronology of later outbreaks, the pathology of the disease, its occurrence among animals, some information about the extent of mortality among its human victims, the disposal of the corpses, the plague's social, economic, and psychological effects, and how it was understood and described by contemporaries.

The main contemporary Syriac account of the first known outbreak of bubonic plague during the reign of Justinian occurs in the second part of the *Ecclesiastical History* of John, Bishop of Ephesus (489–578/9). John was a native of Amida (Diyarbakr) in northern Mesopotamia and was in Palestine when the plague arrived, traveled from there to Constantinople witnessing the plague conditions along the way, and was present in Constantinople during the plague there. The Syriac text of his account is published in the second volume of Land's *Anecdota Syriaca*.[1] This text was largely reproduced by the monastic author of the *Zūqnīn Chronicle*, which was completed at the monastery of Zūqnīn near Amida in 775.[2] John's account is also the basis for the passage in the *Chronicle* of Michael the Syrian, the Syrian Orthodox Patriarch (1166–1199).[3] Both the author of

---

[1] *Anecdota Syriaca*, 2:304–25.

[2] *Incerti auctoris*. John's account is at pp. 79–109. There is an English translation of this account in *CZ*, 94–113.

[3] *Chronique de Michel le Syrien*. The Syriac text is in 4:305–07, the French translation in 2:235–40.

the *Zūqnīn Chronicle*[4] and Michael the Syrian[5] call their source John of
Asia. A summary of this outbreak of plague in the *Chronicle* of Dionysius
of Tel Maḥrē, the Syrian Orthodox Patriarch (815–845), is constructed
of excerpts from John's account.[6] These are all different versions of the
same text, and thus represent a single source, although each of these texts
contains information the others do not, so they all must be consulted.
Material that, in some fashion, goes back ultimately to John of Ephesus
is also found in the eleventh-century Christian Arabic *Chronicle of Séert*,
which is based on earlier Syriac sources.[7] An independent contemporary
Syriac source for the plague in the time of Justinian consists of a short but
extremely valuable paragraph taken from the sixth-century Syriac continuation of the *Historia Miscellanea* attributed to Zacharias Rhetor, bishop
of Mitylene, which ended in 491. This passage is preserved in Michael
the Syrian's text.[8]

References to subsequent outbreaks of bubonic plague occur scattered
throughout the Syriac chronicles, including two particularly informative
contemporary passages. One concerns the plague of 686 in northern
Iraq as described by John bar Penkayē,[9] and the other the widespread
plague of 743–745 recounted in the *Zūqnīn Chronicle*.[10]

The generic term for pestilence or epidemic disease in Syriac is
mawtānā, "mortality," which corresponds to *wabā'* in Arabic, or sometimes simply *mawtā*, "death." It is relevant that *mawtānā* is used for pestilence in the Syriac translation of the Bible (*Peshittā*).[11] A "great plague"
is called a *mawtānā rabbā*. Often, references to "pestilence" occur both
in the Bible and in Syriac literature without any indication of what the
disease was, and this usage predates the outbreak of bubonic plague. The
continuator of Zacharias of Mitylene refers to a pestilence (*mawtānā*) at

[4] *Incerti auctoris*, 2:109; *CZ*, 113.
[5] *Chronique de Michel le Syrien*, 2:235, 4:305.
[6] The text is in *Chronicon ad annum Christi 1234*, 1:197–98. The Latin translation is in
Anonymi auctoris chronicon, 1:155–56.
[7] *Histoire Nestorienne*, 182–86 [90–94].
[8] *Chronique de Michel le Syrien*, 2:240, 4:307–08. See Conrad, "*Ṭāʿūn* and *Wabāʾ*," 305. This
passage appears in Syriac in *Historia ecclesiastica Zachariae*, 2:191–92, a work that corresponds to *CSCO* 84, and in Latin translation in *Historia ecclesiastica Zachariae*, 2:129–30,
which corresponds to *CSCO* 88, and in an English translation in Hamilton and Brooks,
Syriac Chronicle, 313. In these cases, the text in Michael the Syrian was used to reconstitute
that of Zacharias.
[9] The Syriac text is in Mingana, *Sources Syriaques*, 159*–167* with a French translation on
pp. 187*–194*, and an English translation in Brock, "North Mesopotamia," 67–72.
[10] *Incertis auctoris*, 2:179–88; *CZ*, 168–74.
[11] See for example the quotations from Jer. 24:10 and 29:17 in the *Zūqnīn Chronicle* (*Incertis
auctoris*, 2:319).

Amida in 500–501.[12] Sometimes a pestilence is simply called a *kūrhānā*, "disease," or a *shabṭā*, "scourge," a more general term that is used for all sorts of calamities including plagues.

The specific term for bubonic plague in Syriac is *sharʿūṭā*, which refers both to the swellings or tumors and to the disease itself. The correspondence of *sharʿūṭā* to *ṭāʿūn* in Arabic is explicit in the *Chronicle of Séert*[13] and implied in the bilingual *Chronology* of Elias bar Shīnāyā (or Elias of Nisibis, 975–c. 1049), where *sharʿūṭā* in the Syriac text is rendered by *ṭāʿūn* in the Arabic text.[14] But, more often than not, outbreaks of bubonic plague are simply called *mawtānā* in Syriac literature, even when one can tell what it was from the description in the text. For instance, John of Ephesus never refers to the first outbreak of bubonic plague as *sharʿūṭā* but only *mawtānā*, or he uses some other term. To avoid any misunderstanding, the title of the ninth chapter in the table of contents of Book Ten of Zacharias' *Historia Miscellanea* is "concerning the plague of tumors" (*mawtānā dᵉ sharʿūṭā*).[15] It is also the case that during the first pandemic of bubonic plague from 541 to 749 outbreaks of other diseases occurred, which are also called *mawtānā*, so one must pay attention to how these events are described in the text. To form a calque on the Arabic maxim that "every *ṭāʿūn* is a *wabā'*, but not every *wabā'* is a *ṭāʿūn*,"[16] every *sharʿūṭā* is a *mawtānā*, but not every *mawtānā* is a *sharʿūṭā*.

In early Syriac literature, dates are usually given according to the year of the Greeks (AG) or the year of Alexander, that is, the Seleucid Era, in which the year started on the first of October. Thus, any year in the Seleucid Era overlaps two years in the Common Era (CE), from October of the first year through September of the second year. Dates are also sometimes given according to the year of a ruler's reign or, after the rise of Islam, according to the lunar Muslim era (Anno Hegira, AH). Thus, John of Ephesus in his *Lives of the Eastern Saints* says that the outbreak of the great plague (*mawtānā hᵉwa rabbā*) occured in 853 AG (541–542 CE).[17] But at the beginning of his account of the great plague (*mawtānā rabbā*) in his *Ecclesiastical History* John has the year 855 AG (543–544 CE).[18] Michael the Syrian repeats this date and equates it with the sixteenth

---

[12] *Historia ecclesiastica Zachariae*, 2:24.
[13] *Histoire Nestorienne*, 185 [93].
[14] Elias of Nisibis, *Opus Chronologicum*, 1:124. See also Conrad, "*Ṭāʿūn* and *Wabā'*," 305.
[15] *Historia Ecclesiastica Zachariae*, 2:174.
[16] Conrad, "*Ṭāʿūn* and *Wabā'*," 279.
[17] John of Ephesus, *Lives of the Eastern Saints*, 639 (437).
[18] *Anecdota Syriaca*, 2:304. The numbers are spelled out. This is not in the *Zūqnīn Chronicle*; Harrak has inserted this passage from Land in his English translation: *CZ*, 94.

year of Justinian (527–565),[19] which was 542–543. This narrows the year down to 543. Because John tells us himself at the end of his account that it was written three years after the plague began, when the calamities were over,[20] this might very well be the year in which he wrote rather than the year the plague started. Dionysius of Tel Maḥrē put the *mawtānā rabbā* in 857 AG (545–546 CE) but equated that with the sixteenth year of Justinian (542–543),[21] which is clearly inaccurate. In what appears to be an independent source, Jacob of Edessa (died 708) says that the *mawtānā rabbā* arose in Kush (Ethiopia) in 853 AG (541–542 CE) and spread throughout the East in 854 (542–543).[22] A Syriac chronicle that ends in 724 CE also dates the "first plague" (*mawtānā qadmāyā*) to 854 AG (542–543 CE),[23] that is, the sixteenth year of Justinian.

According to the *Chronicle of Séert* the plague (*wabā'*) struck in the tenth year of an unnamed ruler.[24] The context would suggest Justinian, whose tenth year was 536–537. But the tenth year of Khusraw I (531–579) was 540–541, which would agree with John of Ephesus and Jacob of Edessa.

Whenever it began, according to Michael the Syrian's account from John of Ephesus, the scourge of the plague (*shabṭā dᵉ mawtānā*) lasted for three whole years.[25] Outside of its account taken from John of Ephesus, the *Zūqnīn Chronicle* also has the *mawtānā rabbā* lasting for three years, from 855 AG (543–544 CE) until 858 AG (546–547 CE).[26] According to the *Chronicle of Séert* this plague (*al-mawtān*) lasted for three and one-half years.[27]

John of Ephesus was hardly exaggerating when he exclaimed (in two places) that this plague (*mawtānā*) or scourge (*shabṭā*) afflicted the

---

[19] *Chronique de Michel le Syrien*, 2:235, 4:305.

[20] *Incerti auctoris*, 2:109; *CZ*, 113.

[21] *Chronicon ad annum Christi 1234*, 155. The date in this text is written in the Syriac system of using letters of the alphabet for numbers. In this system, 857 could easily be a scribal error for 855.

[22] *Chronicon Jacobi Edesseni*, 5:320; 6:242.

[23] *Chronicon miscellaneum*, *CSCO* 3, p. 143 (text), and *CSCO* 4, p. 111 (translation). The designation of this epidemic as the "first *mawtānā*" is curious because this chronicle has already referred to earlier epidemics as *mawtānā*, such as the pestilence (*mawtānā*) accompanied by famine that occurred in the time of Shapur II in the fourth century, ibid., *CSCO*, 3, p. 130 and *CSCO*, 4, p. 101. The chronicler evidently means that this was the first known outbreak of bubonic plague, although he calls it *mawtānā*.

[24] *Histoire Nestorienne*, 182 [90].

[25] *Chronique de Michel le Syrien*, 2:240, 4:307.

[26] *Incerti auctoris*, 2:112, 119; *CZ*, 115, 119.

[27] *Histoire Nestorienne*, 185 [93].

entire world.[28] Jacob of Edessa says the same thing.[29] The *Chronicle of Séert* knows merely that the plague (*wabā'*) spread throughout Persia, India, and Abyssinia (al-Habasha).[30] According to Michael the Syrian, the plague spread above all in the lands of the south. Michael quotes John of Asia (Ephesus) as saying that it started with the interior (or remote) people of the countries south-east [*sic*] of India, namely Kush (Ethiopia) on the borders of Egypt, Himyar (Yaman), and other places.[31] That the plague visited Yaman appears to be corroborated by the inscription of Abraha on the dam at Ma'rib dated 543 CE, which refers to death and sickness striking the community at Ma'rib; the dam was repaired when the fatal epidemic had passed.[32] Zacharias of Mitylene has the plague starting in Ethiopia on the border of Egypt.[33]

From Ethiopia, the plague spread to Egypt – advancing inexorably, seizing the land like the curved scythe of a harvester – and reached Alexandria.[34] From Alexandria it spread all over the Mediterranean, to Libya, Africa,[35] Italy, Sicily, Gaul, and Spain.[36] It also spread from Alexandria to Palestine via the ports of Gaza and Ashkelon, going from the coast inland to the region around Jerusalem.[37] John of Ephesus was in Palestine when the plague (*mawtānā*) broke out and left for Mesopotamia when the plague was at its worst. On the way he noted the presence of the plague (*mawtānā*) in Syria. During the intensity of the pestilence he traveled with a group of people from Syria to Constantinople. Along the way, he records the spread of the plague to Cilicia, Moesia, Iconium, Bithynia, Asia, Galatia, and Cappadocia.[38] These regions are not mentioned in any order, and, if John went through all of the

---

[28] *Anecdota Syriaca*, 2:304. This is repeated in the *Zūqnīn Chronicle*, by Dionysius of Tel Maḥrē, and by Michael the Syrian.

[29] *Chronicon Jacobi Edesseni*, 5:320, 6:242.

[30] *Histoire Nestorienne*, 182–83 [90–91].

[31] *Chronique de Michel le Syrien*, 2:235, 4:305. From our point of view, the geography is off; these places are actually west of India.

[32] Piotrovski, "L'économie de l'Arabie préislamic," 220.

[33] *Chronique de Michel le Syrien*, 2:240, 4:308; *Historia ecclesiastica Zachariae*, 2:129 [192].

[34] *Chronique de Michel le Syrien*, 2:236, 240, 4:305, 308. According to Procopius, *PW* 2.22.6, pp. 542–45, this plague started with the Egyptians living in Peleusium and spread from there to Alexandria.

[35] Serious plagues that struck both rural and urban areas in Byzantine Tunisia in 543 and 599 may explain reports of labor shortages on the land. See Edis, "Byzantine Era in Tunisia," 56.

[36] *Chronique de Michel le Syrien*, 2:236, 240, 4:305, 308.

[37] *Anecdota Syriaca*, 2:307. This is also in the *Zūqnīn Chronicle* and Michael the Syrian.

[38] *Anecdota Syriaca*, 2:310. This is repeated in the *Zūqnīn Chronicle* and by Michael the Syrian.

regions he names here, he did not take the direct route. The plague may have been spread in these regions by travelers (like John himself) going from Syria and Palestine to Constantinople. The plague reached Constantinople shortly after John arrived.[39] To the places mentioned by John, the continuator of Zacharias of Mitylene adds that the plague struck Phoenicia, Arabia,[40] Antioch, Osrhoëne,[41] and Mesopotamia, and spread little by little among the Persians and as far as among the peoples of the north-east.[42] Bubonic plague appears to have reached China by the early seventh century.[43] This outbreak of bubonic plague lasted longer in the east. At the end of his account of the three years of plague, John of Ephesus remarks that "these same calamities still persist in the eastern territories and are not over."[44] The *Zūqnīn Chronicle* records a pestilence (*mawtānā*) that broke out in Mesopotamia in 858 AG (546–547 CE),[45] and a great pestilence (*mawtānā rabbā*) that broke out at Amida in 869 AG (557–558 CE), where 35,000 people died within three months.[46]

As John of Ephesus describes it, this first outbreak of bubonic plague was slow and moderate until it reached Constantinople. Whenever it invaded a city or village, it fell furiously and quickly upon it and its suburbs as far as three miles. It would not move on until it had run its course in one place. "After becoming firmly rooted, it moved along slowly."[47] This allowed word of the plague to precede its arrival. The people of Constantinople learned about the progress of the plague by hearsay over a period of one or two years.[48]

---

[39] According to Procopius, *PW* 2.22.9, 2.23.1, pp. 454–55, 463–65, the plague arrived in Constantinople in mid-spring of its second year and ran its course in four months.

[40] This is most likely the Byzantine province of Arabia.

[41] This is the territory around Edessa.

[42] *Chronique de Michel le Syrien*, 2:240, 4:308; *Historia ecclesiastica Zachariae*, 2:129 [192]. Procopius, *PW* 2.22.21, pp. 472–73 also says that the plague struck the land of the Persians and visited all the other barbarians.

[43] Twitchett, "Population and Pestilence," 42, 62.

[44] *Incerti auctoris*, 2:109; *CZ*, 113.

[45] *Incerti auctoris*, 2:112; *CZ*, 115.

[46] *Incerti auctoris*, 2:119; *CZ*, 119. Michael the Syrian (*Chronique de Michel le Syrien*, 2:268, 4:323) repeats this. Harrak lists this occurrence under bubonic plague in his index (*CZ*, p. 385).

[47] *Incerti auctoris*, 2:92–93; *CZ*, 103; *Anecdota Syriaca*, 2:313. This is corroborated by Procopius, *PW* 2.22.6–7, 9, pp. 452–55, who says that the plague spread at times favorable to it and seemed to move by a fixed arrangement and stay in each country for a specified time. It always started from the coast and spread inland.

[48] *Incerti auctoris*, 2:93; *CZ*, 103.

The next reference to bubonic plague (*mawtānā dᵉ sharʿūṭā*) is in the month of April (Nisan) 873 AG (562 CE),[49] but the place is not specified. Bubonic plague (*sharʿūṭā*) broke out in Constantinople again in 885 AG (573–574 CE).[50] There was another outbreak of bubonic plague (*sharʿūṭā, ṭāʿūn*) in 911 AG (600 CE), when many houses were left without inhabitants and fields went unharvested,[51] but we are not told where. The Syriac sources do not seem to notice the outbreak of bubonic plague (*ṭāʿūn*) in lower Iraq in 628,[52] but Jacob of Edessa records a severe pestilence (*mawtānāʿazzīzā*) that broke out in all the regions of Syria in 18 AH (639 CE),[53] which coincides with the plague (*ṭāʿūn*) of ʿAmwās in the Arabic sources,[54] and that one was certainly bubonic plague.[55] There is a reference to *sharʿūṭā*, probably in upper Iraq, in the Life of Mar Sabrishoʿ (died 650).[56] The next recorded plague event is the pestilence (*mawtānā*) in northern Mesopotamia in 67 AH (686–687 CE) described by John bar Penkayē,[57] which was clearly bubonic plague. About a decade later, many people perished in an outbreak of bubonic plague (*sharʿūṭā, ṭāʿūnʿazīm*) in Syria in 79 AH (March 698 to February 699), which is equated with 1009 AG (October 697 to September 698) in the text.[58] Evidently, this outbreak occurred between March and September of 698, and it appears to be the same occurrence of bubonic plague (*sharʿūṭā*) recorded in an anonymous Syriac chronicle as happening throughout Syria in 1010 AG (698–699 CE).[59] Either one of these accounts is a year off, or, as is more likely, this plague lasted for two years. There was another great pestilence (*mawtānā rabbā*) in 1016 AG (704–705 CE) that was especially virulent in the region of Serug in northwestern Mesopotamia. The excessive

[49] *Chronicon miscellaneum*, CSCO 3, p. 143 (text), and CSCO 4, p. 111 (trans.).

[50] *Chronicon anonymum*, CSCO 3, p. 230 (text), and CSCO 4, p. 174 (trans.).

[51] *Opus Chronologicum*, CSCO 62, 1:124; CSCO 63, p. 60. Elias says this came from the *Ecclesiastical History* of Āllahāzᵉkhā.

[52] al-Ṭabarī, * Taʾrīkh*, 1:1061.

[53] *Chronicon Jacobi Edesseni*, CSCO 5, p. 330; CSCO 6, p. 257. This is repeated in Elias bar Shīnāyā who says he got it from Jacob.

[54] al-Ṭabarī, *Taʾrīkh*, 1:2511–25.

[55] Conrad, "Arabic Plague Chronologies and Treatises," 87, 69.

[56] Mingana, *Sources Syriaques*, [182] 231.

[57] Brock, "North Mesopotamia," 67–68; Mingana, *Sources Syriaques*, 159*–60*.

[58] *Opus Chronologicum*, CSCO 62, 1:154; CSCO 63, p. 74.

[59] *Chronicon anonymum ad A.D. 819*, CSCO 81, p. 13; CSCO 109, p. 9. This is also translated in Palmer, *West-Syrian Chronicles*, 78. There is also a reference to depopulation caused by plague (*plagae*) in Septimania in 694. See Claude, "Relations between Visigoths and Hispano-Romans," 128. King suggests that plague may have been decisive in the crisis during the last years of the Visigothic Kingdom. See King, *Law and Society*, 170.

mortality on this occasion suggests that this was also bubonic plague.[60] Then from December to February 1024 AG (712–713 CE) there was a great pestilence (*sh'ḥāṭā rabbā*), and many people died without pity. Before it was over there was a destructive earthquake on Monday morning, February 28, 713, in which many people perished in collapsed buildings. The *Chronicle of Disasters*, which records these events, says that the earthquake was followed (i.e., in the spring of 713) by a third affliction (*m'ḥūtā*),[61] another outbreak of bubonic plague (*shar'ūṭā*), when countless people were buried without pity in all sorts of places.[62] In this text, bubonic plague appears to be distinguished from a severe epidemic of some other disease; *sh'ḥāṭā* refers to a "swelling" or a "sore".[63]

There was a great outbreak of bubonic plague from 743 to 745. Dionysius of Tel Maḥrē notes that there was an epidemic (*mawtānā*) in 1054 AG (742–743 CE) in the year that the caliph, Hishām, died.[64] Dionysius also says that the caliph, Yazīd III, died of a tumor (*shar'ūṭā*) that erupted on his head in 1055 AG (743–744 CE).[65] Dionysius then tells of a major epidemic of bubonic plague (*mawtānā d' shar'ūṭā*) accompanied by famine that broke out in Mesopotamia, Bostra, and the Hawran in 1056 AG (744–745 CE).[66] The *Zūqnīn Chronicle* has a detailed account of this pestilence (*mawtānā*) and famine, which it says started in the winter of 1055 AG (743–744 CE).[67] Harrak has pointed out that the Zūqnīn chronicler borrowed many expressions and passages from the account of John of Ephesus to describe this plague in his own time.[68] Thus, the information in the *Zūqnīn Chronicle* that this plague occurred in the territory stretching

[60] *Incerti auctoris*, 2:155; *CZ*, 148. This passage is also translated in Palmer, *West-Syrian Chronicles*, 61.

[61] *M'ḥūtā* can also mean disease, scourge, or plague. See Payne-Smith, *Syriac Dictionary*, 263.

[62] Nau, "Un colloque du patriarch," 254–55 (text), 264–66 (French trans.). There is an English translation in Palmer, *West-Syrian Chronicles*, 45–46. The *mawtānā* of 1024 AG (712–713 CE) is also recorded in another anonymous Syriac chronicle. See *Chronicon anonymum 846*, CSCO 3, p. 233; CSCO 4, p. 177.

[63] Payne-Smith, *Syriac Dictionary*, 570.

[64] *Chronicon ad annum Christi 1234*, CSCO 81, p. 314; CSCO 109, p. 245. Hishām died in 125 AH, which virtually coincided with 1054 AG. The chronicler of Zūqnīn put the death of Hishām in 1055 AG (743–744 CE). See *Incerti auctoris*, 2:177; *CZ*, 166.

[65] *Chronicon ad annum Christi 1234*, CSCO 81, p. 317; CSCO 109, p. 247. This is repeated by Michael the Syrian (*Chronique de Michel le Syrien*, 2:503, 4:464), who puts it in 1056 AG (744–745 CE).

[66] Ibid. This is also repeated by Michael the Syrian (*Chronique de Michel le Syrien*, 2:506, 508, 4:464–66).

[67] *Incerti auctoris*, 2:179, 182; *CZ*, 168, 170. At the end of the second passage, the pestilence is simply called a "disease" (*kūrhānā*).

[68] *CZ*, 21–23, 168.

from the Euphrates to the West, the cities of Palestine, the North and South as far as the Red Sea, and in Cilicia, Iconia, Asia, Bithynia, Lusonia (probably Moesia), Galatia, and Cappadocia[69] merely reproduces John's own list and needs to be confirmed from other sources. Closer to home, the *mawtānā* to which Severus, bishop of Amida, succumbed in about 1058 AG (746–747)[70] may have been bubonic plague.

According to Conrad and Dols, the first pandemic of bubonic plague ended in 749 and the disease disappeared.[71] In partial support of this, Conrad points out that after the mid-eighth century there are no references to *sharʿūṭā* in the Syriac chronicles; continued outbreaks of pestilence are usually called *mawtānā*.[72] This does, in fact, appear to be the case, but the matter is not as simple as that. It should be clear from the chronology of outbreaks of bubonic plague from the mid-sixth to the mid-eighth century that *mawtānā* and especially *mawtānā rabbā* were used to refer to them. If not every *mawtānā* was *sharʿūṭā*, at least some of them were. What prevents the use of *mawtānā* in describing events after the mid-eighth century from also referring to bubonic plague? One should not be a slave to terminology but should pay attention to what is described. Some subsequent outbreaks of epidemic disease are examined here to show that bubonic plague might have persisted after the mid-eighth century along with many other maladies that clearly were not.

An example illustrates the problems. The *Zūqnīn Chronicle*[73] describes how, in 1062 AG (750–751 CE), famine (*kapnā*) drove large numbers of Armenians to flee to Syria bringing various diseases, including *mawtānā*, with them. In Syria the Armenian refugees suffered from the disease (*kūrhānā*) of *shūḥānā* (ulcer or abscess) and then of *karsā* (diarrhoea),[74] obvious symptoms of famine. They were also overcome by *mawtānā*, and most of them died. So many of them died that people were not able to bury them. This is a common way of describing the consequence of bubonic plague. The Syrians also suffered from famine, abscesses (*shūḥānā*), and sores (*shʿḥāṭṭā*), which exterminated them. But there were more victims of famine than of disease. Conrad is somewhat misleading in saying

[69] *Incerti auctoris*, 2:184; *CZ*, 171–72.
[70] *Incerti auctoris*, 2:190; *CZ*, 176.
[71] Conrad, "Arabic Plague Chronologies and Treatises," 53. See also Dols, "Plague in Early Islamic History," 380; and Twitchett, "Population and Pestilence," 63–64.
[72] Conrad, "*Ṭāʿūn* and *Wabāʾ*," 306.
[73] *Incerti auctoris*, 2:204–05; *CZ*, 188.
[74] *Karsā* is literally "belly." *Shʿray karsā* is more properly diarrhea (Payne-Smith, *Syriac Dictionary*, 228), but this is what seems to be intended by the "disease of the belly" here.

that on this occasion plague took a heavy toll at the monastery of Zūqnīn among the monks and "people who had fled there to escape the pestilence."[75] According to the text, forty-two people of the monastery of Zūqnīn died of *sh*ḥāṭā* (not *mawtānā*), not counting the strangers. Because *sh*ḥāṭā* can mean "swelling" as well as "sore,"[76] this could still have been plague, but *sh*ḥāṭā* appears to be a symptom of famine in this passage, not of *mawtānā*. Nor does this text tell us why the "strangers" were at the monastery.

The distinction between *mawtānā* and other diseases is also maintained in the *Zūqnīn Chronicle's* account of how the ʿAbbāsī army attacking the fortress of Qamh on the Euphrates north-east of Melitene in 1078 AG (766–767 CE) suffered from various diseases (*kūrhānē m*shaḥl*pē*) such as dysentery ("the disease of the belly," *kābā d* karsā*) and haemorrhoids (*t*ḥūrā*) as well as *mawtānā* and famine.[77] Here *mawtānā* is again distinguished from afflictions associated with famine.

The fatal disease (*kūrhānā*, *kābā*) and *mawtānā* that broke out in Mawṣil in 1085 AG (773–774 CE) and spread throughout the territory of Mawṣil and upper Mesopotamia as far as Amida accompanied by famine was probably meningitis. The victims' heads swelled, and they died quickly or went into a coma for several days and suffered from abscesses followed by stomachaches, pustules, and pimples.[78] However, the *mawtānā* of 1085 that prevailed in lower Mesopotamia, when more than 1,000 coffins were removed from Mawṣil every day, houses were left without residents, large villages in the district of Nisibis were completely ruined, all the officials died, but mainly priests were killed in cities and villages,[79] could well have been bubonic plague, and Harrak puts it under bubonic plague in his index.[80]

Another *mawtānā* that lasted for two years (841–843 CE), recorded by Michael the Syrian, began in Mesopotamia and spread to Syria, Palestine, and the coast. It left many villages deserted and their fields without harvesters. In a single day, 500 people died at Ramla. Being unable to dig graves, the survivors threw the corpses into long ditches. One-third

[75] Conrad, "Epidemic Disease in Central Syria," 51.

[76] Payne-Smith, *Syriac Dictionary*, 570.

[77] *Incerti auctoris*, 2:230; *CZ*, 207.

[78] *Incerti auctoris*, 2:333, 357–66; *CZ*, 30, 287, 305–10. This would seem to be the same disease (*kūrhānā*) that Michael the Syrian says seized its victims by the head and carried them away quickly; it spread throughout Syria, Mesopotamia, and the territory of Mawṣil (*Athōr*) in 1083 (770–771 CE) (*Chronique de Michel le Syrien*, 2:526, 4:477).

[79] *Incerti auctoris*, 2:367–68; *CZ*, 312.

[80] *CZ*, 385.

of the population of Palestine is said to have perished in this epidemic,[81] which looks like it could also have been bubonic plague.

But, how do we know that? This judgment is based on the detailed description of the symptoms and pathology of the disease and its effects provided in Syriac literature. We are told by John of Ephesus that people would reel and collapse suddenly, without exhibiting any symptoms, wherever they were – in the streets, at home, at harbors, on ships, in churches, at work, or in the marketplace.[82] The *Chronicle of Séert* simply says that a person opened his mouth while walking and fell dead.[83] This may have been a pneumonic form of plague. For these victims, the disease appears to have been concentrated in the intestines. John of Ephesus tells of corpses with their putrefied bellies swollen, their mouths open, eyes staring, and arms stretched upward, that burst open in the streets with their pus running down like water. The bellies of corpses burst open when the bodies landed in the burial pits. The corpses of women sat in their private rooms with their mouths swollen and wide open. The stench was unbearable.[84]

Those who did not die immediately were struck by a painful swelling of the groins, some in one and some in both, from which some succumbed and some survived.[85] At the same time, swellings appeared on the thigh, in the armpit, and on the neck.[86] In some cases, both knees

---

[81] *Chronique de Michel le Syrien*, 3:109–10, 4:543.

[82] *Incerti auctoris*, 2:96–97; *CZ*, 105; *Anecdota Syriaca*, 2:315–16. This is also in Dionysius of Tel Maḥrē (*Chronicon ad annum Christi 1234*, CSCO 81, p. 198; CSCO 109, p. 156). Michael the Syrian (*Chronique de Michel le Syrien*, 2:236, 4:305) repeats this and adds that stretcher-bearers carrying the corpses would fall and perish (Ibid., 2:237, 4:306). This is corroborated by Procopius, *PW* 2.22.14–16, 23, 31, pp. 456–57, 460–61, 462–63, who says that many or most people were struck without warning and died immediately. In this context, he also says that people would get a sudden, low-grade fever, no matter what they were doing, that would last until evening. Many vomited blood without any visible cause and died right away.

[83] *Histoire Nestorienne*, 183 [91].

[84] *Incerti auctoris*, 2:80, 98–99, 101, 106; *CZ*, 94–95, 106–07, 108, 111; *Anecdota Syriaca*, 2:305, 318, 320. But any cause of excessive mortality could result in stinking corpses. We are told that the city of Antioch was pervaded by an unbearable stench because of the multitude of corpses after a great earthquake in 767 AG (455–456 CE). See *Chronicon 724*, CSCO 3, p. 140 (text), and CSCO 4, p. 109 (trans.).

[85] *Incerti auctoris*, 2:95, 187; *Chronicon ad annum Christi 1234*, CSCO 81, p. 198; CSCO 109 p. 156; *Chronique de Michel le Syrien*, 2:236, 4:305; *CZ*, 104, 173–74; *Anecdota Syriaca*, 2:315; *Histoire Nestorienne*, 183 [91].

[86] *Chronique de Michel le Syrien*, 2:240, 4:307; *Incerti auctoris*, 2:187; *CZ*, 174; *Historia ecclesiastica Zachariae*, 2:191–92. A plague among horses in 763–764 CE is said to have been similar to the *sharʿūṭā* that afflicted humans because it struck the animals in the neck. See *Incerti auctoris*, 2:221; *CZ*, 201. Procopius, *PW* 2.22.17, pp. 456–59 also says that swellings developed inside the armpit, beside the ears, and on the thighs.

discharged water, blood, and pus.[87] If three black pockmarks appeared deep inside the flesh in the palm of a person's hand, the victim died within hours. These marks distinguished those who perished from those who survived.[88] In those cases where the groins became inflated and filled up with fluid so that they burst open, creating large, deep abscesses that discharged blood, pus, and water night and day, the victim would survive.[89]

According to the Syriac continuation of Zacharias, those who survived remained staggering and reeling.[90] The chronicler of Zūqnīn says that survivors suffered exhausting fatigue for one, two, five, or six months and up to a year, many others for up to two years, and many never recovered completely. Some went bald and could only be recognized by their clothing. Monks could not be distinguished from priests because they all became bald. As the chronicler put it, "the very few who survived endured."[91]

Conrad points out that bubonic plague was less of an affliction from October to January, and that it frequently struck in the spring, becoming more active in March and lasting until September/October.[92] This does seem to have been the case on several occasions noted in the chronology above, and presumably this had something to do with fleas being dormant during the winter. But Procopius could see no seasonal pattern; the plague attacked some people in the summer, others in the winter, and still others at other times of the year.[93] The outbreak of bubonic plague accompanied by famine in 743–744 described in the *Zūqnīn Chronicle* serves to illustrate the process. During the winter of 743–744 people were first stricken by the disease (*kūrhānā*) of the sore (or "swelling", *shʻḥātā*) and abscess (*shūḥānā*), and most of the heads of households died, but, because it was winter, the dead could not be buried. People were discarded in streets, porches, towers, shrines, and all the houses, suffering

---

[87] *Incerti auctoris*, 2:187; *CZ*, 174.

[88] *Incerti auctoris*, 2:96; *Chronique de Michel le Syrien*, 2:236, 4:305; *CZ*, 105; *Anecdota Syriaca*, 2:315; *Histoire Nestorienne*, 183 [91]. This is corroborated by Procopius, *PW* 2.22:30, pp. 462–63.

[89] *Incerti auctoris*, 2:187; *CZ*, 173. Procopius, *PW* 2.22.37, pp. 464–65 says the same thing.

[90] *Chronique de Michel le Syrien*, 2:240, 4:308; *Historia ecclesiastica Zachariae*, 2:192.

[91] *Incerti auctoris*, 2:185, 187–88; *CZ*, 173–74. Procopius, *PW* 2.22:39, pp. 464–65 adds that the tongues of some survivors were affected; they lisped or spoke incoherently and with difficulty.

[92] Conrad, "Die Pest und ihr soziales Umfeld im Nahen Osten," 104; idem, "Epidemic Disease in Central Syria," 50.

[93] Procopius, *PW* 2.22.5, pp. 452–53.

both from the severe disease and the harsh famine. Those who had food suffered from the disease (*kūrhānā*) more than anyone else. When it began to warm up, bubonic plague (*sharʿūṭā*) was discovered in those who were ill. They began to collapse in the street, and there was no one to bury them.[94]

The initial outbreak of bubonic plague in the time of Justinian also struck domestic and wild animals. John of Ephesus says that one could see "cattle, dogs, other animals, and even mice (*ʿuqbrē*), whose groins were swollen and were cast away and dead."[95] This, of course, provides a clue as to where the fleas were carried. Sometime between the famine of 546 and the twenty-fifth year of Justinian (551–552) there was an epidemic (*mawtānā*) among cattle throughout the regions of the East that lasted for two years,[96] but this could have been something other than bubonic plague. The equine epidemic among horses, mules, and donkeys in 1075 AG (763–764 CE) may, however, have been related to bubonic plague. The Zūqnīn chronicler says that it was similar to the bubonic plague (*sharʿūṭā*) that afflicted humans because it struck its victims in the neck.[97]

Why does bubonic plague seem to disappear after the middle of the eighth century? Perhaps, based on the discussion above, this is only an illusion. But it is also possible that the plague bacillus affected its victims in non-bubonic forms. Pneumonic plague normally occurs in winter and is highly contagious. Is it possible that the great pestilence (*shḥāṭā rabbā*) from December to February, 712–713, and the disease (*kūrhānā*) in the winter of 743–744 were pneumonic plague? Was the bubonic-like epidemic that struck equines in 763–764 a mutant form of bubonic plague? Was the epidemic in 773–774, which Harrak identifies as meningitis, meningeal plague (an inflammation of the membranes of the brain and spinal cord)? If the disease occurred in non-bubonic forms after the mid-eighth century, it would not have been called *sharʿūṭā* but *mawtānā*. If so,

---

94 *Incerti auctoris*, 2:182; *CZ*, 170.

95 *Incerti auctoris*, 2:95–96; *CZ*, 105; *Anecdota Syriaca*, 2:315. This is repeated by Michael the Syrian (*Chronique de Michel le Syrien*, 2:236, 4:305) and summarized by Dionysius of Tel Maḥrē (*Chronicon ad annum Christi 1234*, CSCO 81, p. 81; CSCO 109, p. 156).

96 *Chronicon Jacobi Edesseni*, CSCO 5, p. 321; CSCO 6, p. 243. This is repeated by Michael the Syrian (*Chronique de Michel le Syrien*, 2:245, 4:309). The *Histoire Nestorienne* puts this epidemic (*wabā'*) among cattle in the twenty-sixth year of Justinian (552–53). See *Histoire Nestorienne*, 185 [94].

97 *Incerti auctoris*, 2:221–22; *CZ*, 200–01. The chronicler even says that wise and God-fearing people believed that this pestilence had been sent upon people, but God, in His mercy, had diverted it from humans to animals.

might that help to explain why the bubonic form disappeared temporarily, to reappear a century and one-half later? But, this is pure speculation.

In any case the human mortality was staggering, but was its extent exaggerated by contemporaries? Can we take the numbers recorded in the Syriac sources literally? One cannot discount the presence of rhetorical hyperbole in these accounts, or the fact that the large round numbers they give can only have been estimates at best. There are at least two considerations to remember in dealing with this kind of information. One is that recording the number of fatalities was one of the ways these authors attempted to express the magnitude of the disaster. The other is that the number of fatalities is meaningless in demographic terms without knowing the size of the total population. Percentages are more useful for this than raw numbers. In what follows, the estimations of plague mortality found in the Syriac sources are reported. Whether or not they are useful for demographic history remains to be seen.

Even without offering actual numbers the Syriac accounts speak of depopulation. We are told that during the first outbreak of bubonic plague in the time of Justinian the majority of people in Egypt perished, so that Egypt became uninhabited and deserted. A throng of people succumbed at Alexandria, which became emptied and ruined.[98] John of Ephesus says that the mortality in Palestine was greater than in Alexandria; entire villages and towns were depopulated.[99] We get numbers for Constantinople where John relates that 5,000, 7,000, 12,000, and up to 16,000 corpses of the poor (who died first) would be removed in a day.[100] He knows this because at the beginning, men were stationed at the harbors, straits, and gates to count the number of bodies. They would have counted more than 300,000 bodies removed from the streets, but, when those who were counting reached 230,000, they realized the corpses were numberless and gave up. After that, countless victims were removed.[101]

---

[98] *Chronique de Michel le Syrien*, 2:236–38, 4:306.

[99] *Incerti auctoris*, 2:82–83; *CZ*, 96–97; *Anecdota Syriaca*, 2:307.

[100] *Incerti auctoris*, 2:94; *CZ*, 104; *Anecdota Syriaca*, 2:314. This is repeated by Dionysius of Tel Maḥrē (*Chronicon ad annum Christi 1234*, CSCO 81, p. 197; CSCO 109, p. 155) and by Michael the Syrian (*Chronique de Michel le Syrien*, 2:235, 4:305). This is more or less confirmed by Procopius, *PW* 2.23.2, pp. 464–65, who says that the deaths were a little more than normal at first and then increased until they reached 5,000 each day and even 10,000 or more.

[101] *Incerti auctoris*, 2:14–15; *CZ*, 104; *Anecdot Syriaca*, 2:324–25. This is also repeated by Dionysius of Tel Maḥrē (*Chronicon ad annum Christi 1234*, CSCO 81, pp. 197–98; CSCO 109, pp. 155–56) and by Michael the Syrian (*Chronique de Michel le Syrien*, 2:235–36, 4:305).

What did this mean for that great city? Michael the Syrian says that out of innumerable myriads, only a small number of people remained there.[102] Elsewhere, as it has been mentioned earlier, 35,000 people died in three months in the great pestilence (*mawtānā rabbā*) that struck Amida in 557–558.[103]

Concerning later events of the plague, Michael the Syrian estimated that one-third of the people in the world perished in the great pestilence (*mawtānā rabbā*) of 704–705.[104] During the plague (*shar'ūṭā*) of 743–744 Dionysius of Tel Maḥrē says that 100,000 people died in Mesopotamia alone, while 20,000 died each day for a month at Bostra and in the Hawran.[105] It has already been noted that Michael the Syrian reports that in the *mawtānā* of 841 to 843, 500 people died in a single day at Ramla and that one-third of the population of Palestine perished.[106] Even if this was not bubonic plague, the mortality rate was similar. If such numbers are to be believed, how could the population have recovered? Did it recover? It is not beyond imagination that villages and small towns could have been utterly decimated, but the recurring estimate of an overall mortality rate of one-third seems realistic and believable.[107]

The most immediate concern was the disposal of the corpses. Stinking corpses were cast in corners, the porticos of buildings, churches, and martyria; bodies piled up in the streets without enough survivors left to bury them.[108] Sometimes corpses remained in the streets for days without burial; the stench made the streets impassable.[109] People feared to go

---

[102] *Chronique de Michel le Syrien*, 2:240, 4:307. But Michael's estimate that scarcely one person in one thousand survived is surely hyperbole; 99.9% mortality is difficult to believe for a city like Constantinople. See *Chronique de Michel le Syrien*, 2:240, 4:308.

[103] *Incerti auctoris*, 2:119; *Chronique de Michel le Syrien*, 2:268, 4:323; *CZ*, 119.

[104] *Chronique de Michel le Syrien*, 2:480, 4:449.

[105] *Chronicon ad annum Christi 1234*, CSCO 81, p. 319; CSCO 109, p. 249. It is difficult to imagine that the Hawran had a population of 600,000 in the mid-eighth century. Michael the Syrian repeats this account from Dionysius but gives the number of victims in Mesopotamia as 1,000 (emended by the editor to 4,000, which is still not the number given by Dionysius) and adds that there were innumerable deaths in the East. See *Chronique de Michel le Syrien*, 2:508, 4:466.

[106] *Chronique de Michel le Syrien*, 3:109–10, 4:543. It is worth noting that al-Mas'ūdī, *Kitāb murūj al-dhahab*, 2: 233 reports that, during the plague of Shiroe in 628, more than 100,000 people perished in Iraq, which amounted to between one-half and one-third of the population. Although it is difficult to believe that the population of Iraq was at most 300,000 in the early seventh-century, the fractional estimate is probably valuable.

[107] Twitchett, "Population and Pestilence," p. 53 estimates that in China more than one-half of the population in the affected provinces perished in 806, and 30–40% in 891.

[108] *Incerti auctoris*, 2:80, 100; *CZ*, 94, 107; *Anecdota Syriaca*, 2:304–05, 318–19.

[109] *Histoire Nestorienne*, 183 [91].

out in the streets of Alexandria because of the stench of the corpses and even for as much as twelve *darics* could hardly find anyone to carry them off.[110] On his journey from Syria to Constantinople, John of Ephesus saw devastated villages with corpses lying on the ground with no one to bury them.[111] Wherever a few people survived they would carry the corpses, cast them away, and return, while others would pile up the corpses in a heap and dig graves for them.[112]

At Constantinople, the removal of corpses was more urgent than anything else.[113] Because the poor died first and were cast away in the streets, they were shrouded, given funeral rites and a decent burial. It was they who were escorted out of the city daily by the thousands, counted and deposited in one great common burial before matters got confused. The poor vanished, although a small number of them survived.[114] Anyone who was still alive had to remove the corpses from his own house,[115] but afterwards graves could not be found so bodies were simply collected from streets and carried on stretchers, boards, and biers to the shore, where they were laid out in groups of two or three. Because the corpses were putrid and decaying, some sewed mattings for them, carried them to the shore on biers, and piled them on each other. Bodies piled up along the shore in heaps of 2,000, 3,000, or 5,000, and then countless numbers. At the shore, the corpses were loaded on ships and cast in the straits or like dung (*zeblā*) on the opposite shore. Matters reached the point that there were not enough stretchers or stretcher-bearers, whose numbers were decreasing, and corpses piled up in the streets.[116]

At that point, the Emperor Justinian intervened ordering 600 stretchers to be made and appointing his *referendarius*, Theodore, to take as

[110] *Chronique de Michel le Syrien*, 2:237–38, 4:306.
[111] This part of John's passage is adapted by the Zūqnīn chronicler to describe the plague of 743–44. See *Incerti auctoris*, 2:184; *CZ*, 184.
[112] *Incerti auctoris*, 2:87; *CZ*, 99; *Anecdota Syriaca*, 2:311.
[113] *Incerti auctoris*, 2:97; *CZ*, 106.
[114] *Incerti auctoris*, 2:94–95; *CZ*, 104; *AnecdotaSyriaca*, 2:314. The Zūqnīn chronicler adapted this account of John of Ephesus to describe the plague of 743–744 (*Incerti auctoris*, 2:182; *CZ*, 170).
[115] Procopius, *PW*2.23.3, pp. 464–65 says that each man buried the dead of his own house at first, throwing them into the tombs of others. Afterward, there was complete confusion and disorder.
[116] *Incerti auctoris*, 2:97–100; *Chronicon ad annum Christi 1234*, *CSCO* 81, p. 198; *CSCO* 109, p. 156; *Chronique de Michel le Syrien*, 2:236–37, 4:305; *CZ*, 106–07; *Anecdota Syriaca*, 2:317–19. Procopius, *PW*2.23.12, pp. 468–69 notes that during this phase of disposing of the corpses, the usual burial rites were not observed, the dead were not carried out escorted by the usual procession, nor were the usual chants sung over them.

much gold as necessary and hire people to dig large pits in which to pile the bodies. He was ordered also to fill any grave he could find no matter who owned it. Theodore crossed the Golden Horn to Sycae (Galata) and brought many people from a mountain overlooking the city to whom he offered much gold.[117] He also put men with gold in charge of the diggers to motivate them and to pay people to carry corpses. Corpse-bearers were gradually given five or six and then up to seven or ten *dīnārs* for each load. If someone had more bodies than he could handle, he would go to Theodore and tell him, and Theodore would have the bodies removed. Those who were still healthy would carry corpses, some for high wages, some for low wages, and some for no reward. There appears to have been some profiteering; healthy people who wanted gold would collect up to one pound of gold or up to 100 *dīnārs* on some days. John of Ephesus makes a point of relating two stories about greedy corpse-bearers who died without enjoying their profits. But the city was cleared of corpses.[118]

Theodore had very large pits dug, in each of which 70,000 bodies were laid. He appointed men to bring the corpses down, sort them, and pile them up. These men piled the bodies in rows and trampled them down with their feet like hay.[119] John of Ephesus also uses the image of a "deadly, destructive, and bitter wine press" for the burial pits:

> Men and women were trodden down, and in the
> space between them the young and infants were
> pressed down, trodden with the feet and tramp-
> led down like spoilt grapes... Those who were
> treading corpses were standing, and as soon as
> they laid down a man or a woman, a young man or
> an infant, they trampled them with their feet to
> press him down flat so that a place be made for
> the others.[120]

John provides us with the gruesome image of a body sinking in the putre-faction of the corpses below.[121]

[117] This is also reported by Procopius, *PW* 2.23.6–11, pp. 466–69, except that he says that Theodore went to Sycae, where he took the roofs off of the towers of the fortifications and filled them with bodies.

[118] *Incerti auctoris*, 2:100–01, 104–05; *Chronique de Michel le Syrien*, 2:237–39, 4:305–07; *CZ*, 107–08, 110; *Anecdota Syriaca*, 2:319, 322–33; *Histoire Nestorienne*, 185 [93].

[119] *Incerti auctoris*, 2:100; *Chronicon ad annum Christi 1234*, CSCO 81, p. 198; CSCO 109, p. 156; *Chronique de Michel le Syrien*, 2:237, 4:306; *CZ*, 108.

[120] *Incerti auctoris*, 2:106; *CZ*, 111; *Anecdota Syriaca*, 2:324.

[121] Ibid.

This is not the only example of the organized disposal of the dead during this plague. On the eastern side of the frontier, in the Sasanian empire, the *Chronicle of Séert* cites the *History* of Bar Sahdē to the effect that Yūsuf (Joseph), the catholicos of the Church of the East, exerted himself to bury the corpses that were cast on the ground and in the streets.[122]

During the plague of 686–687 in upper Iraq, John bar Penkayē tells of human corpses strewn in the roads and streets like "dung on the earth" (Jer. 16:4) so that springs and rivers became contaminated. People did not even bury the dead but left them and fled like pagans (i.e., Zoroastrians). Dogs began to eat many people while they were still alive.[123] As noted earlier, during the outbreak of bubonic plague in the spring of 713, numberless people were buried without pity in all sorts of places.[124]

The next most extensive description of the disposal of the dead is in the *Zuqnīn Chronicle*. Although the chronicler depended on John of Ephesus in certain parts of his account, he included details that could not have come from John. He tells us that Arabs and Jews dug holes all over the ground (for the dead), and that the graves of the Christians were all filled so they had to dig holes in the ground too. He reports, along with or from John, that the pestilence (*mawtānā*) started with the poor, which is probably true in any case, and that when the poor had almost all perished, the mortality struck the notables of villages and cities. The survivors could manage to bury only their own family members, but many of the victims lacked relatives and were discarded in the street to be devoured by dogs, with no one to bury them. People were hired to collect the bodies from houses and streets, and human corpses were removed continuously all day. Funeral rites were performed for only a few because of how fast the deaths occurred, the small number of priests, and the large number of countless stretchers. When priests went to one stretcher, 50, 60, and up to 90 and 100 stretchers would be gathered in one place.

[122] *Histoire Nestorienne*, 185–86 [93–94]. Joseph had a bad reputation in the east Syrian tradition, and Bar Sahdē says that he did not know anything else good about him.
[123] Brock, "North Mesopotamia," 68; Mingana, *Sources Syriaques*, 160*. John's reference to dogs resonates with what Agathias of Myrina says about the exposure of the dead by Zoroastrians in the sixth century. See Agathias, *Historiae* 2.23.5, pp. 70–71; Agathias, *Histories*, 57. However, it is with regard to the famine, not the plague, of 686–687 that John says that no one was left to bury the dead because everyone was exhausted from hunger and that "the storage pits that famine had emptied were again filled by the famine with the corpses of human beings." See Brock, "North Mesopotamia," 70; Mingana, *Sources Syriaques*, 163*.
[124] Palmer, *West-Syrian Chronicles*, 46.

The priests organized matters by instructing people to bring their dead relatives to the nearby *tetrapylai* each morning and gather the dead of each place or street in one spot. The stretchers gathered in one place in the morning each contained two, three, or four young people. The priests would divide themselves up each morning and go in all directions to perform mass funeral services. More than 100 stretchers were taken out in a single convoy, with more than 200 or 250 people in them; more than 500 stretchers went out of a single gate each day.[125] This sounds like it was happening in a particular city. Although the chronicler does not identify it, this was most probably at Amida.

Even allowing for exaggeration, it is clear that the mortality was so great that the most immediate focus of concern was simply disposing of the bodies of the dead. Otherwise, the most immediate reaction was one of traumatic shock. People were totally unprepared for the first outbreak of bubonic plague in the time of Justinian. John of Ephesus says that nothing like it had happened since the beginning of the world.[126] Even regarding the *mawtānā* of 685, John bar Penkayē says that "there had been nothing like it, and I hope that there will be nothing like it again."[127]

How did people deal with such excessive mortality? John of Ephesus, in speaking of the outbreak of the earlier plague (*mawtānā*) in 853 AG (541–542 CE), says that "everyone was in perturbation and doubt and confusion."[128] John of Ephesus also says that shocked, agitated, and speechless people were beyond mourning; their hearts grown mute, they treated human corpses like the carcasses of animals.[129] John bar Penkayē says that during the plague of 686–687:

> No brother had any pity on his brother, or
> father on his son; a mother's compassion for
> her children was cut off; she would gaze on
> them as they were convulsed with the pangs of
> death, but she was not willing to approach and
> close their eyes.[130]

---

[125] *Incerti auctoris*, 2:182–83, 185; *CZ*, 170–72.

[126] *Chronique de Michel le Syrien*, 2:235, 4:305.

[127] Brock, "North Mesopotamia," 68; Mingana, *Sources Syriaques*, 160*.

[128] John of Ephesus, *Lives of the Eastern Saints*, 640 [438].

[129] *Incerti auctoris*, 2:102; *CZ*, 109; *Anecdota Syriaca*, 2:320–21. John of Ephesus uses the biblical reference to "the burial of an ass" (Jer. 22:19) in this passage more than once.

[130] Brock, "North Mesopotamia," 68; Mingana, *Sources Syriaques*, 160–61*. In this passage, it is also said that brothers and family members became like dogs and wild animals to anyone who died.

John of Ephesus also used the imagery of drunkenness to describe their dazed confusion,[131] as did the Zūqnīn chronicler in the plague of 743–744.[132] Michael the Syrian adds that during the plague in the time of Justinian people became enraged, attacked each other like mad dogs, or went to the mountains and killed themselves,[133] while the *Chronicle of Séert* says that people fled from place to place in fear of death.[134] The Zūqnīn chronicler also says that people began to wander from one city to another and from one region to the next during the plague of 743–744.[135] Such flight or wandering is also likely to have spread the plague.

Rumor and hysteria were rife. As John of Ephesus put it, "a sane person could no longer be found easily."[136] He relates that as the plague was spreading from Alexandria to Palestine, spectral boats of shining brass were seen, especially at night, in which headless black people were sitting holding poles of brass, heading for Ashkelon and Gaza.[137] At Constantinople, the rumor spread that if pottery were thrown from upper-story windows onto the street the plague would leave the city. Women did that in one neighborhood, and the word spread from one neighborhood to another throughout the city. For three days no one was seen in the streets, because they were all at home driving away the plague by breaking pottery. When people grew tired of breaking pottery and continued to die anyway, the simple and common people got it into their heads that death came in the form of monks and clerics. They would howl at them and run away shouting "We belong to the Mother of God!" or to some martyr or apostle. Among some of them, this lasted for two years after the plague was over.[138]

Some measures were more practical. At Alexandria and Constantinople, no one left home without hanging a written tag on his neck or arm containing his name and district, so, if he should die, his family could

---

[131] *Incerti auctoris*, 2:108; *Chronique de Michel le Syrien*, 2:239–40, 4:307; *CZ*, 112. *The Chronicle of Séert* (*Histoire Nestorienne*, 185 [93]) says that the people of Alexandria became like drunkards from the disease that stupefied their brains.

[132] *Incerti auctoris*, 2:182; *CZ*, 170.

[133] *Chronique de Michel le Syrien*, 2:236, 4:305.

[134] *Histoire Nestorienne*, 183 [91].

[135] *Incerti auctoris*, 2:182; *CZ*, 170.

[136] *Incerti auctoris*, 2:107; *CZ*, 112.

[137] *Incerti auctoris*, 2:82–83; *Chronique de Michel le Syrien*, 2:238, 4:306; *CZ*, 96; *Anecdota Syriaca*, 2:307. Procopius, *PW* 2.22.10–13, pp. 454–57 says that some people were struck by apparitions when they contracted the plague.

[138] *Incerti auctoris*, 2:108–09; *Chronique de Michel le Syrien*, 2:239–40, 4:307; *CZ*, 112–13. John blames demons for misleading people in both cases. These stories are not in Land.

be informed and they could come and bury him.[139] It was simplest just to leave. During the plague of 686–687 in upper Iraq, the survivors scattered like sheep over the mountains to escape it only to be followed and robbed by looters.[140] In 743–744, survivors moved outside the city.[141]

The immediate social and economic effects of the plague are easy to discern because our sources are quite specific about them. The long-range effects are more difficult to assess. In those regions where the plague recurred from the mid-sixth to at least the mid-eighth century there should have been a major, long-term demographic crisis.[142] This was due not only to plague; for more than two hundred years the population of the Levant was repeatedly decimated by epidemic disease, famine, earthquakes, massacre, and deportation. We will return to this issue later. Because the poor (i.e., the working classes) died first, there would also have been a labor crisis among farmers, artisans, and domestic servants. Consumer markets would have been reduced. One would expect economic depression, inflation (there were fewer people and they had access to abandoned wealth), increased wages for surviving working people, changes in landholding and social structure, and so on. We hear about none of these things from the Syriac sources. They do tell us about short-term inflation (often quite steep) caused by famines but not by plague.

Virtually all of our information about the social and economic effects of the plague in the Syriac sources is derived from or influenced by the account of John of Ephesus. It is clear that he favored the interests of the poor and devalued material wealth, as did the Zūqnīn chronicler. It was God's mercy that the poor died first, when the rich were still around to bury them. When the plague struck the rich and powerful, there was no one left to give them a decent burial.[143] Part of the terror of the plague was that it did, in fact, appear to be indiscriminate and arbitrary. It struck ordinary people and notables alike with no apparent reason, while people seemed to survive for no apparent reason. The plague took both servants and masters. There were large houses where everyone died

---

[139] *Incerti auctoris*, 2:102; *Chronicon ad annum Christi 1234*, CSCO 81, p. 197; CSCO 109, p. 155; *Chronique de Michel le Syrien*, 2:237, 4:306; CZ, 109; *Anecdota Syriaca*, 2:321; *Histoire Nestorienne*, 183 [91].

[140] Brock, "North Mesopotamia," 68–69; Mingana, *Sources Syriaques*, 161*.

[141] *Incerti auctoris*, 2:187; CZ, 173.

[142] Dols, "Plague in Early Islamic History," 372–73, 381. Twitchett, "Population and Pestilence," 58 agrees that "epidemics must have had some effect upon demographic trends."

[143] *Incerti auctoris*, 2:95; *Chronique de Michel le Syrien*, 2:235–37, 4:305; CZ, 104; *Histoire Nestorienne*, 183 [91]. The Zūqnīn chronicler applies this also to the plague of 743–774. See *Incerti auctoris*, 2:186; CZ, 173.

and some where a solitary notable survived with just a few other people. John of Ephesus uses a rhetorical reversal of status in saying that those who used to be served had to stand up and serve themselves and their own sick servants. Even the imperial family was reduced to living humbly with only a few people to serve them.[144] The Zūqnīn chronicler adapts this passage to describe the plague of 743–744, but intimates that many large, wealthy families and many tribes were left without a single heir, so that the possessions, fields, and houses of the wealthy were inherited by their friends.[145] According to John of Ephesus, it was useless to make wills when the heirs died before the testators did.[146]

Abandoned property was left unguarded and no one took it. At least John of Ephesus offers some cautionary tales to the effect that people who did try to take abandoned wealth died anyway.[147] John claims that the people of Constantinople, being warned of the plague by hearsay before it arrived, prepared themselves ahead of time by giving alms and distributing their property to the needy.[148] Some of the needy were willing to beg from the living rather than enter the houses of the dead to loot them, but most people refused to take charity from the rich because those who did so died.[149]

At Constantinople, economic life ground to a halt. John of Ephesus says that, "In all respects everything stopped." Buying and selling ceased; there was no one left who could stand up and do their work; all the provisions in the marketplaces ran out; and food was exhausted. This

---

[144] *Incerti auctoris*, 2:95, 101–02; *CZ*, 104–05, 108; *Anecdota Syriaca*, 2:315, 320. But both points are corroborated by Procopius, *PW* 2.23.4–5, pp. 464–67, who says that many houses became completely destitute of human inhabitants and that formerly prosperous men were deprived of the service of sick or dead servants.

[145] *Incerti auctoris*, 2:184; *CZ*, 171.

[146] *Incerti auctoris*, 2:102; *Chronicon ad annum Christi 1234*, CSCO 81, p. 198; CSCO 109, p. 156; *Chronique de Michel le Syrien*, 2:238; 4:306; *CZ*, 109; *Anecdota Syriaca*, 2:321.

[147] *Incerti auctoris*, 2:83; *Chronique de Michel le Syrien*, 2:238, 4:306; *CZ*, 97, 109; *Anecdota Syriaca*, 2:307, 321; *Histoire Nestorienne*, 183 [91]. For the story about the city on the borders of Egypt where everyone perished except seven men and a ten-year-old child, see *Incerti auctoris*, 2:83–84; *Chronicon ad annum Christi 1234*, CSCO 81, p. 197; CSCO 109, p. 155; *Chronique de Michel le Syrien*, 2: 238–39; 4:306–07; *CZ*, 97–98; *Anecdota Syriaca*, 2:307–08; *Histoire Nestorienne*, 184 [92]. For the story about the shop of the silversmith in Constantinople, see *Incerti auctoris*, 2:103; *Chronique de Michel le Syrien*, 2:238, 4:306; *CZ*, 109–10; *Anecdota Syriaca*, 2:321–22.

[148] *Incerti auctoris*, 2:93–94; *CZ*, 103; *Anecdota Syriaca*, 2:314.

[149] *Incerti auctoris*, 2:103; *Chronique de Michel le Syrien*, 2:238, 4: 306; *CZ*, 109; *Anecdota Syriaca*, 2:321.

proved to be a great affliction for those who had other diseases.[150] Such conditions are likely to have been exacerbated by the fact that mortality in the countryside meant that herds went untended and crops unharvested. On his journey from Syria to Thrace, John of Ephesus noted feral herds of sheep, goats, oxen, and pigs wandering about with no one to tend them, and unharvested fields of wheat, fruit crops, and vineyards.[151] During the epidemic among cattle (*mawtānā dᵉ tawrē*) that lasted for two years in the entire East, probably in about 551–552, fields went uncultivated for lack of oxen.[152] According to the *Chronicle of Séert*, during the plague (*wabā'*) that struck cattle in 552–553, people used camels, asses, and beasts of burden for plowing.[153] Elias bar Shīnāyā reports that during the outbreak of bubonic plague (*sharʿūṭā, ṭāʿūn*) in 600, fields went unharvested because of depopulation.[154]

How did people understand such a disastrous experience? Procopius argues that, because it was universal and indiscriminate, and had no (known) natural explanation, the plague must be referred to God.[155] John of Ephesus, according to his antimaterialist agenda, believed there was an angel in charge of the scourge (*shabṭā*) whose job was to make people despise the things of this world.[156] The Syriac continuator of Zacharias of Mitylene says it was well known that the scourge (*mᵉḥūtā*) came from Satan, who had been ordered by God to punish people.[157] John bar Penkayē thought that famines, earthquakes, and plagues were signs of the end of the world.[158] John of Ephesus repeatedly says that

[150] *Incerti auctoris,* 2:97; *CZ,* 105–06; *Anecdota Syriaca,* 2:316. Procopius, *PW* 2.23.18, pp. 470–71 says virtually the same thing: work stopped, artisans abandoned their trades, there was widespread starvation, and the sick died sooner from the lack of necessities.
[151] *Incerti auctoris,* 2:87–88; *Chronique de Michel le Syrien,* 2:240, 4:307–08; *CZ,* 99–100; *Anecdota Syriaca,* 2:311.
[152] *Chronicon Jacobi Edesseni, CSCO* 5, p. 321; *CSCO* 6, p. 243. This is repeated by Michael the Syrian. See *Chronique de Michel le Syrien,* 2:245, 4:309.
[153] *Histoire Nestorienne,* 185 [94]. This could not have come from Jacob of Edessa.
[154] *Opus Chonologicum, CSCO* 62, 1:124; *CSCO* 63, p. 60.
[155] Procopius, *PW* 2.22.25, pp. 452–53.
[156] *Incerti auctoris,* 2:105; *Chronique de Michel le Syrien,* 2:239, 4:307; *CZ,* 111; *Anecdota Syriaca,* 2:323. The *Chronicle of Séert* quotes Ps. 78:49–50 for "the angel of evil." See *Histoire Nestorienne,* 183 [91].
[157] *Chronique de Michel le Syrien,* 2:240, 4:308; *Historia ecclesiastica Zachariae, CSCO* 84, 2:192; *CSCO* 88, pp. 129–30. For the Arab belief that plague was caused by demons and spirits, see Conrad, "Arabic Plague Chronologies and Treatises," 61.
[158] Brock, "North Mesopotamia," 72; Mingana, *Sources Syriaques,* 165*. John of Ephesus comes close to saying this.

people were being punished for their sins.[159] The Zūqnīn chronicler also explained the plagues of 557–558 and 743–744, and much else besides, as punishment for peoples' sins.[160] John of Ephesus actually says that the punishment should be seen as the "rod of God's gentle mercy" and a call for repentance.[161] If this were the case, then it is at least curious that there are no references to rogations to lift the plague in any of the Syriac accounts of bubonic plague as there are for other kinds of disasters. On the contrary, John of Ephesus tells of a city on the border between Palestine and Egypt where people reverted to paganism and worshipped a brass statue to avert the plague.[162]

John's account, of course, is not objective. It fairly bristles with horrified hyperbole, value judgments, lessons to be learned, and biblical quotations. Why did he write it? He says that he wanted to record these events, but his thoughts were blocked by many fears, and he considered giving it up. Using a familiar rhetorical trope, these scenes were beyond the speech and narrative ability of eloquent speakers. Even if they could describe even part of these events, what would be the use, since there would be no one left to read it. He asks rhetorically, "For whom does the writer write?" His answer is that he is writing for future generations. But he wonders if the remnant coming after him will recover from the terrible plague, learn from it, and be saved from future punishment.[163]

John finds his tongue (or more accurately his pen) in biblical lamentation texts, which he quotes profusely. There are no allusions to classical Greek or Latin literature or even to the Church Fathers. In this respect, his writing is a good example of the new Christian literature that became dominant during the sixth century.[164] The Bible furnishes numerous, useful passages about pestilence and lamenting destruction. In many places, John says that he can do nothing better than to quote them. He begins with a virtual jeremiad and a statement about the usefulness of Jeremiah

---

[159] *Incerti auctoris*, 2:81, 82, 92, 99, 107; *CZ*, 95, 96, 102, 107, 112; *Anecdota Syriaca*, 2:305, 306, 318.

[160] *Incerti auctoris*, 2:119, 179; *CZ*, 119, 168.

[161] *Incerti auctoris*, 2:92–93, 99; *CZ*, 103, 107; *Anecdota Syriaca*, 2:318.

[162] *Incerti auctoris*, 2:85; *Chronique de Michel le Syrien*, 2:239–40, 4:307; *CZ*, 98–99; *Anecdota Syriaca*, 2:309. Naturally, John attributed this to devils in the form of angels, the statue was cast down by a whirlwind, and all the people perished. The city is not identified, John's account is full of tendentious details, and this looks like a plague rumor, but it is still suggestive of the possibility that some people might have been attracted to the old religion in a crisis.

[163] *Incerti auctoris*, 2:82; *CZ*, 96; *Anecdota Syriaca*, 2:306.

[164] Cameron, "Images of Authority," 206.

because of his experience in uttering lamentations. But, unlike Jeremiah, John's lament is not over the destruction of only one city, Jerusalem, and only one people, the Jews, but over many cities.[165] Just to give a sense of the flavor of John's writing, in recounting his journey from Syria to Constantinople, he asks rhetorically how could anyone speak or write about the horrible scenes he encountered day after day, except to say with the prophet: "The earth shall sit in mourning and all its inhabitants shall mourn" (Isa. 24:6).[166] He also believes that biblical prophecies are being fulfilled by current events.[167] John recognizes that the outbreak of plague had been preceded by destructive wars, but says that this plague surpasses and is more terrible than all the other disasters combined. It eclipsed them all like the thin cows that ate the pharaoh's fat cows (Gen. 41:18-21).[168]

John uses the imagery of a wine press of Wrath from the beginning of his account to express how the plague squeezed people as if they were ripe grapes. It is not until one gets to John's description of the burial pits at Constantinople that one realizes how literal that image is meant to be.[169] There is also an element of sensationalism in John of Ephesus, with vivid, gruesome images that stick in the mind, not unlike the presentation of disasters in the modern news media. Such are his description of the burial pits and the house with twenty corpses at Constantinople.[170]

The Zūqnīn chronicler used the same techniques as John of Ephesus, and not just to describe the plague of 743–744, for the same purpose: Disasters are caused by human sin and people should repent. Although it is true that he borrowed expressions and passages from John of Ephesus

[165] *Incerti auctoris*, 2:79; *CZ*, 94; *Anecdota Syriaca*, 2:304. John actually quotes Isaiah more than Jeremiah, but this appeal to Jeremiah would have a long life in Syriac literature. John bar Penkayē uses almost the same wording for the plague of 686–687: "We are forced to use the words of Jeremiah: he lamented for a single people, that is Jerusalem alone, but we [lament] for the entire world." See Brock, "North Mesopotamia," 70; Mingana, *Sources Syriaques*, 162*. This is so close to John of Ephesus that it almost had to have come from him, but there is no other indication that John bar Penkayē might have used him.

[166] *Incerti auctoris*, 2:88; *CZ*, 100; *Anecdota Syriaca*, 2:311.

[167] *Incerti auctoris*, 2:88; *CZ*, 100; *Anecdota Syriaca*, 2:311; Witakowski calls this "presentism." See Witakowski, *Historiography*, 114–15, 143–44.

[168] *Incerti auctoris*, 2:89–91; *CZ*, 101–02; *Anecdota Syriaca*, 2:312.

[169] *Incerti auctoris*, 2:79–80, 82, 99; *CZ*, 94, 96, 107; *Anecdota Syriaca*, 2:304, 318. The Zūqnīn chronicler also uses this imagery for the plague of 743–744. See *Incerti auctoris*, 2:183; *CZ*, 171.

[170] For the burial pits see earlier; for the house with twenty corpses see *Incerti auctoris*, 2:101; *Chronicon ad annum Christi 1234*, CSCO 81, 1:198; CSCO 109, p. 156; *Chronique de Michel le Syrien*, 2:237, 4:306; *CZ*, 108; *Anecdota Syriaca*, 2:320.

to describe the plague in his own time,[171] he went further. For instance, the Zūqnīn chronicler began his account of the plague in his own time with multiple quotations from Jeremiah, most of which are not in the extant text of John of Ephesus.[172]

Finally, it needs to be remembered that the first bubonic plague pandemic did not occur in a vacuum. During the two centuries of its recurrence, people also suffered from disasters caused by famine, bad weather, plagues of locusts, earthquakes, and warfare.[173] Outbreaks of plague were often accompanied by famine. The plague epidemic in the time of Justinian lasted only for three years. It was followed by a famine due to crop failure that lasted for eight years, from 858 AG (546–547 CE) to 866 AG (554–555).[174] Famine accompanied plague in 686–687 in upper Iraq;[175] famine and epidemic disease occurred together in 742–743;[176] the plague of 744–745 in Mesopotamia, Bostra, and the Hawran occurred together with famine;[177] and the pestilence (*mawtānā*) of 773–774 also occurred with famine.[178] On at least two occasions in 743–744 and in 750–751 in Syria, we are told that there were more victims of famine than of disease.[179] It is entirely possible that famine reduced the resistance of people to disease.[180]

There were diseases other than bubonic plague. Sometimes people suffered from multiple diseases at the same time. After a famine in 772–773, people ate the herbs of the field in the spring and got stomachaches. They suffered from various diseases such as ulcers, pustules, eye disease, fever, pimples, pleurisy, hemorrhoids, dropsy, and many other unknown

---

[171] *CZ*, 21–22, 30, 168.

[172] These are Jer. 9:10, 18, and 22, and a fuller quotation of Jer. 9:20–21.

[173] It is not the purpose to recount all of these here. For a brief account, see Morony, "Michael the Syrian," paragraphs: 5–8, 16–21, 26, 30–31.

[174] *Incerti auctoris*, 2:114–15, 119; *CZ*, 116–17, 119.

[175] Brock, "North Mesopotamia," 70; Mingana, *Sources Syriaques*, 163*.

[176] *Chronicon ad annum Christi 1234*, CSCO 81, 1:314; CSCO 109, p. 245. Michael the Syrian puts this in 744–45. See *Chronique de Michel le Syrien*, 2:506, 4:464.

[177] *Chronicon ad annum Christi 1234*, CSCO 81, 1:319; CSCO 109, p. 249; *Chronique de Michel le Syrien*, 2:508, 4:466.

[178] *Incerti auctoris*, 2:333; *CZ*, 287. Famine often coincided with plague according to the Arabic sources for this period. See Dols, "Plague in Early Islamic History," 376. According to Twitchett, "Population and Pestilence," 45–52, outbreaks of bubonic plague in China in the seventh century were also often preceded by famine.

[179] *Incerti auctoris*, 2:182, 205; *CZ*, 170–188.

[180] Dols, "Plague in Early Islamic History," 376; Tucker, "Natural Disasters," 218. Tucker also suggests (pp. 215–16, 222) that the stress caused by terror and disorientation due to all sorts of disasters reduced resistance to disease.

diseases.[181] These may not have been fatal, but they can also be expected to have reduced resistance to plague.

Contemporaries lumped all of these afflictions together. John bar Penkayē refers to an unholy trinity of sword, famine, and plague. He says that during the bubonic plague of 686–687 "what the famine had left, the plague devoured, what the plague left over, the sword finished off," and that "when we escaped from plague, famine chased after us, and anything that we had left over was taken away from us by raiders."[182] The Zūqnīn chronicler says that during the bubonic plague of 743–744 if a man went into his house, he was faced by famine and pestilence (*mawtānā*); if he went out into the open countryside, he would be attacked by thieves.[183] If there was a demographic crisis from the sixth to the eighth century, bubonic plague was not its only cause.

Even without resorting to monocausal explanations, common sense assumes that there should have been a long-term decrease in population in the Mediterranean Basin and western Asia in general as a result of plague and other causes of mass mortality, or at least in those places hit the hardest or most often. This is difficult to verify, although Constantinople appears to have been a smaller city in the ninth century than in the sixth. It is also difficult to reconcile excessive mortality in the urban and rural labor force with evidence for the expansion of labor-intensive forms of production from the late sixth century onward, at least in some places, but probably not in Syria and Mesopotamia. In this case it is possible to argue that the importation of Anatolian and Turkish captives and Berber women from North Africa to Syria in the early decades of the eighth century served to replace a labor force lost to plague mortality and to help rebuild the population.

The issue of demographic recovery via reproduction or replacement following excessive mortality involves questions about fertility and birth rates and average life expectancy. We do not really know what these were. But monasticism arguably drove down the birth rate among Christians in general compared to non-Christians.[184] Polygamy and concubinage may have increased the birth rate among some Muslims, but Muslims suffered from plague mortality at least as much as non-Muslims in the

[181] *Incerti auctoris*, 2:357–58; CZ, 305.
[182] Brock, "North Mesopotamia," 70, 71, 73; Mingana, *Sources Syriaques*, 162*, 164*–65*, 167*.
[183] *Incerti auctoris*, 2:181–82; CZ, 170.
[184] However, it must be admitted that there were exceptional cases of monks with female consorts and children.

seventh and eighth centuries. Generally speaking, a presumed short life expectancy and a high infant mortality rate would create a social need for a high birth rate simply to maintain a stable population. What would happen when the fragile balance was upset by excessive mortality? At least two possibilities are suggested by post-disaster physiology. One is that the stress caused by all sorts of disasters reduces resistance to disease;[185] stress might also reduce fertility rates. The other is that fear releases hormones and neurochemicals that stimulate the survival instinct, driving up levels of dopamine and possibly testosterone, thus stimulating the libido and leading to increased sexual activity after disasters.[186] However that may be, it is difficult to reconcile widespread depopulation with the image of demographic growth and economic expansion associated with early Islamic history.

It is equally difficult to identify changes in social structure or economic life that would have been the specific result of excessive mortality. Along with floods, wars, famines, and earthquakes, did plague make any difference? How could the mass mortality caused by all of these disasters not have had an effect? All one can say at this point is that life seems to have gone on around these events. Wars were conducted in the middle of plagues; the Ma'rib dam was repaired after the fatal epidemic was over; Antioch was rebuilt after each earthquake.

The accounts of the first bubonic plague pandemic in Syriac literature thus raise more questions than they answer. These accounts have the most to say about the symptoms and immediate effects of bubonic plague: the excessive mortality and the concern for disposing of the corpses. However, they should not be used alone, but must be combined with accounts in other languages (Greek, Arabic, Latin, and Chinese) to have a more complete picture.

---

[185] See note 180.
[186] Helen Fisher in Kelleher, "Birds & Bees," *Los Angeles Times*, Oct. 1, 2001, p. E3. Fisher is the author of *The Anatomy of Love*.

4

Justinianic Plague in Syria and the Archaeological Evidence

Hugh N. Kennedy

The impact of the plague on the society of the sixth-century Roman Empire remains a subject of controversy. At the heart of the debate lies the question of the size and extent of the mortality. Was it such that it resulted in a significant and lasting demographic decline, or have we been overly impressed by the lurid accounts in the literary sources and imagined a crisis that never really existed? Was this a pandemic on the scale of the Black Death and subsequent visitations? Finding a check on the literary sources is very difficult. Clearly, there are few if any documentary sources to help us out. The only possible moderator for the written accounts would seem to be the archaeological evidence.

In recent years, a number of commentators have pointed out that the archaeological evidence suggests that the literary accounts of mass mortality are greatly exaggerated or, perhaps, that they related to only one small locality and that such evidence should not be extrapolated to include the entire Mediterranean world, or even just the territories under the control of the eastern Roman Empire. Jean Durliat,[1] for example, accuses us of privileging the written accounts and disregarding archaeological material. Discussing the modern literature on the plague, he argues, "All of these studies have in common their privileging of literary sources, and among these, descriptions of the epidemic, whereas specialists in other kinds of documents accord it [the plague] only minor importance. It is from this insufficiently underscored contradiction that indecisive and divergent interpretations stem."[2] He goes on to argue that the plague

[1] Durliat, "La peste du VIe siècle."
[2] Ibid., 107.

was basically an urban phenomenon and that rural areas were largely spared.[3]

More recently, Clive Foss in his survey of Syria from Late Antiquity to Islam has expressed similar doubts about the importance and effect of the plague.[4] He argues against any demographic decline in Syria in the late sixth century. "Evidence [of demographic decline due to plague], he argues, "is ambiguous at best and fails to support any generalised notion of decline or fundamental change," and he later adds that the plague, "was not such a widespread disaster as it has been portrayed . . . its ravages were repaired rather quickly."[5] Other recent commentators, such as W. Brandes, for example, have accepted that the plague, or rather the succession of plagues from the mid-sixth to the mid-eighth centuries, must have had a serious effect on late antique cities, but they have not really pointed a way to reconciling the descriptions of a major catastrophe in the literary sources and the apparent absence of direct evidence in the archaeology.[6]

This essay returns to the archaeological evidence to see what it does, or does not, tell us about the impact of plague on the longer-term development of Syria. Before looking at the evidence, some points should be clarified. We should not expect to find direct evidence of plague mortality. No mass graves or plague pits for example have been confidently identified. In fact, there are virtually no early Christian cemeteries that have been located in Syria, and the absence of plague burials simply reflects this position.[7] However, recent research on inscriptions from Byzantine Palestine may be suggestive. Tsafrir and Foerster in their study of Scythopolis note, "the information has been collected by Leah Di Segni in her comprehensive study of the dated inscriptions in Roman and Byzantine Palestine [not yet published]. The concentration of burial inscriptions in the latter part of 541 is very striking."

So, if we do not find direct evidence such as mass graves or large numbers of epitaphs pointing to plague as a cause of death, what archaeological evidence could there be for the effects of pandemic disease? We should certainly look for demographic stagnation or decline. On the most general level, it will be suggested by the lack of new towns or settlements. Within existing settlements, the process is likely to be most clearly visible

[3] Ibid., 118.
[4] Foss, "Syria in Transition."
[5] Ibid., 260.
[6] Brandes, "Byzantine Cities."
[7] On the absence of cemeteries in the Limestone Massif see Tate, *Campagnes de la Syrie*, 224.

in the lack of newly built dwellings or residential areas. It is much more difficult to determine the period at which existing houses are abandoned, especially in the Syrian context where most abandonment was peaceful and where the dry conditions and thinness of the soil rarely permit the laying down of a deep stratigraphy. Demographic decline need not necessarily be linked to economic decline for the individual households that survive; on the contrary, evidence from the Black Death suggests that the reduction of pressure on land and other resources may actually leave the survivors more affluent than they were before the epidemic. Neither should the building of new churches be taken as an unambiguous sign of demographic expansion. The history of later medieval Europe suggests that church building continued almost unabated through the pandemic of 1348–1349. It is easy to see how a smaller, but perhaps more affluent, or at least less straitened, population would have been prepared to found and build new churches on vacant lands. The same is true of high-status building. In fact, the archaeological record from the Black Death in western Europe suggests that it is virtually imperceptible in the pattern of élite building. It is in the overall size of cities and in the marginal agricultural areas where we might expect to find the signs of demographic decline.

The advent of the plague in the Mediterranean world was a sudden historical event that can be dated to the years 541–544, with subsequent recurrences every fifteen to twenty-five years. The archaeological evidence rarely offers such precision. The pottery, especially the coarse wares in everyday use, cannot be dated with any exactitude. Throughout Late Antiquity and into the early Islamic period, the basic ceramic patterns remained the same. It is only in the case of certain imported wares that we can use the pottery to suggest more precise dates within this period. In most cases it is impossible to say with any confidence whether the ceramics date from before or after the date of the arrival of the plague or the Islamic conquest.[8] The same is broadly true of the masonry and building types that have been dated in the Limestone Massif. It has been clearly shown that there are recognizable differences between the building types of the later fourth and early fifth century, on one hand, and the sixth on the other.[9] However, the indicators are less clear with regard to developments within the sixth century. In most areas of Syria, neither ceramics

---

[8] On the problems of dating the ceramic evidence in this period, see the articles by Sodini and Villeneuve, Orssaud, and Watson in Canivet and Rey-Coquais, *La Syrie de Byzance à l'Islam.*

[9] Tate, *Campagnes de la Syrie,* 85–166.

nor masonry types allow us to say with confidence whether buildings were constructed before or after 540. For the building types in the Limestone Massif of northern Syria, Tate has elaborated a series of criteria based on a combination of masonry types, decorative features, and such epigraphic evidence as is available to produce a typology of building that, he claims, can date domestic structure to within a decade. Though some of this is necessarily imprecise and speculative, it represents the most satisfactory dating mechanism we have. Two caveats, however, have to be used: The first is that it shows only when buildings were constructed or reconstructed and cannot tell us when they fell into disuse. The second is that it is useful only for structures on the Limestone Massif. Buildings from other areas of Byzantine Syria show quite different techniques.

Although we cannot be certain exactly which buildings were constructed before and which after the coming of the plague, the number of buildings closely dated by inscription does at least enable us to make some broad generalizations. Even here, it can be suggested there are problems. The absence of building inscriptions may not in fact demonstrate the lack of new building, but rather the loss of the epigraphic habit, that is to say, people were still building new constructions but were no longer commemorating these in the old way. While building inscriptions certainly disappear, not only in Syria but also in those areas like Anatolia and the Balkans that remained under Byzantine rule in the seventh century, the number of inscriptions on churches and other structures make it clear that the practice continued through the second half of the sixth century, and that while there may have been some decline in the epigraphic habit between 540 and 600, there is no evidence to show that this was the case.

Most of the literary evidence suggests that it was the cities that were most severely hit by the plague, and so it is with the archaeology of the cities that we must begin our inquiry. Antioch was, of course, the most important city in Byzantine Syria.[10] As is well known, however, the archaeological record from Antioch is very scanty. It is clear that great damage was done by an earthquake in 526 and by the sudden Persian conquest of 540. We know from Procopius that Justinian made a major effort to reconstruct the city thereafter, but we also know from the archaeological record that this was done on a significantly smaller scale than before. Some areas, notably the island formed by two branches of the Orontes,

---

[10] For Antioch in Late Antiquity, see the classic account in Downey, *History of Antioch*, 503–78. Also Kennedy, "Antioch: From Byzantium to Islam," and, for a recent overview, Kondoleon, *Antioch*.

previously within the city walls, were now left outside. Some houses in the city were destroyed and not rebuilt. On the other hand, the houses in suburban Daphne do seem to have been reconstructed and used through the late sixth century. The archaeological evidence is not sufficient for us to conclude that people were leaving the plague-infested central areas for more salubrious suburban areas, but it may well point to that.[11]

The archaeological record at Apamea, capital of Syria II in Late Antiquity, is much fuller.[12] Unlike Antioch, the city seems to have been spared from serious damage by both the 526 earthquake and the 540 Persian invasion. In 573, however, it was taken and sacked by the Persians, and much of the evident decline of the city in the late sixth century may be attributable to that. The site has been extensively excavated, and a number of large houses have been explored. In the main, these are high-status dwellings and can be dated with some confidence. There are no newly built houses that can be ascribed to the period after 540. The fate of the houses and shops that had existed then is mixed. The shops on the decumanus near the cathedral have coins of Justin I (518–527) but none later. The Triclinium House built in the fourth century was rebuilt after a fire in 539, and the Pilaster House was rebuilt in the early sixth century. Of the other main houses investigated, the House of the Deer and the House of the Trilobe Columns were repaired at some stage in the sixth century. With the exception of the House of the Consols, they had all been deserted or at least were in a state of decay by the end of the sixth century. How far this was the result of the plague, or of conquest in 573, or of both, is of course impossible to tell.

The urban history of Gerasa in the sixth century is difficult to read. This is partly because very little excavation has been done in the domestic quarters of the city and the only areas of housing that have been explored systematically date from the Umayyad period. We know that church building continued. Whittow sees the building of the Propylaea Church in 565 as a sign of the continuing vitality of the city.[13] However, there are a number of reasons to be skeptical about this. The inscription that gives us the date may refer only to the laying of the small mosaic in the diaconikon,

[11] Foss, "Syria in Transition," 193–94.
[12] Balty, "Apamée au VIe siècle" provides an overview that stresses the continuing prosperity of the city through the sixth century, despite the catastrophe of 573, and paints a melancholy picture of the great proprietors abandoning their spacious and elegant town houses to the incoming Bedouin after the Muslim conquest as they made their way to Constantinople. See also Foss, "Syria in Transition," 210–25, which updates Balty's report and produces a somewhat less optimistic view of continuity through the sixth century.
[13] Whittow, "Ruling the Late Roman and Early Byzantine City."

rather than to the building of the entire church. But even if it does relate
to the whole building, the construction of a church in the middle of
the street not only blocked the street itself but obviously meant that the
bridge over the river that led to the street was abandoned and probably
ruined, leaving, as far as we know, only one bridge to connect the two
sides of the city. Neither the construction of the Propylaea Church nor
the building of the Isaiah Church near the abandoned north theater in
559 tell us anything about the demographic history of the city. They tell
us only that there were still some people with money to construct modest
churches in what had been the heart of the city.

The city on which we have the fullest information is Scythopolis or
Bet Shean. The publication of the excavations by Tsafrir and Foerster
have given us the most detailed and nuanced account of the late antique
history of any city in the Near East, and possibly of any city in the Mediterranean world. The most striking feature of Scythopolis in this period is
the persistence of a tradition of public civic architecture into the sixth
century. Constructions included the building of new streets, the "Silvanus
Street" of 515–516 and the street near the amphitheater of 521–522, the
semicircular sigma, laid out in 506–507. There were also public buildings,
like the large Eastern Baths (499–500 onwards with the latest inscription
dated to 534–535), the Western Baths of 534–535, the basilica attached
to the Silvanus Street development, and work on the city walls carried
out in the reign of Justin I, 518–527. After 541, this pattern almost completely ceases. The only dated structure of importance was a bath for
lepers erected as a work of charity by the Bishop Theodorus in 558–559.

The contrast between the levels of building activity in the city pre- and
post-plague is startling. This does not necessarily mean that the plague
was the primary cause of the change. The major Samaritan revolt in the
city in 529 certainly inflicted considerable damage (although it did not
put an end to building activity). There may have been political factors,
the drying up of government patronage, for example. What seems clear
is that the city was in a period of demographic stagnation, at best, and
probably of decline. Certainly the growth of the early sixth century had
come to an abrupt halt.

It is difficult to make intelligent generalizations about other cities.
Even those like Caesarea and Bostra, where there has been substantial
archaeological work, have not yielded a clear picture of the state of the
cities in the years after 541. However, it is clear that the level of new
building activity, especially secular building, had declined markedly by
the end of the sixth century.

The case of Hama, however, deserves some consideration. Excavations conducted by a Danish expedition in the 1930s have only recently been fully published. Foss has argued that Hama bucks the trend of decline that is observable in other cities in the latter half of the sixth century: "Development", he concludes, "was very different here from Antioch and especially Apamea. No ruralization is evident here: city life in large and comfortable houses apparently continued without interruption."[14] The evidence on which this encouraging vision is based turns out to be very slight indeed. There are the remains of one large house on the citadel that continued to be occupied into Umayyad times, when it appears that the figurative mosaics were damaged by iconoclasts (whether that suggests that the house was lived in by people affected by the new Puritanism or a roofless ruin open to the gaze of the curious and malicious is, of course, quite unclear). There were also a few other houses, "too poorly preserved to describe, [which] also appear to have been in continuous use." We also have an inscription recording restoration work on the cathedral (now the great mosque) in 595. And that is all. To construct a thriving late sixth-century city from such fragmentary materials is a truly imaginative piece of archaeological inventiveness. The city may have been thriving, but the archaeological evidence does not tell us that.

Similar caution must be used in accepting Foss' account of the small city of Tarutia, northeast of Hama, as "continuing to flourish through the sixth century." Certainly an impressive basilical church was built in 505 and a defensive tower in 510, but the latest building inscription found on the site dates from 539. After that, there is silence. Once again, the dangers of assuming that the sixth century was a sort of economic and demographic plateau, and that what is true for the beginning continued until the end, are clearly apparent.

The archaeology of rural settlement in Syria is highly developed. Nowhere else are the villages of the late antique Empire so clearly visible, and nowhere else have they been so rigorously studied. The best-known area is the Limestone Massif, the rocky rolling hill country between Antioch and Aleppo, stretching as far south as Hama. In this area, the pioneering survey work of Georges Tchalenko led to a clear vision of a prosperous rural society, with its houses and churches deserted but still largely intact.[15] Since Tchalenko's work was published, more research has been done on the area and some of his conclusions have been modified. For the

---

[14] Foss, "Syria in Transition," 230–31.
[15] Tchalenko, *Villages antiques de la Syrie.*

purposes of this essay, the most important contributions have been the excavation of several houses in the small village of Dehes[16] and Georges Tate's reassessment of the social and economic bases of the society.[17]

Using both inscriptions, which date some but only a small proportion of the domestic structures, and masonry types, which give a broad band dating of most structures, Tate argues that there were two main peaks of construction, one in the third century when settlement on a large scale was first beginning in these areas and the other in the late fifth and very early sixth centuries. After 540, there is a marked decline in the numbers of inscriptions. Furthermore, most of the inscriptions that do survive on domestic structures relate to just certain parts of the structures, a new portico for example, rather than a whole new building.[18] He concludes, "it is indeed around 550 that the building of houses was interrupted, but that does not mean that all construction stopped." In other words, we see the end of the building of new houses, but not a complete end to the beautifying and improving of existing ones.

The pattern is confirmed by the study of individual settlements. The small but prosperous village of Refada near the shrine of St. Simeon boasts five dated inscriptions from 341 to 516, but nothing after that and no evidence of later construction work.[19] In Déhes, the excavators examined the evolution of three houses in detail. They point out that there are no further architectural developments after the middle of the sixth century but that occupation continued at a lower economic level for several centuries after that.[20] Certainly to judge from the coin finds, the village seems to have continued to be part of a monetary economy. Overall population levels are very difficult to discuss on the basis of so small a sample. The village was clearly no longer expanding after the middle of the sixth century. Whether the population was in decline at this stage is not clear, but if it was in decline, this may be attributable to a number of causes, of which plague is only one.[21]

Unfortunately, work done on other areas of rural Syria have not yielded comparable results. F. Villeneuve's wide-ranging survey of rural life in the Hawran has little to say about changes over time except to note that at

---

[16] Sodini et al., "Déhes (Syrie du Nord)," 1–305.

[17] Tate, *Campagnes de la Syrie.*

[18] Ibid., 167–81.

[19] Tchalenko, *Villages antiques de la Syrie,* 1:194–97.

[20] Sodini et al., "Déhes (Syrie du Nord)," 300–1.

[21] Although it clearly did decline at some stage and the site became deserted during the tenth century.

some time in the Byzantine period, "perhaps in the fifth century," the area saw a return in force of the nomads and that the Muslim conquest, in consequence, did not mark a major break.[22] However, in the same volume, M. Sartre has suggested a pattern of building activity based on the epigraphic material from the area. He notes a great surge of building inscriptions from the early years of Justinian's reign in the cities of Bostra and Gerasa that comes to an abrupt end in 541. He then observes that there are numerous rural churches dedicated in the years after 550. He attributes this pattern directly to the plague, suggesting that the rural church building is a sign of renewed prosperity and recovery from the epidemic. The rural churches may reflect the prosperity that seems to be typical of the southern Hawran and areas like the Balqa in Jordan in the late sixth and early seventh century.

Obviously, the evidence is patchy but we can suggest some tentative conclusions. The first is that the expansion of settlement that had characterized much of rural and urban Syria in the fifth and early sixth centuries came to an abrupt end after the middle of the sixth century. There is evidence that housing starts almost ceased, although renovations and additions to houses did continue in rural areas. Church building, however, continued up to and, in some areas like northern Jordan, beyond the Muslim Conquest. The archaeological evidence is entirely consistent with a pandemic that caused massive loss of life on repeated occasions. It does not prove positively that this was the case, but it does not provide any evidence against it. *Pace* Durliat, Brandes, and others, there is no real tension or contradiction between the archaeological and the written evidence. And, in view of the inarticulate nature of the archaeological record, we are probably right to privilege the written and look to it for guidance.

---

[22] Villeneuve, "L'économie rurale," 128–29.

III

THE BYZANTINE EMPIRE

5

Crime and Punishment

The Plague in the Byzantine Empire, 541–749

Dionysios Stathakopoulos

The inner structure of the plague's deadly itinerary still escapes us. We can reconstruct the dates of its appearance and disappearance, attempt to trace the mortality it caused, and, in a bold moment, even try to discern its effects on the stricken populations, but all in all, we still can produce only a fragmentary prose about its presence in the Late Antique Mediterranean.[1] Nevertheless, the only way to arrive at a full, all-encompassing picture of this complex phenomenon is to separate fact from interpretation and then assemble these facts to produce a balanced view of the plague, avoiding such extreme positions that either deny the pandemic any importance or make it responsible for every change that followed its course.

We have good reason (and the right)[2] to assume that bubonic plague was the disease that entered the realm of the Byzantine Empire in 541 (and, as such, was within the sphere of interest of Byzantine historians) at Pelusium, a small city on the extreme eastern branch of the Nile's mouth.[3] All of the plague's contemporary authors who produced a description of it, long enough to include a symptomatology, name its most characteristic traits: fever followed by buboes in the groin, axilla, or cervical region.[4]

---

[1] See the overview by Horden, "Mediterranean Plague."

[2] Contrary to a current medical revisionism, according to which it is safer and wiser to refrain from any attempt to identify past diseases (retrospective diagnosis) unless based on paleopathogical findings; cf. Leven, "Krankheiten."

[3] Procopius, *BP* 2.22.6, p. 250.

[4] To name but the most important ones: Procopius, *BP* 2.22.17, p. 252; Evagrius, *Ecclesiastical History* 4.29, p. 178, 22–24; Koder, "Ein inschriftlicher Beleg"; John of Ephesus in Pseudo-Dionysius of Tel-Mahrē, *Chronicle*, p. 87; Agathias, *Historiae* 5.10. 3, p. 176; Theophylactus Simocatta, *Historiae* 8.15.2, p. 271; *Megas Chronographos* 9, p. 42, 9–12.

Pelusium was merely a point of entrance for the disease. Its origin in
(Central) Africa is by now well argued for.[5] The same cannot be said for
the moment of the pandemic's outbreak. In 1857, V. Seibel collected a
large number of unusual natural phenomena that preceded and accompanied the Justinianic Plague and that, along with the disease, formed
"an overwhelming revolution."[6] He recorded earthquakes, comets, and
floods that were seemingly omnipresent throughout the first half of the
sixth century and cautiously connected these causally to the outbreak
of the plague. Purely deterministic and in his understanding of the disease hardly different from that of his Byzantine sources, Seibel's views
have not been seriously taken into account. However, in the past years
under the label of "evolved determinism," focus is once again set on such
unusual natural phenomena with the objective to help define why the
plague broke out when it did.[7] D. Keys ascribes this role to the dust-veil
event, an uncommon atmospheric phenomenon that occurred in 536.[8]
The sun dimmed for about one year to eighteen months. As to the causes
of the dust-veil event, there is still no consensus: while Keys argues for
a large-scale volcanic eruption in the southern hemisphere,[9] M. Bailey
favors a huge comet impact in the late 530s.[10] This dreadful portent
caused the destruction of crops throughout the Mediterranean and certainly encouraged the movement of nomadic peoples in search of food
and fodder for their animals beyond their usual radius[11] as well as similar
unusual migratory movements of rodents that could have indeed spread
the plague from a natural focus in East Africa to Byzantine emporia further north.[12]

We reach firmer ground again in dealing with the chronology of the
pandemic's waves. There were about eighteen plague waves in the roughly
two centuries of its presence in the Mediterranean. However, not all of
them are equally well attested or described with the same amount of
detail in the written sources. We have most data on the first and the last

---

[5] See the essay of Peter Sarris in this volume.

[6] Seibel, *Die große Pest*, 2.

[7] Keys, *Catastrophe*, vii.

[8] For an overview, see Stathakopoulos, *Famine and Pestilence*.

[9] Keys, *Catastrophe*, esp. 251–95.

[10] Baillie, *Exodus to Arthur*, esp. 65–88, 125–36, 153–61, 181–99, 205–18, 230–48.

[11] In 536, 15,000 Saracens crossed the border to Euphratensia because of an excessive
drought as recorded by Marcellinus Comes, *Chronicon*, 105; cf. Koder, "Climatic Change,"
275.

[12] This is, in short, Keys' quite plausible theory, *Catastrophe*, 15–23.

visitations of the disease, conforming to a macabre cycle. It is important to view these waves more closely before we can move on to discuss issues such as perception, response, and effects of the pandemic.[13]

After the plague broke out in Pelusium in mid-summer 541, it continued its course in two directions, to Egypt and the north African coast and to Palestine.[14] In the course of 541, it is attested in Gaza, the Negev, and Alexandria, and it reached Jerusalem and Zora in the Hauran shortly after.[15] Some Syrian cities were infected in the spring and summer of 542 along with Myra in Lycia, much at the same time as the pandemic reached Constantinople in mid-spring of the same year.[16] It was probably from Constantinople that the plague reached Sykeon in Galatia some time in the summer of 542.[17] Asia Minor was overrun by the infection as John of Ephesus informs us; he mentions Cilicia, Mysia, Iconium, Bithynia, Asia, Galatia, and Cappadocia.[18] In the fall of 542, the infection had reached the region of Media Atropatene and befallen the Persian army – even the Great King himself.[19] The next possible station of the pandemic is Sicily, where the testimony consists of one tombstone set up for three young boys, possibly siblings, who died in late December 542.[20] This is admittedly weak by itself, but the following, also non-literary data I supply, help to place it in an overall more plausible frame. A short while later,

---

[13] Nevertheless, I refer to these waves as briefly as possible. A detailed presentation of each wave can be found in my *Famine and Pestilence*.

[14] I have published a detailed chronology of the first wave in "Travelling with the Plague," 99–102 and also in Kislinger and Stathakopoulos, "Pest und Perserkriege bei Prokop," 76–98; therefore, I provide only the references to the sources at this point without elaborating on specific details.

[15] Gaza: Glucker, *City of Gaza*, 124–26; Negev: (Nessana) Kirk and Welles, "Inscriptions," 168, 179–81; (Rehovot) Tsafrir, "Greek Inscriptions," 161; (Eboda) Negev, *Greek Inscriptions from the Negev*, 30–31; Alexandria: John Malalas, *Chronographia*, 18.90, p. 407, *Chronique de Michel le Syrien*, 235ff; Jerusalem: Cyril of Scythopolis, "Vita of Cyriacus" in Schwartz, *Kyrillos von Skythopolis*, 10, p. 229; Zora: Koder, "Ein inschriftlicher Beleg."

[16] Antioch: van den Ven, *La vie ancienne de S. Syméon*, 59–60; Epiphaneia or Apameia: Evagrius, *Historia Ecclesiastica* 4.29, pp. 177–78; Emesa: "Leontios of Neapolis," Rydén, *Das Leben des heiligen Narren Symeon*, 151; Myra: *Hagios Nikolaos* 52, pp. 40–41; Constantinople: Procopius, *BP* 2.22.9; 2.23.1–2,18–19, pp. 251, 256, 259; John of Ephesus in Pseudo-Dionysios of Tel-Mahrē, *Chronicle*, 74–93; John Malalas, *Chronographia* 18.92, p. 407 Theophanes, *Chronographia* AM 6034, p. 222.

[17] *Vie de Théodore de Sykéon* 8, pp. 7–8.

[18] John of Ephesus, in Pseudo-Dionysios of Tel-Mahrē, *Chronicle*, 80.

[19] Procopius, *BP* 2.24.5–8, pp. 260–61.

[20] Manganaro, "Byzantina Siciliae," 133. I would like to thank Ewald Kislinger for drawing my attention to that inscription.

in late January–February 543, there are four funerary inscriptions from Sufetula (modern Sbeïtla in Tunisia) set up for young siblings who died one after the other and were buried in the same church.[21] Marcellinus Comes records the presence of the plague in Italy and the Illyricum throughout the year 543.[22] Finally, the vast epigraphic material from the city of Rome provides us with a plausible time frame for the plague's outbreak in the eternal city. There is a group of nine epitaphs for a period of four months, from early November 543 to late February 544, suggesting the disease's presence in the city.[23] No similar frequency could be found in the dated epitaphs of the sixth century in all ten volumes of the most complete repertory we have. On March 23, 544 the Emperor Justinian issued Novel 122 wherein he declared the plague's ravage as terminated.[24] This was the first and best-documented wave of the Justinianic Plague.

The second wave broke out in Constantinople from February to July 558.[25] It is probably connected to a visitation of the plague in Cilicia, Mesopotamia, and Syria in 560–561.[26] The third wave ravaged Italy and Gaul in 571[27] and is attested in Constantinople in 573–574.[28] The following manifestation of the plague occurred in 590–591: Rome was hit in the early months of 591,[29] following Ravenna, Grado, and Istria in 591–592,[30] and Antioch in 592.[31] The fifth wave of the pandemic broke out in Thessalonica in the summer of 597.[32] It was disseminated into Avar territory, which corresponds to modern European Turkey, by the spring of 598,[33]

---

[21] Duval, "Nouvelles recherches," 277–80.

[22] Marcellinus Comes, *Chronikon*, ad annum 543, p. 107.

[23] *Inscriptiones Christianae Urbis Romae*, the references are here given in chronological order by the volume and inscription number: 1.1452, 2.4287, 7.17624, 2.5088, 2.4289, 8.20839, 2.5087, 2.5087, 2.5087.

[24] *Novella* 122 in *CIC*, 3:592–93.

[25] Agathias, *Historiae* 5.10, pp. 175–76; John Malalas, *Chronographia* 18.120, p. 418; Theophanes, *Chronographia* AM 6050, p. 232.

[26] Theophanes, *Chronographia*, AM 6053, p. 235; *La vie ancienne de S. Syméon* 126–29, pp. 112–22; Conrad, "The Plague in Bilād al-Shām," 147–48.

[27] Marius of Avenches, *Chronica*, ad annum 571, p. 238.

[28] John of Biclaro, *Chronica*, ad annos 572–573, pp. 213–14; *Chronicon* ad annum 846, p. 174. Agapius, *Kitab*, 8, 437; *Chronique de Michel le Syrien*, 2.309–10.

[29] *Liber Pontificalis*, 309; Gregory of Tours, *Historia Francorum* 10.1, pp. 406–9; Gregory the Great, *Dialogues* 3.19, 2–3; 4.18, 2; 4.27, 6; 4.37, 7; 4.40, 3, vol. 2, pp. 346–48; vol. 3, pp. 72; 90; 128–30; 140; Paul the Deacon, *Historia Longobardorum* 3.23–24, pp. 104–5.

[30] Paul the Deacon, *Historia Longobardorum* 4.4, p. 117.

[31] Evagrius, *Ecclesiastical History* 4.29, p. 178, 11–16.

[32] Lemerle, *Les plus anciens recueils* 29–46, pp. 57–82.

[33] Theophylactus Simocatta, *Historiae* 7.15.2, p. 271.

then moved on to the Eastern Mediterranean, Syria, Constantinople, Bithynia, and Asia Minor in 599,[34] arriving in Northern Africa and Italy in the course of 599–600,[35] and finally infesting Ravenna and Verona in 600–601.[36] We have some vague information on another wave that hit Constantinople in the times of the Emperor Heraclius, dated to about 618–619,[37] whose presence is then recorded in Alexandria prior to its capture by the Persians in 619.[38]

After this visitation, we are left on the threshold of a period whose sources are characterized as "both limited in number and difficult to use."[39] There is an almost total absence of recorded plague epidemics within the realm of the Empire after 628, when the *Chronicon Paschale*, the last contemporary source, stops. On the contrary, the information flow on the plague from the newly established regions under Islamic rule is rich and derives not only from Arabic sources but also from Byzantine texts. If we were to recount only those visitations of the plague that have reportedly struck the Empire, then the result would be quite meager, and there would appear large chronological gaps between the outbreaks that cannot be accounted for. One might take as a working hypothesis that Constantinople would have been hit by each outbreak of the plague due to what Duncan-Jones has called 'the special vulnerability of the capital.'[40] An example from Tudor England can illustrate this trend; between 1480 and 1580 in a total of twelve epidemics, some major provincial towns were hit between two and eight times (with an average of five times), whereas only London was hit all twelve times.[41] Communication between the Islamic- and the Byzantine-controlled territories existed, both in the commercial and in the military areas.[42] Therefore we may expect that the outbreaks recorded in the Islamic regions will eventually have been disseminated at least in some areas of the Byzantine Empire and would

[34] Elias of Nisibis, *Opus Chronologicum*, ad annum 911, p. 60; Chronique de Michel le Syrien, 2.373–74, p. 171.

[35] Gregory the Great, *Register epistularum* 9.232, 10.20, 2: 814–15, 850–51.

[36] Paul the Deacon, *Historia Longodardorum* 4.14, p. 121.

[37] Nicephorus, *Breviarium* 8, 12, pp. 48, 54; George Monachos, *Chronicon*, p. 669; *Miracula Sancti Artemii* 34, p. 52.

[38] Leontios, *Vie de Jean de Chypre* 24, p. 375; Delehaye, "Une vie inédite de Saint Jean l'Aumonier" 37, p. 53.

[39] Haldon, *Byzantium in the Seventh Century*, xxi; for a survey of these sources see xxi–xxviii.

[40] Duncan-Jones, "Impact of the Antonine Plague," 135.

[41] Slack, *Impact of the Plague*, 61; cf. also the commentary of Biraben, "Rapport," 122.

[42] Lilie, *Die byzantinische Reaktion*; Walmsley, "Production, Exchange and Regional Trade," esp. 321.

have then reached the capital. The silence of the Byzantine sources may not be an insurmountable obstacle that would prevent us from making any hypothesis about this period; nevertheless it enforces a great amount of caution. We can hint at what possibly happened, but will have to refrain from attempting to present a chronologically secure reconstruction of the plague waves of the seventh and early eighth centuries.

Therefore, I restrict myself to providing only a short review of the seventh and later visitations:[43] [7] 626–628 (Palestine, Persia, and Northern China); [8] 639 (Syria, Iraq, and Palestine), [9] 669–673 (Iraq, Egypt, and Palestine), [10] 680 (Rome and Pavia)[44]; [11] 683–687 (Iraq, Egypt, and Syria); [12] 698–700 (Syria and Iraq) – this wave reached Constantinople by water and ravaged the city for four months in 698;[45] [13] 704–706 (Syria and Iraq); [14] 713–715 (Syria and Egypt) – here we also have a possible connection to a recorded outbreak in Crete during the pontificate of Andrew of Crete,[46] although this is both chronologically and historically doubtful; [15] 718–719 (Iraq and Syria); [16] 724–726 (Egypt, Syria, and Mesopotamia); [17] 732–735 (Syria, Egypt, Palestine, Iraq, and Asia Minor).

The plague had nevertheless a grand exit. The pandemic originated in the Islamic world, ravaging Egypt and Northern Africa in 743–744, moving on to Syria, Mesopotamia, and Iraq in the following year.[47] In 745–746, it broke out in Rome, Calabria, and Sicily and was transmitted through the movements of the Byzantine army in southern Greece and the islands of the Aegean.[48] In mid-spring 747, it reached Constantinople and raged in the city for almost a year.[49] Then, in 748–750 it seemed to return to the Orient – or perhaps it never ceased to be present there – and is recorded in Iraq, Syria, and Mesopotamia.[50] The outbreak that

---

[43] The best and most detailed survey is given by Conrad, "Plague in the Early Medieval Near East," 159–292.

[44] Paul the Deacon, *Historia Longobardorum* 6.5, p. 166. For the reference to Northern China, see Dols, "Plague in Early Islamic History," 376, n. 51.

[45] Theophanes, *Chronographia* AM 6190, p. 370; Nicephorus, *Breviarium* 41, p. 98.

[46] *Vita of Andrew of Crete* 9, pp. 177–78; cf. Detorakes, "Ανέκδοτον εγκώμιον εις Ανδρέαν Κρήτης," 93.

[47] Severus, *History of the Patriarchs* 18 in *PO* 5:97, 115; *CZ*, 168–74; *Chronique de Michel le Syrien*, 2:506, 508; *Chronicon ad annum 1234*, pp. 248–49; cf. Conrad, "Plague in the Early Medieval Near East," 294–99.

[48] Theophanes, *Chronographia* AM 6238, pp. 422–23; *Megas Chronographos* 17, p. 45; Letter of Pope Zacharias to St. Boniface, in *Regesta pontificum Romanorum*, 1:265.

[49] Theophanes, *Chronographia* AM 6238, pp. 422–23; *Megas Chronographos* 17, p. 45; Nicephorus, *Breviarium*, 67, pp. 138–40; idem, *Antirrhetikos*, in *PG* 100:496B–497A; Theodore Studites, *Laudatio Platonis*, in *PG* 99, 805B–D.

[50] *CZ*, 184–89; cf. Conrad, "Plague in the Early Medieval Near East," 301–6.

reportedly hit Naples around 767 is counted by some scholars as the last visitation of the disease, but there is reason to suppose that the recorded date may be erroneous.[51]

In a total of 210 years from 541 to 750, there were about eighteen outbreaks of the plague. This amounts to an average of one outbreak about every 11.6 years. This seems to apply to the first six plague waves for which we can compute the inter-epidemic intervals for Constantinople. These range approximately from eleven to seventeen years, with an average of 14.2 years, a fact corroborated by Evagrius, who records that the plague seemingly broke out during the first or the second year of the indiction cycle, indicating a periodicity of roughly fifteen years.[52] The situation appears to have changed during the seventh and eighth centuries, although the meager source material on which we have made our calculations demands particular caution. From the thirteenth to the eighteenth wave, Syria was reportedly hit on all six waves, with inter-epidemic periods ranging from five to nine years and an average of 6.6 years. Given the limitations of the material we may nevertheless assume that it projects an actual trend of "endemization" of the disease as manifested through these quite short inter-epidemic periods.[53]

Plague, as any disease, is both a biological as well as a social entity.[54] To have argued for its identification with the clinically established category of "modern plague" and to have secured the duration and approximate periodicity of its outbreaks covers, in part, only the biological-medical side of the disease. To address its social component, we need to examine such aspects as popular perception and response as well as the effects that the pandemic had. It is uncertain whether populations experienced the different waves of the pandemic as belonging to one and the same cycle – as we do today. The lack of a specific term both in Greek and Latin to denominate solely the plague was certainly not helpful in that respect.[55] Authors who experienced more than one visitation in their lifetime and wrote about them, however, suggest that the same disease returned at frequent intervals.[56]

---

[51] See the essay of Michael McCormick in this volume.

[52] Evagrius, *Historia Ecclesiastica* 4.29, pp. 177, 33–178,2.

[53] For the following section I am indebted to Prof. R. Stichel for a number of valuable suggestions.

[54] See the essay by Hays in this volume.

[55] Stathakopoulos, "Die Terminologie der Pest," 1–7; Bodson, "Le vocabulaire latin des maladies."

[56] Evagrius, *Historia Ecclesiastica* 4.29, pp. 178.11–16; Agathias, *Historiae* 5.10.1–3, pp. 175–76.

The plague, as all epidemic diseases, was perceived in both a metaphysical and a rational way. The metaphysical approach prevailed both in terms of its antiquity and the wide acceptance it enjoyed. According to this approach, plagues were an expression of divine retribution or punishment, the result of human transgression, either individual or collective. This was a notion central to both popular Greek and Jewish thought; as such, it spans the most influential texts of Byzantine culture, namely, Homer and the Old Testament.[57] Although in the New Testament, Christ does not present disease as a necessary result of sin, the Christian interpretation of disease established and stressed categorically exactly this relation.[58] In Byzantine texts dealing with the plague, this was the dominant opinion spanning time, space, and genres. To name but some characteristic examples, we encounter this notion both in secular historiography, chronography, jurisdiction, and hagiography.[59] Collective sin of the people brings about the just divine wrath in the form of the plague. In two polemical instances, this transgression is not presented as collective, but as individual. Justinian, termed "lord of demons" in Procopius' *Anecdota*, is made solely responsible for the plague, as is the iconoclastic Emperor Constantine V by iconophile authors.[60]

Contrary to this divine aetiology, a rational interpretation of disease had been first established by Hippocrates: "I do not believe that the 'Sacred Disease' is any more divine or sacred than any other disease, but on the contrary, has specific characteristics and a definite cause."[61] According to him, epidemic diseases were defined as follows: "When a large number of people all catch the same disease at the same time, the cause must be ascribed to something common to all and which they all

---

[57] Individual sin: Agamemnon in the Iliad (Rhapsody I), King David in the Old Testament (2 Sam 24.1–18); Collective sin: The Philistines (1 Sam 5–6); see von Siebenthal, *Krankheit als Folge*; Parker, *Miasma*, 235–56.

[58] In one instance Jesus even denies that an ailment may be a result of sin: John 9.1–3: "And as Jesus passed by, he saw a man which was blind from his birth. And his disciples asked him, saying, Master, who did sin, this man or his parents, that he was born blind? Jesus answered, Neither hath this man sinned, nor his parents: but that the works of God should be made manifest in him." Röhser, *Metaphorik und Personifikation*, 73–80; Sendrail, *Histoire culturelle de la maladie*, 167ff.

[59] Procopius, *BP* 2.22.1–3, p. 249; Malalas, *Chronographia* 18.92, p. 407; Agathias, *Historiae* 5.10.6, p. 176; Theophylactus, *Historiae* 7.15, p. 271; *CIC*, 3.592; *La vie ancienne de S. Syméon* 69, p. 59; *Hagios Nikolaos* 50–52, p. 40; Lemerle, *Les plus anciens recueils* 30, 41, pp. 76, 79–80.

[60] Procopius, *HA* 18.36ff, pp. 118ff; Theophanes, *Chronographia* AM 6238, p. 423; Nicephorus, *Breviarium* 67, p. 140.

[61] Hippocrates, *De morbo sacro* 1, p. 139.

use; in other words to what they all breathe."[62] This definition was later adopted by the other great medical personality of Antiquity, Galen,[63] and retained its authority throughout the Middle Ages.[64] The malignant air responsible for these outbreaks was called *miasma*.[65]

The picture, however, is more complicated than this obvious duality. Certain patristic authors acknowledged *miasmata* as the causes of epidemics.[66] As early as the fourth century, Basil of Caesarea admits that the air inhaled in unwholesome locations will bring about disease.[67] He does not, however, ascribe the original cause of diseases to natural phenomena; it is God that smites humans with disease, droughts, or dearth to cure sins and evil, as such trials are meant to avert the survivors from the sufferings of eternal damnation.[68] Even more remarkable in this respect is Anastasius of Sinai's *Questions and Answers*, a work written at the very end of the seventh century and, as such, one whose author must have experienced numerous visitations of the plague.[69] Question 114 addresses the topic whether it is possible to escape the plague by fleeing to another location.[70] Anastasius answers with a piece on the origin of plagues. They either break out as a result of divine chastisement or because of corrupt air, vapors, pollution, and stench; in the first case, they cannot be escaped, but in the second, with God's will, flight to a location with healthier air will often help avoid death. This is Anastasius' effort to offer a compromise between "Hellenistic rationalism... and Christian views on direct divine intervention," between a "pre-Christian medical and physiological tradition" and the Judeo-Christian model of disease as "chastisement from

[62] Hippocrates, *De natura hominis* 9.3, p. 188 and *Hippocratic Writings*, p. 266.
[63] Galen, *Definitiones medicae* 153 in *Claudii Galeni opera omnia*, 19:391.
[64] We encounter a practically identical definition of epidemics (*loimoi*) in Hesychius Alexandrinus (5th–6th c.), *Lexicon* 2:992; the *Suidae Lexicon* (10th c.) 3:290; or Gennadios Scholarios (15th c.), *De divina providentia* 4.14 in *Oeuvres complètes*, 4:451.
[65] Hippocrates, *De flatibus* 6.98, vol. 1, p. 109.
[66] This is also implied in the *Suidae Lexicon* 2:270, in which an entry on the lighting of fires (*enauein*) informs us that people used to light fires and kindle pyres in the cities to drive out the corrupting disease of the air. While such an instance is not recorded in any Byzantine historical work, we may assume that the use of fire against *miasmata* may not have been included in the *Suda* for mere encyclopaedic reasons.
[67] Basil of Caesaria, *Quod Deus non est auctor malorum* 9 in *PG* 21:349C.
[68] Ibid., 5 (337Cff).
[69] On this work see Beck, *Kirche und theologische Literatur*, 442–45; Dagron, "Le saint, le savant," 143–55; and especially Haldon, "Works of Anastasius of Sinai," 107–48, with complete references.
[70] *Quaestio CXIV, PG* 89:765C–767B.

heaven ... designed to drive out the evils afflicting the body politic."[71] It would be needless to point out which of these two sides prevailed.

Summing up, we must notice that although the physiological–rational definition of epidemics was current in the Byzantine period, no source referring to the plague names it as the infection's cause. It is only indirectly that we can find traces of it, albeit merely to demonstrate that it was not the correct perception of the disease. The author of the seventh-century *Miracula Sancti Demetrii* describes the outbreak of the plague in Thessalonica in 597 as follows: "Neither babies, nor women, nor the flower of youth, nor men of arm-bearing and city-service age were spared from the disease: only the elderly escaped. God had desired thus so that no one would be able to claim that the epidemic had been a natural phenomenon caused by the corruption of the air, and not a divine punishment."[72]

Alternative theories about the cause of epidemics occupy a marginal position in the source material on the plague. Agathias is the only author to offer such alternative perspectives openly, adopting at the same time an agnostic stance:

According to the ancient oracles of the Egyptians and to the leading astrologers of present-day Persia there occurs in the course of endless time a succession of lucky and unlucky cycles. These luminaries would have us believe that we are at present passing through one of the most disastrous and inauspicious of such cycles: hence the prevalence of war and internal dissension and of frequent and persistent epidemics of plague. Others hold the view that divine anger is responsible for the destruction, exacting just retribution from mankind for its sins and decimating whole populations. It is not for me to set myself up as a judge in these matters or to undertake to demonstrate the truth of one theory rather than the other.[73]

Further testimony for the astrological interpretation of epidemics is given in the life of Symeon the younger Stylite, where a group of pagan astrologers in Antioch claimed that the movement of the stars was responsible for, among other catastrophes, pestilential diseases.[74] This was a common trait of the astrological-prognostic literature in which specific planets and constellations were deemed responsible for the outbreak of

---

[71] Haldon, "Works of Anastasius of Sinai," 129ff., esp. 143–45.

[72] Lemerle, *Les plus anciens recueils* 33, p. 77.

[73] Agathias, *Historiae* 5.10.5–6, pp (176), 145.

[74] *La vie ancienne de S. Syméon* 157, pp. 138–39. On the church's polemic against astrology see Riedinger, *Die Heilige Schrift im Kampf.*

epidemics.[75] Procopius also acknowledges this option without giving it too much credit.[76] However, judging from the vast amount of astrological texts that enjoyed wide circulation in Late Antiquity, we are inclined to believe that this view was much more popular than the above testimonies would have us believe.[77]

There is yet another, even more general level in which epidemics were perceived in the early sixth century. Consistent with the three prevailing world eras the completion of the year 6000 from the creation of the world fell between 492 and 508.[78] This was the year that Christians held as the advent of Judgment Day.[79] According to the synoptical Apocalypse (Matt 24, Luke 21, and Mark 13), the end of days would be preceded by wars, famines, pestilences, and earthquakes; these would be the *signs* of Jesus' coming. There is now consensus among scholars that this eschatological anticipation was the reason for the unusually large number of meticulously recorded catastrophes in late-fifth- and sixth-century sources, the plague certainly playing a prominent part among them.[80] As the plague was ravaging Egypt and Alexandria in September 541, crowds in Constantinople gathered round a woman who had gone into ecstasy and was claiming that in three days time the sea would rise and swallow everything.[81] This is one of the few testimonies that bear witness to the eschatological climate that must have been dominant at the time.

The perception of a phenomenon dictates the popular response to it. As the metaphysical-eschatological approach was prevalent, reactions to the plague were predictably situated mostly at that level. At first, people tried to dispel the demonic visions that seemed to be infecting them with the disease by uttering holy names and seeking sanctuary in churches.[82] As the plague's mortality rose more people turned to various saints and

[75] Boll et al., *Sternglaube und Sterndeutung,* esp. 86, 134.

[76] Procopius, *BP* 2.22.5, p. 250.

[77] Material collected in Cumont et al., eds., *Catalogus Codicum Astrolorum Graecorum.* A quick search in this series and in the relevant works in the *Thesaurus Linguae Graecae* online database yielded more than 100 instances of untoward constellations that caused disease and epidemics.

[78] See the discussion with all past references in Brandes, "Anastasios ho dikoros": 24–63, esp. 53ff.

[79] Vasiliev, "Medieval Ideas of the End"; Kötting, "Endzeitprognosen zwischen Lactantius und Augustinus"; Alexander, *Oracle of Baalbek*; Daley, *Hope of the Early Church.*

[80] Brandes, "Anastasios ho dikoros," 44–46 and the excellent survey by Magdalino, "History of the Future."

[81] Malalas, *Chronographia* 18.90, pp. 406–7.

[82] Procopius, *BP* 2.22.10–12, pp. 454–57; similar in Lemerle, *Les plus anciens recueils* 37, p. 78. For the church as sanctuary and healing place, *Vie de Théodore de Sykéon* 8, pp. 7–8.

holy men asking them to intercede with God for the cessation of the scourge and cure them of it. This was a matter of the local cult of holy men; not one particular saint was invested with the power to stop plague throughout the Eastern Empire, as it happened with Sebastian and Roch in the (late) medieval West.[83] In Antioch, people turned to Symeon the younger Stylite for help, in Thessalonica, to St. Demetrius, in Sykeon, young Theodore was brought to the church of St. John the Baptist where he was cured by dew drops that fell from an icon of Christ, while a young girl in Constantinople was saved by St. Artemius, who appeared in her sleep.[84] The role of church dignitaries in this respect as documented in the sources is marginal: St. John the Almsgiver, archbishop of Alexandria in the early seventh century, visited the sick and cared for the burial of the deceased, while Andrew of Crete offered fervent prayers to God to terminate an epidemic of plague in the early eighth century.[85] There is no record of organized processions aiming to illustrate public penance and inspire divine mercy, as in the West,[86] nor any liturgical writings reflecting a response or reaction to the plague.[87]

On the personal level, people obviously resorted to medicine and doctors when faced by the disease. Reference to this is minor and as a rule intended to illustrate the inability of medical science to cure the infection or at least comfort its symptoms.[88] In the medical literature of the period, there is no trace of a reflection on the epidemic. Although authors such as Aetios of Amida (sixth century) and Paul of Aigina (seventh century)

---

[83] Sigerist, "Sebastian – Apollo"; Pesci, "Il culto di San Sebastiano a Roma"; Zeller, *Rochus: Die Pest und ihr Patron*; Köhler, "Pest, Pestheilige, Blutwunder und andere Begebenheiten." The role of helper against the plague was assigned to S. Charalampus, but no written or pictorial evidence for this survives from before the seventeenth century; cf. Papastratos, Χάρτινες Εικόες.

[84] *La vie ancienne de S. Syméon* 69, 127, pp. 59–60, pp. 113ff.; Lemerle, *Les plus anciens recueils* 39–45, pp. 79–82; *Vie de Théodore de Sykéon* 8, pp. 7–8; *Miracula Sancti Artemii* 34, pp. 51–55.

[85] Leontios, *Vie de Jean de Chypre* 24, p. 375; Delehaye, "Une vie inédite de Saint Jean l'Aumonier" 37, p. 53; *Vita of Andrew of Crete* 9, pp. 177–78.

[86] For the seven-fold litany organized by Pope Gregory the Great in 590 see the essay in this book by Alain Stoclet.

[87] The only possible hint can be found in a text replete with eschatological fervor, namely, Romanos the Melodist's hymn *On the Ten Virgins*, written around 550, in Romanos, *Hymnes*, 272–327, esp. strophe 4: "Nothing is missing of what Christ has told, and as he has foretold, so shall it be. Famines and pestilences and constant earthquakes, and nation rising against nation." See Magdalino, "History of the Future," 5–6. On the contrary there is ample material from the late Byzantine period; cf. Goar, *Euchologion*, 627–36; and prayers or homilies for the deliverance from the plague by Gregory Palamas, Kallistos I, Philotheos Kokkinos, and Theophanes of Nicaea.

[88] Procopius, *BP* 2.22. 29–35, pp. 254–55; Lemerle, *Les plus anciens recueils* 38, p. 78.

certainly experienced at least one outbreak of the plague, when dealing with that disease (or at least what they term *loimos*), their approach is
encyclopaedic and not based on observation. Both of them merely repeat
verbatim a section on this disease by Rufus of Ephesus (late first century),
as Oribasius (fourth century) had done in his turn.[89]

Because of the massive mortality it caused, the plague created also a
number of practical problems that had to be dealt with ad hoc. This is
the official level of reaction to the disease. Procopius informs us about
the measures taken by Justinian to make sure that the numerous bodies
of the plague-stricken were swiftly and (more or less) properly buried.
He appointed the *referendarius* Theodorus as responsible for this task and
provided him with money and personnel from the palace guard to this
effect.[90] Similar measures were also taken in later visitations of the plague,
although the sources do not state this expressly, probably because of their
opposition to the iconoclastic emperor who took them.[91]

In addition to the above, there were other ways of reacting to this
large-scale crisis. J.-N. Biraben writes of three fundamental psychological
reactions of society facing a major danger: flight, aggression, and projection.[92] Did the early Byzantine society correspond to this scheme? The
answer for the last of these, projection, that is, the production of literary
or artistic works devoted to the plague, can be stated plainly: There is no
trace of the disease and its impact in any Byzantine work of art.

Flight to or from a locality in times of crisis was one of the most common
and immediate reactions of pre-modern societies. While people fled to
the urban centers when faced with subsistence crises, it was the other
way round when epidemics broke out in those urban centers; those who
could afford it fled the cities en masse. The aphorism attributed to Galen
dictated the course of action: "I urge you to go far away and don't come
back soon (*Cito, longe fugas et tarde redeas*)."[93] As we have already seen,
Anastasius of Sinai deemed flight from an infested locality as compatible
with divine will and, as such, a fitting Christian reaction to epidemics.
Contrary to Procopius' testimony that the inhabitants of Constantinople

---

[89] Aetius of Amida, *Libri Medicinales V–VIII* 5.96, pp. 82–83; Paul of Aigina, *Epitomae medicae*
2.35, pp. 108–9; Orebasius, *Synopsis ad Eustathium* 6.25 in *Oribasii Collectionum*, 3:199–200.

[90] Procopius, *BP* 2.23. 5–9, pp. 256–57.

[91] Theophanes, *Chronographia* AM 6238, pp. 423–24; Nicephorus, *Breviarium* 67, pp. 138–
40.

[92] Biraben, "Essai sur les réactions des sociétés éprouvées," 372.

[93] Unfortunately I have not been able to identify this passage in Galen's works. The quotation is taken from: Zimmermann, "Krankheit und Gesellschaft," 9. In later plague
epidemics, the collective wisdom advised: *cede mox* (flee immediately), *recede longe* (stay
far away), and *redi tarde* (be late in returning); see Bailey et al., *Hope and Healing*, p. 16.

remained in the capital to tend for the sick and the dead, there is ample evidence to suggest the opposite.[94] Evagrius records flight from afflicted cities, and the Patriarch Nicephorus mentions that not only common people had fled Constantinople during the last wave of the Justinianic Plague in 747–748, but that the Emperor Constantine V himself had moved to Nicomedeia and was being informed of the grave situation in the city through official dispatches.[95] There is even one instance where the mechanism was somewhat reversed. When the plague broke out in Myra, the farmers of its hinterland refused to enter the city to bring foodstuffs and other products to its market fearing that they might be infected with the disease.[96]

As Biraben suggests, flight need not be merely spatial; it can be expressed as inner mechanism, as escapism towards charlatans, talismans, wonder-working saints, and their relics. We have already discussed popular resort to astrology or their search for solace from the plague at the hands of holy men. Apart from the group of astrologers in plague-stricken Antioch (mentioned earlier), there is no record of people trying to take advantage of the public fear in cities ravaged by the disease. Agathias, however, allows us an insight into an analogous case that occurred in Constantinople in 557 as the city had been visited by a devastating earthquake. Certain individuals claiming to be prophets or possessed by demons began announcing even worse catastrophes that were to come, aggravating the already tense situation in the city; "It is usual for men of this sort to swarm in times of trouble."[97]

The same applies to the use of talismans against the plague. While there is no written testimony to corroborate this fact, the great popularity of apotropaic talismans against disease and the large number of archaeological findings of such objects from this period suggest that they would have been in use to protect people from the plague, as they had been used against all other diseases throughout Antiquity and the Middle Ages.[98]

---

[94] Procopius, *BP* 2.23.17, p. 259.

[95] Evagrius, *Historia Ecclesiastica* 4.29, p. 179; Nicephorus, *Breviarium* 67, p. 138; idem, *Antirrheticus, PG* 100:496B.

[96] *Hagios Nikolaos* 52, pp. 40–41.

[97] Agathias, *Historiae* 5.5, pp. 169–70; Magdalino, "History of the Future," 6.

[98] On talismans in general see Bonner, *Magical Amulets*; Eckstein and Waszink, "Amulett"; Engemann, "Zur Verbreitung magischer Übelabwehr"; on the objects themselves see Russel, "Archaeological Context of Magic"; cf. also the essay by Alain Stoclet in this volume.

As far as aggression during the disease's visitations in Byzantium is concerned, the evidence we have at our disposal does not seem to conform to Biraben's thesis. There is no mention of the persecution of individuals or groups on account of either social, ethnic, or religious reasons connected causally to an outbreak of plague.[99] It may be argued that some of Justinian's measures against groups considered as heterodox (Jews, Samaritans, pagans, and heretics) and /or homosexuals may be chronologically connected to the presence of the infection. In 545/46, John of Ephesus conducted a witch-hunt of pagans as a result of which many prominent believers of the Old Way were seized, imprisoned, and tortured.[100] Justinian, however, had taken similar actions in 529, long before the plague.[101] The same can be said of a legal text issued in March 545 that included particularly severe restrictions prohibiting the sale or lease of land belonging to the church to any heretics (Jews, Samaritans, pagans, Montanists, and Arians).[102] Justinian legislated repeatedly against such dissident groups throughout his reign; the plague may have, if at all, merely provoked yet another imperial measure, nothing more, nothing less.[103]

The picture is somewhat different regarding a decree that Justinian issued in 559 against homosexuals.[104] In this text, addressed to the inhabitants of Constantinople, the emperor wrote, "We are all praying for the Lord's philanthropy and clemency, above all now that we have enraged him in many ways because of the multitude of our sins; he has threatened us and has shown what we are worth because of our sins, but has had mercy upon us and postponed his anger waiting for our repentance, since he does not desire the death of us, the sinners, but correction and life." The allusion to the divine anger, which had been expressed recently, must refer to a scourge felt in the capital. Indeed, the plague of February–July 558 was a recent enough catastrophe that had definitely visited the city, so an allusion to this is quite possible. Other possible phenomena that could have been meant include the earthquake of December 557,[105] the

99 As for example the persecution of the Jews during the Black Death, cf. Ziegler, *Black Death*, 85–111.
100 John of Ephesus in Pseudo-Dionysius of Tel-Mahrē, *Chronicle*, 71; see Whitby, "John of Ephesus and the Pagans."
101 Malalas, *Chronographia* 18.42, p. 180; Theophanes, *Chronographia* AM 6022, p. 180.
102 *CIC*, 3:654–64.
103 Evans, *Age of Justinian*, 240–52; Noethlichs, "Heidenverfolgung," 1169–71; Seyberlich, "Die Judenpolitik Kaiser Justinians I," 73–80.
104 *CIC*, 3:703–4; cf. Pitsakes, "Η θέση των ομοφυλοφίλων στη βυζαντινή κοινωνία," 207–18.
105 Guidoboni et al., *Catalogue of Ancient Earthquakes*, no. 225.

attack of the Cotrigurs against Constantinople and their raids in Thrace
and continental Greece,[106] or even a combination of the above. In any
case, this *novella* shows a causal connection between divine chastisement
and the emperor's actions that would assure that the cause of the former
be eradicated.

All this has been, in a way, an abstract way of dealing with the pandemic.
As historians of the period, we are asked to quantify the impact of the
infection by discussing its results. Now, the plague is quite a rewarding
and convenient projection-surface for speculation. It is securely dated,
long lasting, well documented – at least partly so – and yet vague enough
for various theories to be connected with its course. The most important
feature of the infection, the one that is most inherently responsible for
its immediate, short-term effects is the mortality it caused. In a rather
absolute way, I would like to stress the fact that in no visitation of the
pandemic can this be computed. The number of victims recorded by
various sources is to be viewed with extreme caution. We are inclined
to be skeptical about such figures, and our disbelief rises with the rising
number of victims. It is highly unlikely that contemporary societies had
the means to count the dead amidst such widespread crises. Furthermore,
as any trustworthy information on the population levels of these cities
at any period within our chronological frame is lacking, we are unable
to draw any reliable conclusions. In spite of the exaggerated rhetoric
applied by our sources, the clear context they convey is that of a sharp
demographic decline brought about by these outbreaks.[107] Their resort
to exaggeration may also be perceived as an attempt to describe what in
their eyes must have seemed as beyond definition or description.

How can we estimate the loss of life caused by the plague without
knowing the volume of the affected population or the approximate mortality and morbidity rates of the infection in that period? Some scholars
attempt to overcome this obstacle by computing the plague-induced mortality on account of modern epidemiological models. This is, to say the
least, a risky enterprise, as it is based on the assumption that the infection has not changed since the sixth century. To name just one example,
Hollingsworth used mathematical models to do so and arrived at the
precise number of 244,000 victims of the disease in Constantinople during the first wave,[108] a dubiously accurate figure considering that the

---

[106] Kislinger, "Ein Angriff zu viel."
[107] For an overview, see the essay by Peter Sarris in this volume.
[108] Hollingsworth, *Historical Demography*, 365–67.

magnitude of the city's population could have been well under the 508,000 estimated by that author. The recent publication of the genome sequence of its causative agent has shown, however, that *Yersinia pestis* "has undergone large-scale genetic flux" and "shows that chromosomal rearrangements are common in vivo."[109] By that, I certainly do not want to be "revisionistic" by implying either that the sixth-to-eighth-century plague did not have catastrophic results or that we should not use modern epidemiology to shed light on its impact, only that we should be cautious in not accepting percentages and numbers a priori only because they would make our work easier by complying to either modern epidemiological data or the rhetorical zeal of our sources. It seems safe to suggest that loss of life because of the plague was considerable, both in the urban centers and in the countryside.

Massive mortality equates a shortage of manpower, expected to be evident in agriculture, the military, and state finances, as a result of limited production and tax revenues. As P. Sarris has offered a masterful and innovative look at the possible effects of the plague in state finances, I limit myself to discussing them regarding agricultural production and the military.

After the first outbreak of the infection both rural and urban production broke down. In a society whose economic existence depended on agriculture and whose agricultural regime, furthermore, was defined by a command on natural resources in width and not in depth,[110] massive mortality signified foremost a lack of manpower for these activities.[111] John of Ephesus describes in haunting images the deserted and desolate countryside, while Procopius does the same for Constantinople.[112] At the same time, this breakdown brought about inflation as a result of the lack of manpower for certain services.[113] The result was in many cases a vicious circle in which one crisis provoked the next: plague caused mortality, the ensuing manpower shortage brought about the breakdown of production provoking in its turn another crisis.[114] A few examples illustrate this.

---

[109] Parkhill, et al., "Genome Sequence of *Yersinia Pestis*," 523; see the essay by Robert Sallares in this volume.

[110] Lounghis, Επισκόπιση βυζαντινής ιστορίας, 37.

[111] See Bryer, "Means of Agricultural Production".

[112] John of Ephesus in Pseudo-Dionysius of Tel-Mahrē, *Chronicle*, 80–81, 88; Procopius, *BP* 2.23.17–21, pp. 258–59.

[113] John of Ephesus in Pseudo-Dionysius of Tel-Mahrē, *Chronicle*, 88; *CIC*, 3:592–93.

[114] See the essential work by Carpentier, "Autour de la peste noire," 1078 ff; and for the period of the Justinianic Plague, cf. Patlagean, *Pauvreté économique et pauvreté*, 77–92.

In 542, as the plague raged in Constantinople, a famine occurred as a result; yet another subsistence crisis followed in 545–546.[115] Again in the autumn of 597 a severe shortage took hold of Thessalonica barely after the city had experienced an outbreak of plague and an Avaroslavic siege.[116] Finally in 618–619, a famine ravaged Constantinople followed immediately by the plague,[117] while the same succession of phenomena took place in the same year in Alexandria.[118]

In the military, the shortage of manpower was also evident. During the first wave of the pandemic, in 542–543, military campaigns were remarkably low-key.[119] In post-plague years, the Byzantine army faced recruitment shortages culminating in 558, because in the course of the second plague wave only a very small force was put together to defend Constantinople by the aging Belisarius against the assault of the Cotrigurs.[120] Notwithstanding these shortages, we must stress that after the mid-540s the Byzantine Empire fought successfully on different frontiers: in Lazica (549–557), defeating the Moors in Africa (546–548), and wiping out the Ostrogoths in Italy (550–561).[121]

As far as the short-term effects are concerned, the picture seems clear. It is when scholars turn to the alleged long-term effects of the pandemic that we experience the placement of the Justinianic Plague in extreme contexts. It is either made responsible for every negative aspect of the late- and post-Justinianic period or classified as harmless and relatively unimportant. We can look briefly into the works of two authors who serve as examples of such extremes positions: J. C. Russell and M. Whittow.[122]

Russell's views on the plague represent an overly simplistic view of history and historical change, ascribing to the disease the most important and formative role in the transition from the late antique Roman Empire to the Byzantine state of the seventh century onward. He argued that the demographic and economic situation of the Empire before the plague had been thriving, as most regions and important cities prospered and

---

[115] Procopius, *BP* 2.23.18–19, pp. 545–46: Malalas, *Chronographia* 18.95, p. 408; Theophanes, *Chronographia* AM 6038, p. 225.

[116] Lemerle, *Les plus anciens recueils* 68–72, pp. 101–3.

[117] Nicephorus, *Breviarium* 8, 12, pp. 48, 54.

[118] Leontios, *Vie de Jean de Chypre* 11, 24, pp. 357–59, 375; Delehaye, "Une vie inédite de Saint Jean l'Aumonier" 7, 26, 37, pp. 22, 36–38, 53.

[119] Teall, "Barbarians in Justinian's Armies," 315–19.

[120] Agathias, *Historiae* 5.15–19, pp. 183–90; cf. Kislinger, "Ein Angriff zu viel," 50–51; cf. also Fotiou, "Recruitment Shortages."

[121] Rubin, *Das Zeitalter Justinians*, 1:345–73 [Lazica]; 2:44–58 [Africa], 181–200 [Italy].

[122] Russell, "That Earlier Plague" and Whittow, *Making of Orthodox Byzantium*, 66–68.

enjoyed a period of population growth, concluding that Justinian's *Reconquista* would have been an easy task were it not for the plague, as "morale was excellent, money was abundant, and manpower was sufficient."[123] All this was destroyed by the plague. What Russell is actually doing is using only partial evidence that supports this picture of dramatic decline, while leaving out any elements that might point in the opposite direction. It is contradictory to assume that a population loss of the magnitude of 20%–25% took place as a result of the first outbreak and, at the same time, ascribe the military accomplishments of the late 540s and 550s to a "short economic revival" between the first two waves of the plague or merely a "momentum" as he does.[124] The monocausal attribution of the failure of the Reconquista to the plague is equally questionable, as it does not take into consideration such factors as the exhaustion of resources due to long-lasting warfare and the extraordinary building activity practised under that emperor.

Russell's grim picture of the plague as a destroyer of the late Roman order needs to be reconsidered, but hardly so by resorting to the diametrically extreme position held by Whittow, who claims that "the economy of the Roman Near East in the years after the plague seems to indicate business as usual."[125] The author, influenced perhaps by J. Durliat's work,[126] dismisses information on the plague in literary sources as rhetorical and exaggerated, while noting that archaeological and papyrological data "provide no indication either of an economic crisis or even of population decline." P. Sarris has discussed such views and has clearly demonstrated numerous weak points in their argumentation.

One final question that must be discussed in this context concerns the fate of cities and whether their decline was favored or not by the plague's repeated outbreaks. Contrary to Russell's view, urban prosperity and decline coexisted in the fifth-to-seventh centuries, albeit in different regions and at different periods. While some cities seem not to have survived past the mid-540s, numerous others did so until the Arab conquests one century later, although perhaps past their peak of prosperity.[127] The plague was certainly *one* of the factors that lead to urban

---

[123] Russell, "That Earlier Plague," 178.
[124] Ibid., 180–82.
[125] Whittow, *Making of Orthodox Byzantium*, 66.
[126] Durliat, "La peste du VIe siècle."
[127] See the excellent survey by Liebeschuetz, *Decline and Fall of the Roman City*, esp. 53–75, 390–410

decline, but not necessarily the gravest one. Warfare and enemy incursions (Persians, Avars, Slavs, and Arabs) often accompanied by massive deportations, other natural catastrophes such as earthquakes and floods, the gradual strangling grip of the centralist Constantinopolitan power centers over city finances, the lack of interest by the Church to prolong and promote the pagan-oriented city-culture – all these are important factors that need to be taken equally into consideration.[128] The plague should not be viewed as the primary cause of historical change, but rather as a catalyst for changes that had, in part, already begun to manifest themselves.

The first half of the eighth century marked the beginning of a period of imperial strength, both ideologically and militarily, and of a move toward economic prosperity.[129] Whatever our overall view of the Justinianic Plague and its effects, the survivors ultimately mastered the situation.

---

[128] Cf. Brandes, "Die Entwicklung des byzantinischen Städtewesens," 21ff and Liebeschuetz, *op. cit.*

[129] Haldon, *Byzantium in the Seventh Century*, 31; idem, "Production, Distribution and Demand"; Rochow, *Kaiser Konstantin V*, 35–42.

6

Bubonic Plague in Byzantium

The Evidence of Non-Literary Sources

Peter Sarris

In the year 540, or shortly thereafter, as part of an on-going campaign to eradicate from the Byzantine Empire the final remnants of classical paganism, the Emperor Justinian ordered that the temple to Isis, at Philae in southern Egypt, be destroyed.[1] According to Plutarch, among the many civilizing skills that mankind had been taught by Isis was that of how to cure disease.[2] That the following year Egypt should have fallen victim to an outbreak of bubonic plague may have struck many adherents of the old gods as a sure sign of the folly of imperial policy. According to the contemporary historian Procopius, the plague first manifested itself at the *entrepôt* of Pelusium, before spreading to Alexandria, the rest of Egypt, and to Palestine.[3] A harrowing account of the ravages of the plague within Egypt is preserved for us in the writings of John of Ephesus, who witnessed the effects of the disease while traveling to Constantinople via Palestine and Syria in the early 540s.[4] John reports that "it was told about one city on the Egyptian border [that] it perished totally and completely with [only] seven men and one little boy ten years old remaining in it."[5]

---

[1] Procopius, *BP* 1.19.35, p. 106 and *PW* 188–89. This article is based on a paper first delivered to the Oxford University Byzantine Studies Seminar in 1994 and subsequently to the Ancient History and Mediterranean Archaeology Seminar at U.C. Berkeley (1998) and the Pre-Industrial Seminar, University of Durham (1999). I would like to express my thanks to those who attended these seminars for their comments and suggestions. It was first published as "The Justinianic Plague: Origins and Effects" in *Continuity and Change* 17.2 (2002): 169–83.

[2] Guirand, *New Larousse Encyclopedia of Mythology*, 18.

[3] Procopius, *PW* 2.22.6, pp. 452–54.

[4] Conrad, "Plague in Bilad al-Sham."

[5] Preserved in Pseudo-Dionysius of Tel Mahrē, *Chronicle*, 77.

By the spring of 542, the disease had reached the imperial capital of Constantinople, where it was believed to have laid low the emperor himself.[6] That same year the plague reached Antioch, Illyricum, Africa, and Spain. By 543, the pestilence had further extended its reach to embrace Atropatene, Italy, and Gaul, before also eventually arriving in the British Isles.[7]

The subject of this so-called "Justinianic" Plague of Late Antiquity, which was to recur until the mid-eighth century, has been hotly and, at times, fiercely contested in recent years.[8] Debate has focused on two questions: the origin of the plague on the one hand, and, on the other, its effects on the Mediterranean world in general, and the Byzantine Empire, in particular. That the plague as it afflicted the sixth-century Mediterranean was bubonic in character has not been strongly contested. The description of buboes in our narrative sources, and the close similarity between accounts of the Justinianic Plague and those of later bubonic outbreaks, render this identification as close to certain as is possible on the basis of written sources, although bubonic plague would not appear to have been the sole component of the pandemic.[9] This similarity between the Justinianic Plague and later recorded outbreaks is particularly significant given the great antigenic stability that would appear to characterize *Yersinia pestis*, the *bacillus* regarded as the causative agent of bubonic plague.[10] Moreover, both in terms of climate and the character of the native rodent population, the late antique Mediterranean would have served as a highly suitable *locus* for the disease.[11]

The question of the origin of the plague will never be settled with any certainty on the basis of the historical evidence alone, but some hypotheses are more convincing than others. Today, there exist a number of plague "basins" where the disease is endemic to the rodent population. Most of these *foci* of plague activity are of rather recent origin. Some, however, are of more ancient pedigree, with those in the foothills of the Himalayas, in the vicinity of the Great Lakes in Central Africa, and lastly, that scattered across the Eurasian Steppe from Manchuria to the Ukraine

---

[6] Procopius, *PW* 2.22.9–23.21, pp. 454–73; *SH* 4.1, p. 42.

[7] See the chronology in Biraben, *Les hommes et la peste*, 1:27–32. For the plague in Britain, see the chapter by John Maddicott in this volume.

[8] See the excellent bibliographical survey by Stathokopoulos, "Justinianic Plague Revisited."

[9] Allen, "'Justinianic' Plague," 7–10.

[10] Scott and Duncan, *Biology of Plagues*, 51–53.

[11] Ibid., 53–60.

being commonly accepted as the most ancient.[12] In terms of epidemiology, the Justinianic Plague must have come to the Mediterranean from one of these three *foci.*

The Steppe Basin, favored by Russell as the origin of the Justinianic Plague, can be excluded from the equation on chronological grounds.[13] There exists no evidence for bubonic plague on the Eurasian Steppe prior to the late-sixth century at the very earliest or, arguably, until the Black Death.[14] One is thus obliged to choose between India and Africa. In the case of India, the origin favored by Allen, there would appear to be no record in the extant Sanskrit sources for any great demographic cataclysm in the sixth century, but then given the scarcity of Sanskrit historiography for the period, this argument ought not to be pushed too far.[15]

An Indian origin to the Justinianic Plague is plausible, especially given the fact that Byzantine trading relations with the Indian subcontinent are well attested for the early sixth century. The mid-sixth century *Christian Topography* of the (apparently Nestorian) author later known as Cosmas Indicopleustes describes trade between the Byzantine world and the east via Taprobane (Sri Lanka). The author of the *Topography* would not himself appear to have traveled beyond the Red Sea, but claimed to have known a fellow-merchant of Alexandria, by the name of Sopatros, who had visited the island some thirty-five years earlier.[16] Likewise, the Red Sea Port of Clysma (Arsinoë), situated near the emperor Trajan's Nile–Red Sea Canal, is described in the sixth-century *Itinerarium Antonini Placentini* as "*civitas modica... ubi etiam de India naves veniunt.*"[17] Crone has argued correctly that our sixth-century Byzantine sources often confuse India for Ethiopia.[18] The term "India" would appear to have been used with something of the looseness of "America" in Modern English, signifying any area bordering onto the Indian Ocean or its appendage, the Red

---

[12] McNeill, *Plagues and People,* 139.

[13] For Russell's opinion, see Dols, "Plague in Early Islamic History," 373.

[14] McNeill, *Plagues and People,* 139 and 161–207 for the later date, and also Dols, "Plague in Early Islamic History," 373. Note, however, that the Chinese sources appear to record an outbreak of plague among the nomadic Turks in 585: Theophylactus Simocatta, *History,* p. 45, note.

[15] I am grateful to Professor Alexis Sanderson for information on the Indian sources. Allen, "'Justinianic' Plague," 19.

[16] *Topographie Chrétienne* 11.17–19, 3:348–50.

[17] *Itinerarium Antonini Placentini,* 216. Ships from India are also mentioned as docking at Aila on the Red Sea "cum diversis aromatibus," ibid., 212.

[18] Crone, *Meccan Trade,* 31.

Sea.[19] Nevertheless, that Byzantine traders reached the Indian subcontinent in the early sixth century is further suggested by the discovery there of Byzantine coinage from this period.[20]

That the Justinianic Plague probably did not, however, originate in India is suggested by two further details. First, there is every reason to believe that trading relations between India and China were considerably more frequent than those between India and Byzantium, a natural reflection of the greater economic sophistication of the Chinese world at this time.[21] One might thus reasonably have expected a plague originating in India to have arrived in China rather sooner than it would have reached the Mediterranean. Yet, there would appear to be no mention of bubonic plague in China until the year 610.[22] That said, in navigational terms, the sea routes between the Near East and India were, of course, considerably more straightforward than those between India and China, so a certain amount of caution is advisable here.[23] A similar case can be made with rather greater force in relation to the Sasanian Empire of Persia, which also enjoyed healthy and frequent trading relations with the Indian subcontinent.[24] Yet, once again, Byzantium would appear to have been affected by plague before Persia. The Persian army was struck by the disease in Atropatene in 543, and the so-called "Plague of Shirawayh," which beset the Sasanian capital of Ctesiphon in 627/8, was probably the result of the arrival of Persian or even Byzantine troops from the West.[25]

The case against India having served as the origin of the plague is further strengthened when one surveys the positive evidence for an African origin. The Byzantine church historian Evagrius, in the fourth book of his *Ecclesiastical History*, claimed that the plague originated in Ethiopia.[26] This proposition has been rejected by Allen, who wrote that "Evagrius' assertion that it began in Ethiopia can be attributed to a traditional prejudice

---

[19] *Chronicle of John Malalas* 18.56, pp. 268–69; an embassy to Ethiopia is described as one to "India." Note also *Topographie Chrétienne*, 1:17.

[20] Narasmahmurthy, "Numismatic Studies," 3; Ghosh and Ismael, "Coins from Excavations," 16.

[21] Hudson, "Medieval Trade of China."

[22] McNeill, *Plagues and People*, 147.

[23] I owe this point to Mr. T. F. Stone of All Souls College, Oxford, who provided invaluable assistance in the composition of this essay.

[24] Howard-Johnson, "Two Great Powers," 204–05.

[25] Procopius, *PW* 2.24, pp. 472–78; Dols, "Plague in Early Islamic History," 376. For the military context, see Howard-Johnson, "Heraclius' Persian Campaigns."

[26] Evagrius, *Ecclesiastical History* 4.29, p. 177.

that diseases came from that region."[27] Thucydides attributed the origin of the Athenian pestilence to Ethiopia, and Evagrius' claim must therefore be understood, it is argued, within the context of a "classicizing discourse." Yet Evagrius does not mimic Thucydides. Indeed, he points out to the reader the fact that the plague through which he lived, although, like the Athenian pestilence, said to have originated in Ethiopia, was, in terms of its symptoms, very different. He is aware of the coincidence in terms of attributed origin, and comments on it. He goes no further.[28] Moreover, had there existed an ancient prejudice against Ethiopia as a source of disease, it would have been fully justified. Throughout the medieval period, the extant Arabic sources record that both Ethiopia and the Sudan were rife with plague.[29]

Moreover, an African origin to the bubonic plague of the sixth century makes sense both chronologically and geopolitically. The revival of warfare between Byzantium and Persia in the year 502–503 led the Byzantines in the early sixth century to establish ever closer military, diplomatic, and economic relations with the Christian Ethiopian rulers of Axum, using them as a counterweight to Persian influence in southern Arabia.[30] At the same time, the Ethiopians are recorded as having maintained close economic contact with the inhabitants of inner Africa, thus providing an effective vector for the disease.[31] This geopolitical context of the early sixth century was arguably the crucial prerequisite for the transmission of the plague from Africa to Byzantium.[32] Although the question can never be settled definitively, that the Justinianic Plague originated in Africa seems most probable, as both Brown and Keys have recently agreed.[33]

---

[27] Allen, "'Justinianic' Plague," 6.

[28] Evagrius, *Ecclesiastical History* 4.29, p. 177. Evagrius writes that the plague was "en tisi men sumpheromenon toi hupo Thoukudidou graphent, en tisi men polloi dialatton. Kai erchthai men ex Aithiopias kai nun elegato." On the Athenian pestilence, see Scott and Duncan, *Biology of Plagues*, 2–5.

[29] Dols, "Plague in Early Islamic History," 372–73.

[30] Procopius, *PW* 1.19–20, pp. 178–94; *Chronicle of John Malalas* 28.15, 56, pp. 251, 268–69; Greatrex, *Rome and Persia*, 73–115 (revival of war) and 225–39 (machinations in southern Arabia).

[31] *Topographie Chrétienne* 2.54–56, 1:365–81 and Kobischanov, *Axum*, 176–81.

[32] Within inner Africa, an important, original, and convincing mechanism for the transmission of the disease from rodent to human, occasioned by globally well-attested climate change in the 530s, is provided by Keys, *Catastrophe*, 15–27 and 251–64.

[33] Brown, *Rise of Western Christendom*, 125 and Keys, *Catastrophe*, 15–27. Both in response to an unpublished version of this article delivered to a seminar in Oxford in 1994 – see Keys, *op. cit.* p. 308, note 9 – although the paper is misdated by a year; Keys describes it as "the first clear historical exposition of the African rather than an Asian origin of the sixth-to-seventh century plague pandemic."

If historians have differed as to the origin of the sixth-century plague, the question of the disease's impact on Byzantium and the Mediterranean world has occasioned still greater controversy. At first, this might appear perplexing. The contemporary narrative sources available to the historian, be they from East or West, written in Latin, Greek, Syriac, or Arabic, speak with one voice in describing the plague as having had a major demographic impact on communities, urban and rural alike. Thus, for example, the historian Procopius, who was present for the arrival of the plague in Constantinople in 542, describes how at one point it struck down 10,000 victims in a single day.[34] Similarly, John of Ephesus describes "villages whose inhabitants perished altogether."[35] As he passed through Syria, John records having witnessed "houses and waystations occupied only by the dead, corpses lying in the fields and along the roadside, and cattle wandering untended into the hills."[36] Evagrius, whose own family was reduced by the disease, and who was himself afflicted with it as a boy, described how the plague, like the fiscal indiction, returned in a fifteen-year cycle to lay low each new generation.[37] Similarly, the pre-Islamic Arabic poet Hassan Ibn Thabit records the pestilence, described as "the stinging of the *jinn*," devastating the rural population of the empire's eastern fringes.[38] In relation to Frankia too, Gregory of Tours describes a high rate of mortality.[39]

In short, as Conrad has noted, the historian is presented with a wide range of contemporary accounts, written by authors from quite distinct geographical, cultural, social, and religious milieux.[40] These accounts concur that the bubonic plague hit the Mediterranean world like a hammer blow. The sources would suggest that the arrival of the plague did much to weaken the Eastern Empire in the decades leading up to the final dramatic phase of Byzantine-Persian warfare in the early seventh century and, one might infer, limited the empire's capacity to respond to the emergent challenge posed by the forces of Islam in the 630s and 640s.[41] Such, certainly, was the argument made by historians who turned their attention to the subject of the Justinianic Plague in the 1960s and 1970s. Thus Biraben and Le Goff, for example, "pointed to the power vacuum

---

[34] Procopius, *PW* 2.23.1–3, p. 464.
[35] Preserved in John of Ephesus in Pseudo-Dionysius of Tel Mahrē, *Chronicle*, 75.
[36] Conrad, "Plague in Bilad al-Sham."
[37] Evagrius, *Ecclesiastical History* 4.29, p. 177.
[38] Conrad, "Epidemic Disease in Central Syria."
[39] Gregory of Tours, *History of the Franks* 4.5 and 4.16, pp. 199–200, 212.
[40] See Conrad, "Epidemic Disease in Central Syria," 56.
[41] See the excellent account in Whittow, *Making of Orthodox Byzantium.*

caused by the decrease in population due to plague, which facilitated the descent of the Slavs, the advent of Mohammed, and the gradual shift of power away from the Mediterranean toward the north of Europe."[42]

In recent years, however, a marked tendency has emerged to seek to downplay the effects of the late antique bubonic plague, and argues that eyewitness accounts of the disease are hysterical in tone and misleading in effect.[43] This revisionist tendency can be dated back to the publication in 1989 of Durliat's "La peste du VIe siècle, pour un nouvel examen des sources byzantines."[44] This article, characterized at the time by Biraben as "une polémique constructive," has greatly influenced subsequent writing on the sixth century.[45]

Durliat proposed that reliance upon the literary sources had led scholars to exaggerate the impact of the plague on the Byzantine Empire. The testimony of the literary sources for the plague having had a dramatic impact on imperial fortunes and, in particular, on population levels within the empire was, he suggested, gainsaid by the rather more mute and hitherto ignored testimony of the non-literary evidence. In particular, Durliat argued, statistical analysis of the epigraphic data in relation to funerary inscriptions demonstrated no sudden increase in the rate of mortality through the course of the sixth century.[46] The rich seam of papyrological evidence from Egypt – the only region of the empire for which extensive collections of documentary texts survive – showed no sign of the plague's impact.[47] Nor did the numismatic record suggest any fiscal instability on the part of the Byzantine state, such as might be attributable to the advent of the plague.[48] The legal evidence for the impact of the plague Durliat dismissed as paltry.[49] These claims have been widely accepted but have never been explicitly tested, although the general hypothesis has been questioned by both Conrad and Whitby.[50]

---

[42] Allen, "'Justinianic' Plague," 20.

[43] Whittow, *Making of Orthodox Byzantium*, 66–68.

[44] Durliat, "La peste du VIe siècle."

[45] Biraben, "Rapport," 120.

[46] Durliat, "La peste du VIe siècle," 109.

[47] Ibid., 109–10.

[48] Ibid., 110–11.

[49] Ibid., 112. Durliat also raises the spectre of lack of archaeological evidence, while having to admit that "l'archéologie urbaine enregistre ... à partir du milieu du VIe siècle, un déclin assez net de l'urbanisme." For discussion of the problematic nature of the archaeological evidence, see Ward-Perkins, "Land, Labour and Settlement," 322–27.

[50] Conrad, "Epidemic Disease in Central Syria"; Whitby, "Recruitment in Roman Armies," 93–99.

The argument that the epigraphic evidence of extant and discovered funerary inscriptions appears to record no sudden rise in mortality in the Byzantine Empire through the course of the sixth century is a powerful one. The problem with this argument is that our eyewitness accounts inform us that the rate of mortality associated with the advent of the plague and its recurrences was so high that traditional funerary practices had to be abandoned, with bodies being buried *en masse*. Thus Procopius wrote in relation to Constantinople in 542:

> And when it came about that all the tombs which had existed previously were filled with the dead, then they dug up all the places about the city one after the other, laid the dead there, each one as he could; but later ... those who were making these trenches, no longer able to keep up with the number of dying, mounted the towers of the fortifications in Sycae (Galata) and tearing off the roofs, threw the bodies in there in complete disorder.[51]

Likewise, John of Ephesus also records Justinian ordering the digging of mass graves at Galata, and further suggests that considerable problems were encountered in disposing of corpses at Jerusalem and the cities of Palestine. John claims even that many corpses in Constantinople were simply thrown into the sea.[52] Given such circumstances, it would have been perfectly possible for a sudden increase in the rate of mortality not to be evident from the epigraphic sequence.

Durliat arguably had unrealistic expectations of the epigraphic record, given the circumstances in which the inscriptions on which he is dependent would appear to have been made. A similar criticism can, and should, be leveled with regard to the papyrological and legal sources. While it is true that the papyrological evidence for Egypt furnishes the social and economic historian of Late Antiquity with much fascinating and rewarding material, it nevertheless remains highly fragmentary. The papyri simply do not provide the economic historian with the sort of population cohorts, traceable through time, such as the documentary sources for late medieval England provide and on which historians of the Black Death are so reliant. Likewise, the claim that Justinian's legislation subsequent to the advent of the plague in 541 demonstrates little interest in the supposed impact of the disease is rather disingenuous. Imperial legislation in general diminishes in frequency after 541, perhaps partly as a result of the death in 542 of Justinian's *Quaestor* Tribonian, and the exiling in 541

---

[51] Procopius, *PW* 2.23.9–10, p. 466.
[52] Allen, "'Justinianic' Plague," 12.

of the Praetorian Prefect John the Cappadocian.[53] Rather than continuing with the audacious program of administrative and legal reform that had characterized the 530s, Justinian, in Brown's evocative phrase, "sank himself into a dogged routine of survival."[54]

That is not to say, however, that our more "mute" sources are necessarily uninformative. It has already been noted that our narrative accounts describe the plague as having had a dramatic impact on both urban and rural populations. Procopius complains in his *Secret History* of how Justinian was so cruel as to refuse to remit taxes to landowners, in spite of the fact that most of their agricultural laborers had been wiped out by the disease.[55] This testimony as to the impact of the plague on the countryside is highly suggestive. Had the countryside been left largely untouched by the pestilence, the rapid repopulation of affected cities would have been relatively unproblematic, and the long-term consequences of the disease accordingly slight. In spite of Durliat's assertion, the claim that the plague occasioned large-scale agrarian depopulation would appear to be strongly corroborated by the numismatic, legal, and papyrological evidence.

This evidence is at its most striking in relation to the monetary history of the Empire in this period. As Jones pointed out, the vast majority of the fiscal revenues of the late Roman and early Byzantine state were derived from taxes paid on the land and those who worked it.[56] Given that the 540s witnessed no shrinkage in the size of the Byzantine Empire, and no relaxation in the demands made on the state by warfare on both eastern and western frontiers, any substantial diminution in the agrarian population is likely to have occasioned a fiscal crisis – the demand for tax revenues remaining constant, but the source-base for such revenues declining dramatically. It is thus highly significant that, in spite of Durliat's claims, the advent of the Justinianic Plague and its subsequent recurrences coincided with a period of major instability in the imperial coinage – our best measure of the condition of imperial finances.

In Book XXII of his *Secret History*, Procopius launches a vicious attack on Peter Barsymes, first as *Comes Sacrarum Largitionum*, and second as Praetorian Prefect of the East, each one a post that he held twice, initially serving as Praetorian Prefect in 543–546. Peter is accused of unashamedly depriving soldiers on campaign of their pay, and of conducting the sale of

---

[53] Stein, *L'Histoire du Bas Empire* provides an excellent account for this period; see 2:747–56.

[54] Brown, *World of Late Antiquity*, 155. For reform legislation, see Sarris, "Economy and Society," 235–54.

[55] Procopius, *SH* 23.19, pp. 274–76.

[56] Jones, *Later Roman Empire*, 2:770.

offices with scant regard to the interests of the emperor's subjects. During Peter's second period as Count of the Sacred Largesses, from 547–550, Procopius records that he sought to reduce the annual expenditure of the state on pensions, while himself embezzling the tax revenues and forwarding only a portion of them to the emperor. Although, in keeping with the personalizing genre in which he was writing, Procopius attributes these policies to the malice and corruption of an individual, it is clear that he is describing an attempt on the part of the state to retrench expenditure and alludes to an apparent shortfall in fiscal income.[57]

Most significantly, Barsymes is accused, as *Comes*, of "making the gold coinage smaller," something that, Procopius claims, had never been done before.[58] This charge is made quite distinctly from a later one contained within the *Secret History* that Justinian altered the rate of exchange between the gold and the copper coinage: an innovation not blamed on Peter Barsymes and normally dated to the year 538 due to a series of heavy copper coins issued in that year.[59] The two policies, as stated, are described separately, and should not be presumed to have been instituted concurrently.

How, then, does one account for the charge that Barsymes, as *Comes Sacrarum Largitionum* made "the gold coinage smaller"? The accusation is most readily explicable as a reference to the series of "light-weight" *solidi* issued under Justinian, some of which weighed as little as twenty *siliquae* rather than the customary twenty-four. This policy is normally dated to the year 538 on the basis that both the heavy copper coins issued in that year and the light-weight *solidi* show a fully facing bust of the emperor, rather than the three-quarter facing bust normally associated with the *solidus*, and the profile bust that hitherto had characterized the *follis*.[60] Yet this iconographic affinity provides one with little more than a *terminus post quem* for the reform of the gold coinage. As an accurate dating for the light-weight *solidus*, 538 is unsatisfactory. Procopius clearly attributes the policy to Peter Barsymes as *Comes Sacrarum Largitionum* – a post he is first attested to have held in March of 542 and that he had vacated by July of 543.[61]

The light-weight *solidus* is thus most likely to have been issued either in the year 542–543, or during Peter's second period of tenure as *Comes*

[57] Jones et al., *Prosopography of the Later Roman Empire*, 2:999–1002.
[58] Procopius, *SH* 22.38, p. 266.
[59] Ibid., 25.11–12, pp. 294–96.
[60] Hendy, "Light Weight Solidi," 58, note 2.
[61] Jones et al., *Prosopography of the Later Roman Empire*, 2:999–1002.

between 547–550. That is to say, the policy would appear to have coincided with the first ravages of the bubonic plague. In this context, the introduction of the coin makes sense as a measure by which the state sought to respond to a major shortfall in income occasioned by the disease, exacting payments in full *solidi*, while disbursing the lighter coins, just as, amidst the crisis of the early seventh century, the Emperor Heraclius would appear to have decreed that the government was to make payments in the form of silver coinage and was to receive in gold.[62]

Further evidence for the frailty of state finances in the immediate aftermath of the plague is evident from the copper coinage. While great emphasis is often placed on the creation of the heavy *follis* in 538, one should not lose sight of the subsequent history of the coin. As Metcalf noted, the year 542, and those that followed, witnessed a remarkable instability in the weight of the copper coinage, which brought to an end the long period of stability that had been inaugurated by the Anastasian reforms. Between 538 and 551, Metcalf's study records the weight of the copper coinage to have declined by some 23%.[63] Similarly, Hahn's numismatic reconstruction shows the standard weight of the *follis* to have declined from 18.19 grams for the years 512–538, and 24.95 grams between 538 and 542, to 13.64 grams by 570.[64]

Numismatic metrology is, of course, a far more imprecise science than its name would suggest. Nevertheless, the instability of the copper coinage, taken alongside the appearance of the light-weight *solidus*, provides substantial evidence for a crisis in state finance which coincided exactly with the appearance of the plague, and which is most readily explicable in terms of the fiscal consequences of agrarian depopulation.

Agrarian depopulation in the mid-sixth century is further suggested by the legal evidence. Thus in June 545, Justinian legislated on the reallocation of the fiscal dues incumbent upon deserted agricultural lands (*agri deserti*), providing what Teall described as "the definitive form of the *epibolē.*"[65] Moreover, in any economy, a sudden decrease in the overall adult population that is largely uniform in its social distribution, potentially increases the ability of those who sell their labor to demand higher wages, or to negotiate lower rents. To what extent they make such demands, and how successful they are in their attempts, is determined

---

[62] *Chronicon Paschale*, 138–39, note 441.
[63] Metcalf, "Metrology of Justinian's Follis," 210–19.
[64] Banaji, "Rural Communities," Table 5.
[65] Novella 126 in *CIC*, 3:636–64; Teall, "Barbarians in Justinian's Armies," 318.

by the scale of the depopulation, the pre-existing relationship between the availability of labor and demand, and the balance of social forces within that society. The greater the coercive power of those who employ labor, and the more fragmented and insecure the communities of those who supply it, the less likely it is that demographic attrition will lead to a substantial alteration in the character of social relations, or to a redistribution of wealth.[66] Given that the agricultural workforce of the late antique Eastern Empire would appear to have been characterized by its chronic legal and economic insecurity, it is thus highly significant that, after the arrival of the plague, the legal and papyrological sources record just such demands to have been made by agricultural workers, and such negotiations to have been successful at least on the part of lessees.[67]

Thus, in the April of 545, Justinian issued an edict to the Praetorian Prefect of the East and to the Urban Prefect of Constantinople – a measure, thus, of imperial-wide effect. In this edict, Justinian complains of how, in the wake of the plague, tradesmen, artisans, and agricultural workers had given themselves over to avarice and were demanding twice or even three times the prices and wages that had hitherto been the norm.[68] The emperor decreed that those responsible for issuing wages and stipends to building workers, agricultural workers, or any other group of workers were not to credit them with anything more than their customary remuneration. Likewise, Banaji's statistical analysis of Egyptian land-leases recorded among the papyri would appear to record a marked improvement in the security of tenure enjoyed by lessees from the middle of the sixth century onward. From the first half of the sixth century to the second, the proportion of leases of indefinite duration increased from 17.2% to 39.4%. The proportion of leases of only one year's duration declined over the same period from 29.3% to 9.1%.[69]

Naturally, many of these lease-holders recorded in the Egyptian papyri are likely to have been individuals of relatively high social standing, paying rent on extensive plots. Moreover, on the basis of the available papyrological evidence, the extensive leasing of land would not appear to have played a central role in the domestic economy of the great landowning families – members of the imperial aristocracy, whose estates tended to

[66] Brenner, "Agrarian Class Structure."
[67] Sarris, "Economy and Society," 105–34.
[68] Novella 122 in *CIC,* 3:592.
[69] Banaji, "Rural Communities," Table 20.

be cultivated by a centrally-directed agricultural workforce paid, at least in part, in coin.[70] That those owners of land who did rent out holdings, however, were obliged from the mid-sixth century to do so, from their perspective, on ever more disadvantageous terms, would still indicate that, in the context of a plague-ravaged society, a new premium had come to be placed on ensuring the continuous cultivation of land.[71]

That the demands for higher wages made by that proportion of the agricultural and non-agricultural workforce remunerated in coin may also have been successful is suggested perhaps by the trends in the rate of exchange between the gold and copper coinage evident from the mid-sixth century. Given that the poor were generally paid in small-denomination coinage, but prices and taxes were reckoned in gold, any devaluation in gold vis-à-vis copper inevitably benefited the more humble members of society to the disadvantage of their nominal superiors. It is thus perhaps significant that Hahn's reconstruction of the exchange rate between gold and copper shows the number of *folles* per *solidus* to have declined from 210 between 538 and 542 to 180 between 542 and 550.[72]

The non-literary numismatic, legal, and papyrological evidence can thus be seen to concur with the testimony of our contemporary eyewitness accounts for the late antique bubonic plague. Not only urban but also agrarian depopulation would appear to have been widespread; the effects of this on the finances of the Byzantine state would appear to have been considerable. This must necessarily have had an effect on the empire's military capability, as the Byzantine army was the main recipient of imperial revenues.[73] It should come as little surprise that the reigns of Justinian's successors witnessed ever greater fiscal and military frailty on the part of the Byzantine state. Thus Justin II declared upon his accession to the throne in 565 that he "found the treasury burdened with many debts and reduced to utter exhaustion."[74] In 588, the imperial authorities were obliged to reduce military pay by 25%, leading to a major mutiny on the empire's eastern frontier.[75] Further military resentment at imperial economies culminated in the 602/3 with a coup against the Emperor Maurice, his replacement by Phocas, and the

[70] Sarris, "Economy and Society," 105–34.
[71] For a similar tendency in post–Black Death England, see Keen, *English Society*, 53–57.
[72] Banaji, "Rural Communities," Table 5.
[73] Treadgold, *History of the Byzantine State*, 277.
[74] Novella 148 in *CIC*, 3:722.
[75] Jones, *Later Roman Empire*, 1:304.

empire's subsequent descent into a protracted and bloody civil war that opened the way to Persian invasion.[76]

The implications of plague-induced depopulation for the structures of the empire are one thing. What such depopulation meant in terms of human misery can scarcely be estimated. Historians have a duty to question the sources on which they are dependent for their knowledge – such skepticism is a necessary component of the historical craft. In relation to the Justinianic Plague, however, such skepticism has perhaps gone too far: Evagrius' claim as to the origin of the plague is attributed to prejudice; our narrative accounts of the plague are dismissed as hysterical. It is perhaps worth pausing to consider that those who wrote our sources lived through the events they describe, and we did not. Such being the case, and other things being equal, we ought, perhaps, to give them the benefit of the doubt.[77]

---

[76] Ibid., 315. The Byzantine Empire's response to the Persian invasion arguably so exhausted the state as to leave it incapable of meeting the new challenge posed by the Arabs in the 630s and 640s. See Howard-Johnson, "Heraclius' Persian Campaign," 34–35.

[77] That social and economic historians should be more trusting of contemporary accounts of the impact of epidemic disease has also recently been argued in relation to the Black Death by both Hatcher and Horrox: see Hatcher, "Aftermath of the Black Death" and Horrox, *Black Death*, 234.

IV

THE LATIN WEST

7

Consilia humana, ops divina, superstitio

Seeking Succor and Solace in Times of Plague, with Particular Reference to Gaul in the Early Middle Ages

Alain J. Stoclet

The words plucked from Livy for the title of this essay are not all his own. However, by adding *superstitio* to Thucydides' "catalogue" of human reactions to the plague, Livy yet again confirms in the eyes of this reader his status as a matchless historian with an uncanny gift for perceptive analysis.[1]

The invention of this new category coincides with a turning point in Livy's *Roman History*, when the manly mores of old, the cornerstone of Rome's greatness, started to slacken, through contact with foreign customs. In order to "allay the wrath of the gods," which was believed to have unleashed the plague in 364 BC, games were held and, for the first time, included theatrical performances as were already common in Etruria, Umbria, and Greece. To no effect. Not only were the Romans not "reconciled with the gods," but "their own consciences were not freed": The plague continued unabated as did the Romans' feeling of guilt, for they were certain that some past action of theirs had caused the gods to mete out this most severe of chastisements.

Livy's emendation of Thucydides confers paradigmatic value to his behavioral typology. I use this typology as an organizing principle for the materials I have assembled. I feel, however, that this requires a word of explanation.

---

[1] For the references to Livy in the title and in the first five paragraphs of this essay, see Livy, *Ab urbe condita* 7.2–3, vol. 3:358–67. On Livy's well-known debt to Thucydides, *Peloponnesian War*, 2.47.4, vol. 1:341–43, see Oakley, *Commentary on Livy*, 2:39.

For Martin Heinzelmann on the occasion of his 65th birthday: this essay is a version of my 1998 article "Entre Esculape et Marie," at once considerably shorter and different in emphasis since it incorporates much new material.

When threatened by premature though natural death, man has always – whatever the time and place – sought to escape his fate. In doing so, he has been guided by reason or by faith, which latter comes in two varieties: one ordinary and dignified, the other literally extraordinary as well as pitiable. Reason would translate as hygiene, sanitary measures, medicine, or to put it in Livy's own words, "the cure of the sick," as opposed to "the desire to appease peoples' consciences through an exculpatory rite." In the first of its two guises, faith exists within the confines of established religion. Its other visage looks to supernatural powers outside the recognized or dominant canon, and invokes them in various ways. More often than not, as again Livy observes, the sheer scale and wantonness of epidemic disease make but short shrift of reason: faith prevails and divine intercession is solicited by means of public rituals of atonement or appeasement.

In choosing to focus on the agents, whether human or divine, from which solace or succor was sought, I am only slightly straying from Livy's path, again for the sake of convenience.

GODS – *OPS DIVINA*

One of the more fascinating aspects of the Justinianic Plague is that it occurs at a time when Christianity, while progressing steadily, does not reign supreme and has not, in many instances or places, grown roots so deep that it cannot be swept away by the winds of panic. At one end of the spectrum, we find Anglo-Saxon England and its recently converted peoples, in 664:

> At the same time, the kings Sighere and Sebbi succeeded Swidhelm, of whom I have spoken, as rulers of the East Saxons under Wulfhere, King of the Mercians. While the plague was causing a heavy death-toll in the province, Sighere and his people abandoned the mysteries of the Christian Faith and relapsed into paganism. For the king himself, together with many of the nobles and common folk, loved this life and sought no other, or even disbelieved in its existence. Hoping for protection against the plague by this means, they therefore began to rebuild the ruined temples and restore the worship of idols. But Sebbi his fellow-king and colleague held with all his people loyally to the Faith they had accepted, and, as will appear later, remained faithful and ended his days happily.[2]

---

[2] Bede, *EH* 3.30, p. 323. Compare *Beowulf* 166b–167 and 170–188 (reproduced in the appendix to this essay), an epic whose nuclei, both historic (Hygelac's Frisian expeditions against the Merovingian Franks) and textual (if one follows Lapidge, "Archetype of Beowulf," pp. 5–41, but, as is well known, the dating issue is much debated), belong to the period of the Justinianic Plague and whose monstrous protagonist, rising as it does from the marshes, might well embody the miasmas that were deemed by some to carry the plague. See note 46 and Stoclet, "From Baghdad to Beowulf," pp. 169–71.

At the other end of the spectrum, Byzantium a little over a century earlier or four years into the epidemic (546): Justinian, we are told, is frantically hunting down the remnants of paganism among the medical profession with the assistance of John of Ephesus, patriarch of Constantinople, whose *Ecclesiastical History* records this most pointed of inquisitions.[3] Gaul in the second half of the sixth century exhibits shades of all the above symptoms: royal endeavors to control public physicians as well as healers – although the ends appear to be very different from Justinian's, but more about this next – and contrasting loyalties to the new faith. It is well known that Gregory of Tours does not thrive on nuance – his *Histories*, after all, are not what we would expect from such a title, but rather a kind of apocalyptic treatise, a strong warning issued to the flock in view of the impending doom.[4] Nevertheless, his portraits of Chilperic, the bad king, and Gunthram, the good one, ring true, up to a point: that is, they ought to be placed firmly within their regional context, that of Burgundy for Gunthram, of northern Gaul for Chilperic. Gunthram's subjects were predominantly Gallo–Roman and as Catholic as anyone in the post-Roman world; Chilperic's were Franks and, like himself, third-generation Christians, at best. Accordingly, we read about Gunthram organizing and leading a rogations procession at Saint-Symphorien d'Ozon, south-west of Lyons, to combat the plague, and working a miracle on a child beset by fever. Meanwhile, Chilperic, a figure of Antichrist, orders the arenas in Soissons and Paris to be restored, a truly pagan initiative that bears close resemblance, for instance, to the Romans' response to the plague in 364 BC. Moreover, it is also at Chilperic's behest that a most unorthodox healer shows up in Paris, only to clash with the bishop, whose liturgical progress through the streets of the Cité he interrupts with his own, equally well-attended procession and beseeching not Christ but, in all probability, Apollo Medicus, at once the god of plague and Paris' ancient tutelary divinity.[5]

Indeed, engulfed by a harrowing epidemic, Chilperic's Paris seems briefly under his aegis to have experienced a last revival of its pre-Christian beliefs and rituals. These are, to quote Gregory, drawing upon Matthew

[3] Text in Nau, "Analyse de la seconde partie inédite de l'Histoire ecclésiastique de Jean d'Asie"; the relevant passage is at pp. 481–82.

[4] See Heinzelmann, *Gregory of Tours: History and Society.*

[5] On arenas and games: see Navarre, "*Ludi Publici*," here at 1370b, and Piganiol, *Recherches sur les jeux romains*, 137–49, especially p. 148. Gregory of Tours, *Historia Francorum* 5.17, 9.6, 21, pp. 209, 361–63, 379–80. Apollo Medicus: see further along in this essay and my demonstration in "Entre Esculape et Marie."

24:7–8, 11, "the beginnings of the pains," that Christ, addressing his disciples, had foretold:

There will be plagues, famines and earthquakes in various places, and false christs
and false prophets will rise and they will make signs and prodigies in the sky so
as to induce the chosen into error, as has happened nowadays.

The Book of Revelation 19:20 shows what fate awaits such wizards and
their ilk:

The beast was caught up with and the false prophet also, who had made signs
before it, with which he had mislead those who had received the beast's mark
and those who had prostrated themselves before its likeness; both were thrown
alive into the lake of fire, the lake that burns with sulfur.

Thus also did Chilperic perish, at least in Gunthram's vision if not in
reality. And Paris was cleansed first through the removal of the bronze
idols thought to protect it – a small rodent and a snake, attributes of
Asklepios, that is to say of Apollo Medicus, for they are one and the
same – then through a truly apocalyptic fire that reduced the city island
to ashes, sparing only the just and the innocent.[6]

   If nothing else, the Justinianic Plague conference venue would justify
me in taking leave for a moment from Gaul and turning to Rome. The
date is 590:

At this time, there was a deluge of water in the territories of Venetia and Liguria,
and in other regions of Italy such as is believed not to have existed since the
time of Noah [. . .] In this outpouring of the flood the river Tiber at the city of
Rome rose so much that its waters flowed in over the walls of the city and filled
great regions of it. Then through the bed of the same stream a great multitude of
serpents, and a dragon also of astonishing size, passed by the city and descended
to the sea. Straightway a very grievous pestilence called inguinal followed this
inundation, and it wasted the people with such great destruction of life that out
of a countless multitude barely a few remained. First it struck pope Pelagius [II],
a venerable man, and quickly killed him. Then when their pastor was taken away
it spread among the people. In this great tribulation, the most blessed Gregory,
who was then a deacon, was elected to pope by the common consent of all. He
ordained that a seven-fold litany should be offered [. . .][7]

To get at the meaning of Paul the Deacon's curious tale, we must once
again delve into Rome's ancient history, into one of its early encounters

---

[6] Gregory of Tours, *Historia Francorum* 6.46, 8.5, 33, 10.25, pp. 286–87, 328–29, 348–50,
381–82.
[7] Paul the Deacon, *Historia Longobardorum*, 3.24, pp. 104–5; *History of the Lombards*, 127. An
earlier version is found in Gregory of Tours, *Historia Francorum* 10.1, p. 406, and a later
one (873) in John the Deacon, *Vita sancti Gregorii Magni* 1.34–43, in *PL* 75:77–81. The
three versions differ only in minor details. I quote Paul the Deacon's because it is the
most terse.

with the plague, that of 293 BC. On that occasion, a desperate embassy was sent to Epidauros, to seek Asklepios' succor, just as the Athenians had done half a century earlier, to their entire satisfaction and relief. The god obliged and, assuming the shape of a serpent (Greek *drakôn*), as he was wont to do, he traveled to Rome and took up residence on the Tiber Island.[8] The Romans expressed their gratitude by erecting a large temple on the site that would remain in use for centuries, its fame spreading far and wide. Many also kept domestic snakes, so many indeed that, following the elder Pliny, "nothing in the world could halt the increase in the numbers [of these creatures] if the occasional fire did not destroy their seed" (*Natural History*, 22). Against this background, it is easy to make sense of Paul the Deacon's narrative – or rather that of his source, to see that it carries the same fundamental import as Gregory of Tour's, while expressing it somewhat more transparently, more dispassionately. As in Paris, so in Rome, paganism's unexpected if opportunistic resilience would have been a thorn in the Church's side. What Paul's reptilian exodus signifies, in effect, is that Asklepios and his minions are deserting the city. Thereupon, Gregory the Great ascends to the throne of Saint Peter; he ordains that a seven-fold litany should be offered, thus obtaining from the one true God the cessation of the epidemic.

Let us now return to Paris. According to local lore reported by Gregory (8, 33), the brazen effigies harked back to an ancient consecration of the city. We hear nothing more regarding this concept of consecration until the end of the ninth century, when Abbo of Saint-Germain-des-Prés, in his famous poem on the Viking siege of Paris, attributes the foe's final defeat to the miraculous intervention of the Virgin Mary and to the mindful watch she keeps over her city: *urbs in honore micat celsae sacrata Mariae*, "the city," he says, "considers itself honored to be consecrated to almighty Mary."[9] It is my contention that as, probably, in Constantinople, the cult of Mary was introduced and fostered early on, during the Justinianic Plague, to provide the terrified populations with an object of devotion more fathomable or more proximate – and in some ways also more familiar – than Christ himself and thereby to prevent them from lapsing back into devilish superstition.[10] Mary in fact became the *tychè* or

---

[8] Livy, *Ab urbe condita* 10.47, vol. 4:540–43; further sources quoted and discussed by Besnier, *L'Île Tibérine dans l'Antiquité*, 152–83.

[9] Gregory of Tours, *Historia Francorum* 8.33, pp. 348–50; Abbon, *Libri duo bellorum Parisiacae urbis* 2.327, pp. 40–41.

[10] This hypothesis in no way contradicts Vasiliky Limberis' fundamental findings regarding the cult of Mary in Constantinople, to wit, that it was an almost single-handed creation of Empress Pulcheria (c. 450): an amalgamation of elements of the imperial cult and of several tutelary divinities (Limberis, *Divine Heiress*).

tutelary "divinity" of both cities, displacing her pagan forerunners while at the same time inheriting some of their characteristics.[11] As such, she is victory-bringing (*nikèphorè*), against both visible and invisible enemies, hence the invocation to her in the fifth- or early sixth-century Akathistos hymn, "the oldest continuously performed Marian hymn used in the Eastern Orthodox Church":[12]

> Hail to you, through whom trophies of victory are assured,
> Hail to you, through whom enemies are vanquished,
> Hail to you, who are the healing of my body,
> Hail to you, who are the salvation of my soul.[13]

Responding as she does to the prayers of the besieged by dispatching a Viking attacker and releasing the captives he was threatening to execute, so that "falling into the bonds of death, he himself let go those he was holding in chains" (2, 322), Abbo's Mary calls to mind the women in the *First Merseburg Charm*:

> Once they sat; sat here and there.
> Some made fetters; some restrained the hostile army;
> Some loosed the fetters;
> Free yourself from the fetters, escape the warriors![14]

The *Merseburg Charms* are of far greater antiquity than the manuscript containing them, which was written in Abbo's own days or shortly thereafter.[15] Michael Enright has this to say about the lines just quoted:

This charm is much disputed for it may refer to actual physical battle but may also, alternatively, refer to a warding off of the hordes of disease invading the body. In either case, warfare is the central concept and women are involved because the binding and loosing of knots in the sunken weaving hut are interpreted as the magical equivalent of the binding and loosing of warriors on the battlefield.[16]

A number of examples from the Germanic tradition are then adduced in support of this assertion, which need not detain us here, although it

---

[11] Constantinople: Limberis, *Divine Heiress*, chapter 6.
[12] Ibid., 88, favoring an early-fifth-century date as against Grosdidier's late-fifth- to early-sixth-century date.
[13] Verse 23, Limberis, *Divine Heiress*, 94.
[14] Abbon, *Libri duo bellorum Parisiacae urbis* 2.322, p. 40. The translation of the *Charm* is in Enright, *Lady with a Mead Cup*, 117.
[15] De Vries, *Altgermanische Religionsgeschichte* § 451 and Adams and Mallory, "Medecine," p. 376 b, re. the *Second Charm*. Brief commentary on the *First Charm*, not bearing on date, De Vries, *Altgermanische Religionsgeschichte* § 230.
[16] Enright, *Lady with a Mead Cup*, 117.

should be noted that "the idea of women weaving fate"[17] is also found among other Indo–European peoples.[18] Abbo applies the metaphor to Mary without clearly relating it to weaving. However, according to other medieval sources, she excelled not only in this craft but also in several related *opera muliebria*.[19]

The clearest statement of Mary's prophylactic powers in Paris dates to the mid-tenth century – some fifty odd years after Abbo, when ergotism, the scourge of the High Middle Ages, first appears:

In the county of Paris as in the surrounding counties, peoples' limbs were stricken with a burning ailment; they were devoured by its slow progression until death, at last, put an end to their sufferings. A few, who had made for the holy places, stayed clear of these torments. Many were healed in Paris, in the church of Mary, holy Mother of God, so much so that all who were able to visit it, claimed to have been freed from this plague. Duke Hugues gave them their daily victuals. Some, believing the fever had burnt out, were eager to head home; struck by a new bout, they returned to the church and were healed.[20]

The origins of Notre-Dame are riddled with uncertainties. Mary is first mentioned in 775 as one of the patron saints of the church of Paris, in the institutional sense of the word, along with Etienne and Germain. But in the Carolingian period, the cathedral consisted of two adjoining edifices: Saint-Etienne and Notre-Dame. Both are probably much older.[21] A well-informed and attractive hypothesis gives credit for the foundation of Notre-Dame to Bishop Eusebius (591–594), a contemporary of Gregory of Tours and a Syrian, like many of the city's merchants.[22] Byzantine influence must have been particularly strong during his tenure, and there can be little doubt but that the impetus for the cult of Mary was one of its features.[23]

Early Modern examples may help us to grasp more readily what actually happened in Paris in the late sixth century. Both Venice and Lyon were visited by the plague in 1630 and 1643, respectively. In Venice, thanksgiving for its subsiding took the form of a magnificent basilica that still dominates the southern entrance to the Canalazzo: Santa Maria

---

[17] Ibid.

[18] Adams and Barber, "Textile," *s. v. *dek-*, mention the Greek *Moirai* and the Latin *Parcae*.

[19] Herlihy, *Opera Muliebria*, xiii, 76–77, 97.

[20] Flodoard, *Annales*, anno 945, 100.

[21] Duval, Périn, and Picard, "Paris," 109–13.

[22] Périn, *Catalogues d'art et d'histoire*, 41, n. 5, 144, and 808–9.

[23] This is stated in general terms, without any reference to Paris, by Signori, *Maria zwischen Kathedrale, Kloster und Welt*, 56–57, 60. The four feasts of the Virgin – Presentation, Annunciation, Assumption, and Nativity – were added to the liturgical calendar of the church of Rome by a Syrian pope, Sergius I (687–701).

della Salute. The magistrates of Lyon consecrated their city to the Virgin, hoping – rightly, as it turned out – that she would rid it of the disease. Year after year, in Lyon as well as in Venice, ceremonies commemorate these events: a blessing of the city by the archbishop on the feast of the Nativity of the Virgin (September 8) and a procession across the Canalazzo atop a temporary pontoon-bridge to La Salute on the feast of Mary's entrance into the temple (November 21).[24]

KINGS – BETWEEN *OPS DIVINA* AND *CONSILIA HUMANA*

Domald took the heritage after his father Visbur, and ruled over the land. As in his time there was great famine and distress, the Swedes made great offerings of sacrifice at Upsal. The first autumn they sacrificed oxen, but the succeeding season was not improved thereby. The following autumn they sacrificed men, but the succeeding year was rather worse. The third autumn, when the offer of sacrifice should begin, a great multitude of Swedes came to Upsal; and now the chiefs held consultations with each other, and all agreed that the times of scarcity were on account of their king Domald, and they resolved to offer him for good seasons, and to assault and kill him, and sprinkle the stalls of the gods with his blood. And they did so.[25]

Anyone familiar with Arthur Maurice Hocart's anthropological writings on kingship[26] will know that the ancient Swedes of Snorri Sturluson's *Ynglinga saga* were anything but unique in believing that a strong connection existed between king and cosmos. This connection underlies a recurring explanation for plague, namely, that it was a direct consequence of the king's sexual misconduct, specifically in its most extreme form of incest:

The third [of four questions that the emperor Domitian puts to his prisoner, Apollonius, the sage of Tyana, hoping to trip him] related to the plague in Ephesus; 'What motived [sic],' he said, 'or suggested your prediction to the Ephesians that they would suffer from a plague?' 'I used,' said Apollonius, 'O my sovereign, a lighter diet than others, and so I was the first to be sensible of the danger; and if you like, I will enumerate the causes of pestilences.' But the emperor, fearful, I imagine, lest Apollonius should reckon among the causes of such epidemics his own wrong-doing, and his incestuous marriage, and his other misdemeanours, replied: 'Oh, I do not want any such answer as that.'[27]

---

[24] Hahn, "Lyon" and Trenner, "Venedig" in *Marienlexicon*, 4:196–97, 6:583–84. Dionysios Stathakopoulos kindly supplied the Marian identification for the second date, for which I am most grateful.

[25] Sturluson, *Ynglinga saga*, 18.

[26] Hocart, *Kings and Councillors*.

[27] Philostratus, *Life of Apollonius of Tyana*, 2:281.

Philostratus' *Life of Apollonius of Tyana* is from the early third century AD. A much earlier and far more famous instance of the notion that it illustrates is found in Greek mythology. This is, of course, the story of Œdipus, who inadvertently kills his own father, king Laius of Thebes, thus fulfilling an earlier prophecy, then marries the widow, Queen Jocasta, his own mother, and begets four children. A plague ensues, for which Tiresias, a soothsayer, blames the new king's "sin."[28] Although the following example was completely overlooked by Biraben in his catalogue of occurrences of the Justinianic Plague, it quite likely relates to the very same episode that is known to have affected central and northern Italy as well as Provence in and around 654:[29]

In that time Clovis [II] cut off the arm of blessed Denis the martyr at the instigation of the devil. And throughout the same period [or: during his reign] the kingdom of the Franks was laid low by pestiferous ills [*casibus pestiferis*]. This Clovis was given to all manner of filth, he was a fornicator, a defiler [or: deceiver] of women and could think of nothing save food and drink. History has nothing good to say regarding his death or his end. Writers reprove his end with censure, but not knowing the extent of his evil, in their uncertainty about him they relate some things for others.[30]

Note that Clovis' sexual improprieties are rather unspecific and that sacrilege, another of the king's misdemeanors, is given causational primacy, or so it seems. However, one should perhaps not read too much into the order of sentences so obviously cobbled together in a most careless fashion, through mere juxtaposition of what appear to be snippets culled from a variety of sources.

---

[28] As Parker, *Miasma*, acknowledges, the nature of the sin is never specified, so that either incest or parricide could be meant. I am indebted, yet again, to Dionysios Stathakopoulos for this reference. As for the difficult question of the influence of Œdipus' legend, I cannot pronounce on it other than by referring to Edmunds, *Oedipus*. Of the seventy-six European, Middle-Eastern, Asian, and African analogues that he studies (seven medieval, the rest modern), only one exhibits the plague motif, i.e., "Turkish 1," "The Sultan's Son," p. 36.

[29] Biraben, *Les hommes et la peste*, 30, penultimate and antepenultimate entries.

[30] *Liber Historiae Francorum* 44, p. 316: *Eo tempore Chlodoveus brachium beati Dionisii martyris abscidit, instigante diabulo. Per id tempus concidit regnum Francorum casibus pestiferis. Fuit autem ipse Chlodoveus omne spurcicia deditus, fornicarius et inlusor feminarum, gulae et ebrietate contentus. Huius mortem et finem nihil dignum historiae recolit. Multa enim scriptores eius finem condempnant; nescientes finem nequitiae eius, in incertum de eo alia pro aliis referunt.* I have emended Gerberding's translation, *Rise of the Carolingians*, 175. I disagree in particular with his rendering of *casibus pestiferis*, "disastrous circumstances": though *pestifer* may indeed mean "disastrous," its other, narrower acceptation seems preferable in this context. The *LHF* is from the first half of the eighth century. Gerberding, it should be noted, is not interested in the Justinianic Plague and may even be unaware of its existence.

If the end of an epidemic could boost a new dynasty's claims to legitimacy, as seems to have been the case with the Islamic Abbasids in the mid-eighth century,[31] conversely, the outbreak on a large scale of just such a life-threatening malady might have the opposite, destabilizing effect. The early Capetians found themselves in precisely this situation. Flodoard's account, quoted above, shows Hugues Capet's father assisting the victims of ergotsim – known locally as "mal Notre-Dame"[32] – in its incipient stages. Hugues Capet's first and third successors, his son Robert II and his great-grandson Philip I, fell out with the Church over their marriages, which were deemed incestuous according to canon law and publicly branded as such.[33] It is surely no coincidence that precisely these kings are the first to have purportedly possessed the much-celebrated miraculous healing powers[34] that would soon become a major constituent of the dynasty's hallowed status, displayed on solemn occasions from the thirteenth to the eighteenth century. These preternatural faculties were not primarily, as is so often alleged, a political prop designed to enhance the sovereign's weak position vis-à-vis the much more powerful territorial princes, but a clever rebuttal of popular finger-pointing. A thaumaturgic king could not possibly bring death and desolation to his people. In the same way, Mallory's (admittedly much later) Lancelot, after failing in the quest for the Grail on account of his adulterous affair with Queen Guinevere, manages to salvage his reputation as "noblest knight of the land" by means of a healing miracle, performed to the benefit of Sir Urry.[35] The Capetians soon had rivals in this unusual sphere, for the kings of England claimed to be similarly endowed. The earliest text to say so unambiguously dates to the late twelfth century and has them healing not only scrofula, like their French counterparts, but also, more intriguingly, *pestis inguinaria*, bubonic plague!

I believe that it is a sacred duty to assist the lord king, for he is the Lord's anointed and, as such, he is sacred. It is not in vain that he received the sacrament of royal

---

[31] Conrad, "Epidemic Disease in Central Syria," 20, n. 28.

[32] Bauer, *Das Antonius-Feuer*, 19, quoting Henri de Mondeville, Philip the Fair's surgeon. No doubt the emergence of ergotism was linked to the rather sudden increase in production of rye, which, up to the tenth century had represented a negligible fraction of the grain crop of Western Europe. On cereal output in the early Middle Ages, see Devroey, *Economie rurale*, 1:104–5.

[33] Barthélemy, *L'ordre seigneurial*, p. 82.

[34] Robert: Helgaud de Fleury, *Epitoma Vitae regis Rotberti Pii* 27, pp. 128–29. Philip: Guibert de Nogent, *De sanctis et eorum pigneribus*, 1, lines 157 to 166, p. 90.

[35] Thomas Mallory (†1471), *The Book of Sir Launcelot and Queen Guinevere*, chapter 5, pp. 663–69.

unction, whose efficiency, were it not known or were it put in doubt, would be amply attested by the cessation of the inguinary plague and by the healing of scrofula.[36]

By virtue of its very anachronism – *pestis inguinaria* disappeared from western Europe c. 750 – this reference ceases to be an insoluble enigma,[37] and adds fuel instead to the present argument. The English evidence shows more clearly even than the French that the royal touch is a response to the age-old suspicion that first attached to Œdipus. Or it could be that what Peter of Blois means is not that the sacred rite of unction has rendered the reigning king of the moment, *Henry II*, capable of vanquishing *the plague*, but that, having indeed produced this remarkable effect at some unspecified time in the past through the agency of an unnamed king, there was no reason to doubt that it might easily impart potency over a lesser complaint such as scrofula to Peter's Plantagenet lord. The "unnamed king" Peter has in mind would have to be Pippin the Short, for it is he who was reigning when the Justinianic Plague finally ran its course in the West, and he as well who was the first king of the Franks to be anointed.

BISHOPS – *CONSILIA HUMANA*

In the West, as also in Byzantium, bishops had a central role to play in times of plague. Their pastoral duties, the *cura animarum*, would have kept them busier than usual. So too, more surprisingly to the modern mind, the *cura corporum*. Indeed, some practiced medicine themselves,[38] but most, including perhaps Gregory of Tours, would have hired a public

---

[36] Peter of Blois, *Epistolae* 14, in *PL* 207:440D: *Fateor quidem, quod sanctum est domino regi assistere; sanctus enim et christus Domini est: nec in vacuum accepit unctionis regiae sacramentum, cujus efficacia, si nescitur, aut in dubium venit, fidem ejus plenissimam faciet defectus inguinaria pestis, et curatio scrophularum.* Translation and commentary (including verification of the words *inguinaria pestis* against the manuscript tradition): Jacques Le Goff, preface to the 1983 edition of Bloch, *Les Rois thaumaturges*, xiii and footnote 1, and Bloch himself, p. 41.

[37] As in Bloch, *Les Rois thaumaturges*, 41 and Le Goff, ibid., xii–xvi.

[38] T. S. Miller, *Birth of the Hospital*, 57–58, numerous Byzantine instances: Basil of Caesarea in the 4th C., patriarch Photios in the 9th C., etc. A good example from the West is the *Life of S. Brigid of Kildare*, as quoted by Herlihy, *Opera Muliebria*, 29–30, from *Vitae sanctorum Hiberniae*, p. 29: "Though she worked many cures, Brigid was not learned in the medical arts. When she herself developed a severe headache, she went to see a bishop, 'for he both by learning and by practice understood both the types of diseases and their cures.'" In the eighth century, responding to Boniface's inquiries, pope Zachary advises him on matters pertaining to public health (leprosy and rabies): *S. Bonifatii et Lulli epistolae* 87, pp. 197–98.

physician to care for the sick within the confines of the *civitas*. This they did in their capacity as heirs to the late-Roman municipal governments or *curiae*. The institution of the public physician or *archiètros* – a name that applies equally, and somewhat confusingly, to court physicians – was a venerable one, dating back at least to the sixth century BC.[39] It was almost as old, it appears, as professional medicine and the debate over access to care, which it was meant to address. Abuses were frequent, for the appointment brought notoriety and, hence, many opportunities to get rich. It was not until the fourth century AD that gratuity for the *archiètros'* ministrations was passed into law by the first Christian emperors.[40] Several such specialists are attested in sixth-century Gaul, as we shall see, and their continued presence in the Frankish realms ensured that their Greek name found its way into Old High German by the ninth century at the latest: *archiètros* became *arzât*, Modern German *Arzt*.[41]

Leafing through Gregory of Tours' *Histories*, we come across two public physicians (as well as several anonymous court physicians). One, Reovalis, trained in Constantinople, was practicing in Poitiers, probably under the authority of the local bishop. About the other, a certain Marileif, Gregory tells us, first, that he was from the same town, second, that he had originally been in the employ of the church (there or elsewhere, he does not say), third, disapprovingly, that he had been appointed to the court of Chilperic, there to become immensely wealthy and, fourth, with barely contained satisfaction, that having been robbed of his possessions he was forced back into the service of the church. Gregory's interest in this character led me to believe that the church he served was not Poitiers but Tours, that by piecing together these and other shreds of information scattered throughout the contemporary sections of the *History*, it was possible to make out a tug of war between Gregory and Chilperic.[42] Each was trying to hold on to the precious physician or to retrieve him, all the more desperately because of the plague – probably the 588 episode, which we know reached Lyons and may have spread much further, or the previous one, which visited Narbonne and Albi (although, again, it may not have been confined to these localities) in 580, 581, and 582, on the heels of a European-wide epidemic of smallpox (550–580). Chilperic

39 T. S. Miller, *Birth of the Hospital*, 44.

40 Ibid., 44–49 and 72; Stoclet, "Entre Esculape et Marie," 702–3, n. 77.

41 Lloyd and Springer, *Etymologisches Wörterbuch des Althochdeutschen*, 1:358–60; Stoclet, "Entre Esculape et Marie," 702–3, n. 77.

42 Stoclet, "Entre Esculape et Marie," 724. Gregory of Tours, *Historia Francorum* 5.14, 7.25, 10.15, pp. 203, 306, 426.

was acting for his own sake – or so the story goes – Gregory was acting to protect his flock, not against the epidemic, for it could hardly be stopped, but against charlatans whose supposed remedies were far less harmful in his view than the false doctrines that they were wont to spread. One, for instance, Desiderius by name, claimed to be in contact through a messenger with the apostles Peter and Paul, or worse still, to be their equal.[43] Returning to the question of which church Marileif would have served, both before and after his stint at the court, three answers seem possible: Poitiers – likeliest – Tours – doubtful – or both, for, on the face of it and given the circumstances, it would seem rather appropriate that neighboring dioceses should have shared priceless human resources.

Cases that the *archiètros'* scientific or Hippocratic brand of medicine could not cure might be referred to the other division of the "health system," which was also subject to episcopal control and addressed itself less to the flesh than to the psyche. I am referring, of course, to the monasteries, where recovery was besought from the saints – especially, in the Byzantine Empire, from the *anargyroi* or "penniless" saints, a most telling epithet – through rituals of incubation very similar to those that had for many centuries been the hallmark of the sanctuaries of Asklepios.[44] It is possible that, in Gaul as in the East, the Justinianic Plague brought ever-larger crowds to these monastic shrines. To no avail, as Procopius observes.[45]

TALISMANS – *SUPERSTITIO*

Superstitio is in the eye of the beholder. To Livy, reviewing the events of 364 BC, it is a stigma that attaches to non-native novelty in matters of religion or public ritual. To Gregory of Tours, on the contrary, it is the past, in refusing to die, that carries the woeful stain.

In most traditions, talismans are suspect because they are created from inanimate objects in which demons are made to reside through specific manipulations.[46] In the period under consideration, however,

---

[43] Occurrences of the plague, 580–588: Biraben, *Les Hommes et la peste*, 28, 29, 42. Gregory of Tours, *Historia Francorum*, 9.6, p. 361.

[44] Byzantium: T. S. Miller, *Birth of the Hospital*, 62–67. Some pointers concerning the West: Stoclet, "Entre Esculape et Marie," 701–2.

[45] Procopius, *PW* 2.22.11, pp. 454–57.

[46] C. Blum, "Meaning of *stoicheion* and its Derivatives"; Stoclet, "Entre Esculape et Marie," 713–14.

monumental talismans are on conspicuous display in the great cities of
Constantinople and Antioch, which they are supposed to protect from
various nuisances and vermin: snakes, insects, scorpions, and flooding
from the local river.[47] In form and function, the Paris effigies are strikingly similar, but this they may owe less to original intent – about which,
see earlier – than to the interpretation given upon their discovery not by
Gregory himself but, in all likelihood, by his informant, Bishop Eusebius
of Paris, who was, as we know, a Syrian, perhaps from Antioch. These
brazen animals are not said to neutralize the plague, but the disasters
and pests that they do purportedly avert, that is, fire, snakes, and small
rodents, are common enough periphrases for the disease.[48] To Gregory,
they are above all the symbol of perdition, the song of the pagan siren in
the storm of death.

[47] Dagron, *Constantinople imaginaire*, 107–10. A few lines from an article by Andy Newman
in *The New York Times Magazine* of July 30, 2000 attest to the resilience of like customs:
"While most towns try to stamp out their pests, others have embraced them. Hidalgo,
Texas, where killer bees first entered the country, has erected a monument to the yellow
menace."

[48] It grips whole towns in its flames, Livy 10. 47, and see Kerenyi, *Der göttliche Arzt*, 4.
Ancient medicine recommends using fire to disperse the miasmas from which the plague
is thought to arise, and this is precisely what the sixth-century inhabitants of Sens do,
Biraben, *Les hommes et la peste*, 46 and n. 29. Fire is also, as it were, the cradle of Asklepios: Apollo rescues his son from the womb of Coronis, his unfaithful wife, whom he has
sentenced to die at the stake.

Procopius follows Hippocrates in stating that the plague "is caused by a venom that
corrupts the air," according to Biraben, *Les hommes et la peste*, 46. Gregory of Tours, *Historia Francorum* 4.31, p. 168 compares the open sores or bubos whereby the infection
becomes visible to a snake's bite, and the vector of the fatal illness to venom.

Equating rats and plague is contingent upon the knowledge that the former carry
the latter. It is by no means certain that such a knowledge obtained throughout the long
history of mankind's confrontation with the pestilence. Few texts are as wonderfully
explicit as 1 Kings 6:4–5, where the Philistines are told that their afflictions will cease
once they have returned the Ark of the Covenant to its lawful owners and as soon, furthermore, as they have dedicated to the god of Israel golden images of their tumors and
of the "mice" that ravage their land (see Gregoire et al., *Asklèpios, Apollon Smintheus
et Rudra*, 168–71). Strabo, in the first century BC, certainly made the connection
(*Geography*, 3, 4, 18), as MacArthur, "Identification of Some Pestilences," 170, n. 2,
observes. Gods of the plague, which they both cause and cure (Gregoire et al., *Asklèpios,
Apollon Smintheus et Rudra*, 165–68), Apollo and Asklepios "are" rodents: Smintheus, one
of Apollo's epithets, means "mouse," and the name Asklepios is related etymologically to
the word for "mole." The mouse, or rat, or mole is their attribute, as is a small cone, often
interpreted as an *omphalos*, more convincingly as a molehill or as the molehill-shaped *tho-
los*, the central feature of Asklepios' sanctuary at Epidauros, but which, bearing 1 Kings
6 in mind, could equally represent a bubo (Gregoire et al., *Asklèpios, Apollon Smintheus et
Rudra*, 171, n. 1, after Krappe, "Apollon Σμίνθεύς," 40–56). Immunity from plague, (acci-
dental) fire, and rats is granted by St. Columba or Colum Cille: Picard, "Adomnán's Vita
Columbae," 17–20.

APPENDIX

Beowulf, ll. 166b–67, 170–88 (see note 2)
[Grendel] occupied Heorot, the jewel-adorned hall, in the dark
nights. [...] That was a great misery and heartbreak for the
Scyldings' friend. Many a powerful man often sat in council,
sought a plan, what action would be best for a stout-hearted man to
take against the terror of sudden onslaught. At times they vowed at
heathen temples hommage to idols, asked in words that the spirit-
slayer grant them succor against their dire distress. Such was their
custom, the hope of heathens: they recalled hell in their hearts.
They did not know the Creator, the Judge of deeds, nor did they
recognize the Lord God, nor truly did they know how to praise the
Protector of the Heavens, the Ruler of Glory. It shall be woe for
the one who must through cruel enmity thrust his soul into the
fire's embrace, not hope for comfort, or any change; it shall be
well for the one who may seek the Lord after his death-day, and
ask for protection in the father's embrace.[49]

[49] *Beowulf,* ll. 166b–67, trans. Liuzza, 58; ll. 170–74, trans. Swanton, 43; ll. 175–88, trans.
Orchard, *Critical Companion,* 152.

8

Plague in Spanish Late Antiquity

Michael Kulikowski

As with so much of Spanish history in Late Antiquity, tracing the Justinianic Plague in Spain is a matter of guesswork and extrapolation from a very small body of evidence. The amount of evidence at our disposal has expanded dramatically in recent years because of improvements in the quality and quantity of Spanish archaeological research.[1] Reliable archaeological data is now much more plentiful than is the evidence of more traditional historical sources. One might therefore expect the archaeological record to shed light on plague in sixth- and seventh-century Spain, and it does seem to do so. We must, however, begin from the literary sources for the plague in Spain for a simple methodological reason: Nothing in the material record unambiguously demonstrates the existence of plague in late antique Spain. The literary evidence, by contrast, states explicitly that the peninsula was struck by the plague of 541–543, and that during the next century and a half there were at least three further outbreaks.[2] We must in consequence begin from these explicit attestations of plague and then move on to other sorts of evidence that might bear some relationship to them.

We have only a single literary source for the initial outbreak of the Justinianic Plague in Spain, an anonymous Spanish annotator whose marginal notations are traditionally referred to as the *Chronicle of Zaragoza*. That title is a misnomer, as the so-called chronicle is in fact a set of

---

[1] Short introduction to the topic in Kulikowski, "Interdependence of Town and Country"; a larger discussion of the evidence in Kulikowski, *Late Roman Spain*.

[2] References to all the literary evidence are collected in García Moreno, *El fin del reino visigodo de Toledo*, 52–53, 112–115, though it misses the Toledo homiliary discussed next.

annotations on the chronicle of Victor of Tunnuna and his Spanish continuator John of Biclar and was never transmitted separately from them.[3] The Spanish annotator had Victor's important statement about the plague before him when he wrote, and to it he added a statement to the effect that *his diebus inguinalis plaga totam paene contrivit Hispaniam*.[4] Because of difficulties in the chronology of both Victor and the Spanish annotator, it is unclear whether plague struck Spain along with the eastern Mediterranean in 542 or only in the following year, 543, when plague is first attested in Italy.[5] General consideration of the extensive mercantile ties between the Greek East and Spain's main port cities would suggest that plague struck Spain before the end of the sailing season in 542, but there is no way to be certain.[6] The effects of the outbreak are not

[3] Mommsen confused the issue by editing the annotations as a separate chronicle in *MGH, AA* 11, following the suggestion of Hertzberg, *Die Historien und die Chroniken des Isidorus*, that it represented the lost work of Maximus of Zaragoza. Collins, "Isidore, Maximus and the *Historia Gothorum*," proved that this was impossible in terms of both genre and content, and the text has now been re-edited by C. Cardelle de Hartmann under the title *Consularia Caesaraugustana*, alongside the chronicles of Victor and John: see *Victoris Tunnunensis Chronicon*. This edition, based on new manuscript work, supercedes not only Mommsen's, but also the more recent separate editions of Victor: *Vittore da Tunnuna: Chronica*, and John: *Juan de Biclaro obispo de Gerona*.

[4] *Consularia Caesaraugustana*, ad a. p.c. Basili II, in *Victoris Tunnunensis Chronicon*, p. 44, where the editor assigns a date of AD 542 to the consular entry. This follows, and may indeed be based on, Victor's entry for that year: *Horum exordia malorum generalis orbis terrarum mortalitas sequitur et inguinum percussione melior pars populorum vexatur* (ibid., p. 43).

[5] Printed editions confidently assign *anno domini* dates to the entries of Victor and John, and by association those of the Spanish annotator as well, but the chronologies of both authors are actually quite problematical. There were gaps in the consular *fasti* from which Victor worked, and he omitted eight years from his chronology altogether (viz., 445, 452, 472, 478, 481, 493, 503, 547). Victor's dates are thus subject to dispute in and of themselves; it is, for instance, unclear whether Victor thought he was dating the outbreak of plague to 542 or 543. Still more worrying is the fact that our Spanish annotator was quite unaware of the flaws in Victor's chronology. We do not know what independent chronological framework he worked from, and we do not how he correlated this framework to the chronology he found in Victor. To make matters worse, where we can check his chronology against independent sources, our annotator is almost invariably wrong.

[6] Mercantile ties between the East and parts of Spain, particularly the Guadiana and Guadalquivir valleys and the cities of Catalonia and the Levant, remained quite intense until the 550s and 560s, or so the distribution of ceramics would seem to suggest. Regardless of the precise course of its progress, the plague struck Constantinople in May of 542 (Stein, *Histoire du Bas-Empire*, 2: 759–60), which is to say right in the middle of the year's sailing season (on which see Casson, *Ships and Seamanship*, 270–72, with the exceptions to this general rule tabulated in Saint-Denis, "Mare clausum," and Rougé, "La navigation hivernale sous l'Empire romain.") Given that, it would be rather surprising if plague had not reached Spanish port cities some time before October of 542. On the other hand,

accessible to us from the literary sources, but two sites do provide archaeological evidence that might reasonably be attributed to plague.

The most impressive of these is Valencia, the Roman city of Valentia.[7]
Situated in the Spanish Levant, Valencia was one of several eastern cities
in constant contact with both North Africa and the eastern provinces of
the empire. These ties were chiefly economic, and their continuation
into the first half of the sixth century is documented by the quantity of
ceramic remains at Valencia and nearby sites. Valencia differs from other
big Spanish cities in having adopted the practice of intramural burial
very early. In most of the peninsula, the Roman prohibition on intramural burial was observed until the later sixth or the seventh century. At
Valencia, however, we can document intramural burials from the later
fifth century at two separate urban excavations that lie very near to one
another in the Calle del Mar and the Plaza de Almoina. Both sites lie above
what had been the heart of the Roman city, including the forum in which
the Diocletianic martyr Vincent was thought to have been condemned. It
is likely that some sort of martyrial monument prompted the creation of
Valencia's urban cemetery, although the extant remains of a late antique
basilica are certainly later than the earliest burials.[8] These began as a
series of low-status burials from the late fifth century, while in the late
sixth or the seventh century, a series of higher status burials in well-built
mausolea occupied a large section of the Plaza. It is, however, a series
of burials intermediate in date that concerns us here. Several collective
graves, dug in ditches with no attempt at organization and no detectable
funerary rite except for an attempt to orientate the cadavers from east
to west, can probably be dated to the middle parts of the sixth century.
One such grave, located in the Calle del Mar, held the remains of at least
eleven individuals. Two mass inhumations from the Plaza de Almoina held
five and fourteen bodies, respectively.[9] Although there are no probative

Greek armies were engaged in a grueling Italian war in precisely these years, and plague
appears not to be attested in Italy before 543 (Marcellinus Comes, *Chronikon*, s.a. 543),
which suggests that we cannot press our inferences about the Spanish situation too far.

[7] See in general Ribera and Soriano, "Enterramientos de la Antigüedad tardía"; Soriano,
La arqueología cristiana; Escrivá and Soriano, "El área episcopal de Valentia"; Escrivá and
Soriano, "El área cementerial"; Soriano, "Las excavaciones arqueológicas"; Soriano, "Los
restos arqueológicos"; Soriano, *Cripta arqueológica*; Marín, Piá, and Rosselló, *El foro romano*;
Marín, et al., *L'Almoina*; Ribera and Rosselló, *L'Almoina*; Albiach, et al., "Las últimas
excavaciones."

[8] Albiach, et al., "Las últimas excavaciones," corrects earlier chronological assumptions.

[9] For the Calle del Mar: Ribera and Soriano, "Enterramientos de la Antigüedad tardía,"
153–60. For the Plaza de Almoina: Escrivá and Soriano, "El área episcopal de Valentia,"
349; Albiach, et al., "Las últimas excavaciones" refrains from comment.

grounds for associating these collective burials with plague victims, the ceramic evidence for a mid-sixth-century date and the extreme disorder of the bodies within their simple graves offer strong circumstantial grounds for thinking that the thirty or so Valentians deposited in these simple ditches died of plague. One other site allows for similar inferences. At the cemetery of San Antón, which lay along the chief road north out of Carthago Nova, modern Cartagena, there is a great density of burial from a concentrated period in the first half of the sixth century. To the site's excavators, this suggests some connection to epidemic mortality, although we must note that the typology of the graves at Cartagena is conventional and deliberate, unlike the ditch burials at Valencia.[10]

For recurrences of the plague, we have once again to fall back on literary evidence. The plague is likely to have struck Spain again in 584, at the same time as it did Narbonne and Albi, inasmuch as both cities lay within the Gothic kingdom in those years.[11] The plague that attacked Marseilles in 588 certainly did affect Spain, given that Gregory of Tours reports its having reached the Gallic city from Spanish ports.[12] According to Gregory, a Spanish merchant had brought the disease to Marseilles along with his cargo, and the city as a whole was rapidly infected. Spain's Mediterranean trade had shrunk to a small trickle by the 580s, so it is likely that Gregory's ship worked the cabotage routes between Catalonia and Narbonensis. Indeed, Gothic Narbonensis may have remained peculiarly subject to the disease, given that when we next have evidence for plague it is likewise concentrated in the Gallic part of the Gothic kingdom.

The Mozarabic chronicle of 754 records that, during the reign of King Egica (687–702), the kingdom was struck by bubonic plague: *plaga insuper inuinalis huius tempore inmisericorditer inlavitur.*[13] The anonymous chronicler is imprecise about the date of the outbreak, but contemporary ecclesiastical documents allow for greater precision. In the royal law with which he confirmed the acts of the sixteenth council of Toledo,

[10] Berrocal and Laiz, "Tipología de enterramientos."
[11] The evidence is Gregory of Tours, *Historia Francorum* 6.33, pp. 273–74: *"Per loca enim lues vastabat sed maximae apud urbem Narbonensim validius desaeviebat et iam tertio anno quod ibidem adpraehenderat et requieverat; populique revertentes a fuga, iterum morbo consumpti sunt. Nam et Albigensis civitas maximae ab hoc inquomodo laborabat."* This does not make any specific reference to plague in the Iberian portion of the Gothic kingdom but does state that Carpetania – the part of the old Roman province of Carthaginiensis that fell within the Visigothic kingdom – had been devastated by locusts.
[12] Gregory of Tours, *Historia Francorum* 9.22, p. 380: *"Nam superius diximus, Massiliensis urbis contagio pessimo aegrota quanta sustenuerit, altius replecare placuit ... Interea navis ab Hispania una cum negotio solito ad portum eius adpulsa est, qui huius morbi fomitem secum nequiter deferebat."*
[13] *Cronica Mozárabe de 754* 41, p. 58.

Egica stated that the bishops of Narbonensis had been unable to travel to Toledo because of the outbreak of bubonic plague; he therefore ordered them to hold a local synod at Narbonne and there subscribe to the written record of the Toledan council.[14] The year was 693. At the seventeenth council of Toledo, held in the following year to intensify the royal campaign against Spanish Jews, Egica had again to make special arrangements for Narbonensis, exempting Narbonensian Jews from enslavement on the grounds that the region was already almost depopulated because of foreign invaders and the bubonic plague.[15] This outbreak under Egica seems to have been followed rapidly by another recurrence. An Arabic source, the *Akhbar Majmu'a*, records that plague and famine destroyed half the population of Spain between 707 and 709, just two years before the Arab conquest of 711.[16] The text is quite late, dating from the eleventh century, but if we accept its testimony, it would seem that plague had become endemic in the peninsula by the second half of the seventh century.

The problem with such a statement lies in epidemiology. Endemic plague is a density-dependent disease and the population of Spain was simply too small, even in the largest cities, for a density-dependent disease to reproduce itself endemically.[17] The peak of Spain's Roman population has been estimated at between five and ten million, and the third and fourth centuries had almost certainly been a period of demographic expansion, inasmuch as a great deal of land that had been uncultivated in the early empire was brought under the plough between 200 and 400.[18]

---

[14] XVI Toledo. *Lex edita in confirm.* (*Concilios visigóticos*, 515–16): *"Et quia ingruente inguinalis plaguae vastatione ad Narbonensem sedem pertinentes episcopi nequaquam sunt in hac sancta synodo adgregati, ideo per hanc nostrae mansuetudinis legem instituentes iubemus, ut omnes ad eiusdem cathedrae [diocesim] pertinentes episcopi in eadem urbe Narbona cum suo metropolitano adunentur et cunctis huius concilii capitulis vigilaci ab eis indagatione perlectis accedant ordinibus debitis subscriptores."*

[15] XVII Toledo. *Tomus regis*: *"... illis tantumdem hebraeis ad presens reservatis qui Galliae provinciae videlicte infra clausuras noscuntur habitatores existere vel ad ducatum regionis ipsius pertinere, ut quia delictis ingruentibus et externae gentis incursu et plagae inguinalis interitu pars ipsa ab hominibus desolata dinoscitur (Concilios visigóticos, 525)."*

[16] The *Akhbar Majmu'a* records that in the years 88, 89, and 90 of the *hijra*, Spain was struck by a plague that destroyed more than half the population. See *Ajbar Machmuâ*.

[17] Sallares, *Ecology of the Ancient Greek World*, 221–93, for epidemiology, with 262–70 on plague.

[18] The pioneering work of Fernández Corrales, *El asentamiento romano*, on the spatial analysis of ancient settlement in Extremadura has revolutionized our understanding of the distribution of ancient population. Although confined to a single modern Spanish *autonomía*, Fernández's results are borne out in a variety of more restricted contexts: Aguilar et al., "La ciudad antigua de Lacimurga"; Reynolds, *Settlement and Pottery*; Gómez Santa Cruz, "Aproximación al poblamiento rural hispano-romano"; González Conde, *Romanidad e indigenismo*; Salinas de Frías, "El poblamiento rural antiguo."

The chronic instability of the fifth century is likely to have arrested population growth, even if it did not precipitate any major demographic crisis. By the first decades of the sixth century, one can perceive the gradual fading of late Roman villa culture and a substantial decline in the number of known rural sites.[19] In part, this impression reflects methodological problems in detecting sixth- and seventh-century sites, but the collapse in numbers is dramatic enough to suggest a genuine demographic decline by the start of the sixth century. Even at its peak, however, the Spanish population was not large enough to sustain density-dependent diseases endemically. Outbreaks would therefore depend upon constant reintroduction of infection from outside the peninsula. That epidemiological conclusion might seem to be borne out by the explicit attestations of plague in late antique Spain, which, as we have seen, document at most four separate outbreaks.

Yet one underexploited literary source does suggest a more constant presence of plague in seventh-century Spain.[20] This is a Toledan homiliary of the seventh century, which survives in an eleventh-century manuscript from the monastery of Silos.[21] Among 118 homilies from a wide variety of patristic sources, four unique sermons treat the progress of plague toward a city and the responses that it behooves Christians to take in the face of it.[22] In the first sermon, the preacher tells his congregation that the plague is approaching from afar. What has hitherto remained in the distance is now approaching, and God's wrath is its cause.[23]

---

[19] The corpus of Roman villas by Gorges, *Les villas hispano-romaines*, is now badly out of date, and the dating of many of the sites listed in it has been substantially revised in recent years. For patterns of rural population, see the works cited in note 18, as well as the results of the Ager Tarraconensis survey in Carreté et al., *A Roman Provincial Capital and Its Hinterland*.

[20] The text is virtually unused, cited in Orlandis, *Historia del reino visigodo español*, 214, with no consideration of its implications, summarized in Orlandis, "Homilías visigóticas de Clade," and missed in García Moreno, *El fin del reino visigodo de Toledo*.

[21] Now located in London, British Library, Add. 30,853. First treated in Morin, *Liber comicus*, 406–25, its contents are inventoried in Grégoire, *Les homéliaires du Moyen Âge*, 161–85, with an edition of the otherwise unpublished sermons at 197–230.

[22] These four homilies appear in an English translation by Anna Langenwalter in an appendix to this essay.

[23] *Sermo* 57, *de clade*, lines 1–8. (Grégoire, *Les homéliaires du Moyen Âge*, 214): "*Ecce, dilectissimi fratres, luctuosa nos perterruit nuntiorum relatio quae fines terrae nostrae infestos pestilentia narrat, quae vicinam nobis cruentam mortem insinuat. Inguinalis etenim pestilentiae plaga que hucusque a longe nobis et nuntiata peccatis nostris ingruentibus iam vicinat. Iam etenim terrae nostrae depopulat et que longe a nostris finibus eferbebat praeproperis gressibus adpropinquat. Ecce quae a longe audivimus, iam prope facta sunt nobis.* Ibid., lines 18–19: *Exurgite, rogo, exurgite a somno corporis et preparate vos ad vincendum divine animadversionis iram.*"

It comes to urge repentance on the reprobate congregation, and the sermon gives us the words in which reprieve is to be sought: "Tibi, domine, peccavimus...Remobe iam a nostris finibus plagam. Lues inminentis plage dispereat, mucro pestilentie seviens et in his quibus grassatur deficiat et ad nos te propitiante non transeant." The second sermon preaches true conversion of the heart as the only adequate response to the plague, and the third urges the congregation simply not to carry on in its iniquity if God should chance to spare them the plague's visitation. The fourth returns to the theme of penitence and chastisement.

The question, of course, is whether we can take this set of plague homilies as evidence for the general prevalence of plague in seventh-century Spain, or whether they are an artefact of a single outbreak, included in the Toledo homiliary for literary reasons. The latter option might appear to have a certain plausibility, insofar as homiliaries are compilatory works. On the other hand, homiliaries do tend to be compiled with a utilitarian end in view, and this was certainly the case with our Toledo homiliary. Its sermons were selected for practical use across the liturgical year, with no repetition of occasions. Moreover, many sermons, the plague cycle among them, are clunky and pedestrian beside the Caesarian and Augustinian homilies that surround them and are thus unlikely to have been selected solely for their literary merits. From these indications, we should probably conclude that the plague sermons were included in the Toledo homiliary because they were expected to be needed – that, some time in the course of his career, the homiliary's compiler expected to need to admonish his flock in the face of impending bubonic plague. That, in turn, suggests that plague, and the expectation of its visitations, had become an established part of life in seventh-century Spain.

Our consideration of the Toledo homiliary nearly exhausts the positive evidence for plague in Spanish Late Antiquity.[24] Only a single epitaph from the period attests to death from plague.[25] We must next ask whether any sixth- and seventh-century historical developments might bear a relationship to the plague and its impact. Such speculation is problematic when working from as small an evidentiary basis as we are constrained to do. Nevertheless, there are a number of historical changes

---

[24] It is sometimes said that the Gothic capital at Toledo was stricken in 573, e.g., Orlandis, *Historia del reino visigodo español*, 214, on the basis of John of Biclar, ad a. VII Iustini/V Leovigildi: *"In regia urbe mortalitas inguinalis plagae exardescit in qua multa milia hominum vidimus defecisse."* This is, however, a reference to an outbreak in Constantinople, where John was a resident at the time of the outbreak.

[25] *Corpus Inscriptionum Latinarum* 2/7:667: *"ab inguina/li plaga o/biit er/a DC/XLVII"* (i.e., AD 609).

that do seem to bear the imprint of the plague. In economic terms, the later sixth century witnessed the rapid acceleration of trends that had existed since the later fifth century. In particular, we may note the effective ending of regular commerce between Africa and Spain by the 560s, as witnessed by the almost total absence of African fine ware from Spanish sites after those dates. This change affected the whole of the peninsula, including the most accessible maritime and fluvial ports, and even those that lay within the areas occupied by Byzantine armies after 552. With this decline of African imports, coastal towns now conformed to a pattern that had begun at interior sites by the middle of the fifth century. The rhythm of trade with the eastern empire, which had been vigorous right into the first half of the sixth century, likewise slowed dramatically in the second half, trickling to a halt some time early in the seventh century. Again, it is striking to note that the Byzantine province in southeastern Spain fared no better than did the rest of the peninsula. Carthago Nova itself was the only partial exception to this rule.[26]

Evidence for trade between Gaul and Spain is less good because the typologies of south Gallic ceramics are less developed than are those of Africa and the East. On the other hand, there is some evidence that the flourishing late Roman towns along the coast of Biscay, as well as those in the Ebro Valley, experienced similar declines in imports. In other words, the second half of the sixth century seems to have witnessed a very general contraction of wealth throughout Spain. Because this contraction is so general, and is not obviously linked to any of the political upheavals that affected the peninsula in our period, one is tempted to interpret it in terms of larger economic or demographic problems. Perhaps part of the reason for the decline in Spain's capacity to absorb imports was the death of a substantial part of the surviving market for imports, a market that existed in precisely those coastal and fluvial cities that were most likely to have had the earliest and harshest experience of plague.

Another consequence of demographic change that is probably connected to the impact of plague is the disruption of the rural labor force. In the last decades of the Gothic kingdom, we find a large number of laws regulating rural labor, and particularly servile labor.[27] Under Kings

---

[26] The findings of Reynolds, *Settlement and Pottery*, have been confirmed by more recent specialist work.

[27] Because the shape of Visigothic law before the mid-seventh century is a matter of intense controversy, and because the attribution of earlier laws to their correct era of promulgation is difficult, one cannot use the texts from before the 640s with any confidence; only the seventh-century laws of Chindasuinth, Reccesuinth, Ervig, and Egica can be placed in a firm chronological context and used as evidence accordingly.

Ervig and Egica, a great deal of effort was expended in attempts to ensure
that slaves stayed bound to the land, that those who were so bound produced the maximum amount that could be extracted from them, and
that landlords who harbored runaways for their own purposes suffered
appropriate chastisement.[28] There was, evidently, a severe labor shortage,
which the kings tried futilely to correct through compulsion. Whether the
scarcity of rural labor was the result of plague or other demographic crisis
is impossible to say, but plague must certainly have played some role. If
nothing else, it will have severely exacerbated the effects of the famines
that are known to have preceded the plagues of the late seventh and early
eighth centuries.[29]

We are unlikely ever to know the full extent of sixth- and seventh-
century mortality in Spain, irrespective of its causes.[30] We can, however,
detect changes to the way in which the living related to the dead that are
likely to be the result of the high mortality associated with plague. The
process by which death came to be Christianized during Late Antiquity
is well studied, and in Spain the growth of specifically Christian burial
sites is detectable archaeologically from the beginning of the fourth century. On the whole, the Spanish population took a very long time to
alter its late Roman funerary habits. With only the rare exception like
Valencia, the practice of extramural burial was maintained until the late
sixth century, while at important cities like Tarragona and Ampurias, it
was maintained until after the Arab conquest.[31] The typological range
of late Roman burials was likewise maintained very consistently until the
later sixth century, by which point most of the more complicated forms of

---

[28] See especially *Leges visigothorum* 9.1.6; 9.1.9; 9.1.12; 9.1.16; 9.1.21. Of these, the most
significant is 9.1.9.

[29] For the famines, *Cronica Mozárabe de 754* 41, p. 58: "*plaga insuper inguinalis huius tempore
inmisericorditer inlauitur.*"

[30] Neither do we have much idea of the main causes of mortality because of the absence
of biomedical studies on human remains from late antique Spain. Such palaeoanthro-
pological work as has been done suggests that the laboring population, both male and
female, tended to die before reaching forty, suffering from arthritis and with teeth badly
decayed from a diet of very hard grains, while women were disproportionately likely to
die during their child-bearing years. Sites where serious work has been done on excavated human remains include the Parc de la Ciutat at Tarragona, on which see TED'A,
Els enterraments del Parc de la Ciutat, a small portion of the enormous late antique cemetery of Tarraco excavated and largely destroyed in the 1920s and 1930s, on which see
del Amo, *Estudio crítico de la necrópolis paleocristiana*; and the rural cemetery of Goges
on the River Ter not far from Girona, on which see Agustí et al., "La necrópolis de les
Goges." Valuable, though unsystematic, evidence is available from Toledo (Rojas and
Villa, "Consejería de Obras Públicas.")

[31] In general, Kulikowski, *Late Roman Spain*, 232, with references.

deposition – under *tegulae,* in marble or lead sarcophagi, or in graves shaped out of marble slabs – disappeared. It seems likely that plague acted as a powerful solvent of old burial habits, if for no other reason than the scale of death in a short space of time. In such circumstances, the old distinction between an intramural world of the living and a sub-urban world of the dead may have become much less important.

Another change in the relationship between the dead and the living that may be tied to the effects of plague is the increasing acceptance of multiple burials, not the elaborate familial mausolea that had been a feature of elite Roman burials, but rather the consecutive burial of many bodies in single graves, or the simultaneous burial of more than one body in a larger grave. Such burial customs, very hard to document before the sixth century, gradually came to be quite normal. A parallel development is the regular superimposition of new burials on top of old ones. In ear-lier times, it was not unusual for one burial to bite into another one more or less by accident, but from the later sixth century, the consecutive deposition of many individuals in the same grave is frequent.[32] At Santa Eulalia in Mérida, some graves appear to have received as many as eight occupants over the years.[33] Both of these changes represent a real trans-formation away from Roman habits and values, and a corollary of them was an increased tolerance for the physical intrusion of the dead upon the living. Mausolea built entirely above ground, and exposed ossuaries in churches, are impossible to document before the middle of the sixth century, not at all uncommon thereafter. In the same way, above-ground tombs unsealed with mortar or plaster are documented for the first time after the plague years, and their mode of construction implies a tolerance for the sites and smells of decomposition entirely absent in the Spanish past.

There are undoubtedly other aspects of Spanish social history that one might relate to plague, although the changing attitude toward the physi-cal presence of the dead is probably the most striking. Some episodes of peninsular politics may likewise have been shaped by the plague, although here connections become more tenuous. Nevertheless, it is a noteworthy coincidence that two of the worst crises within the ruling elite of the Goths came shortly after outbreaks of plague. Some have gone so far as to suggest that the manifold effects of plague were the single most

---

[32] Serrano and Alijo, "Una necrópolis de época hispano-visigoda" for a case at Peñarrubia (Málaga).

[33] Mateos, *La basílica de Santa Eulalia.*

important factor in the collapse of the Gothic kingdom.[34] So sweeping
a generalization is probably unwarranted, but as our short survey of the
evidence shows, one cannot doubt the importance of plague to Spanish
Late Antiquity. The positive evidence is limited, certainly not enough to
allow us to assess the relative impact of plague on Spain by comparison
to other parts of the western Mediterranean world. But it is clear that
plague was a decisive stimulus in the transition from Spain's fundamen-
tally Roman Late Antiquity to its new and more limited horizons in the
early Middle Ages.

APPENDIX: FOUR ANONYMOUS SERMONS ON THE PLAGUE
FROM THE TOLEDO HOMILIARY

Translated by Anna Langenwalter, University of Toronto

A Sermon on the Catastrophe, to be Read
on the First Day (Grégoire, *Les homéliaires*, 214–17)

Behold, most beloved brothers, the mournful tale of the messengers terrifies us, as it describes the borders of our land afflicted with pestilence,
and introduces bloody death as our neighbor. For the groin wound of
the pestilence, which before was far from us and was announced for our
sins, now draws near. For it now depopulates our land, and that which
seethed far from our borders approaches with quick steps. Behold, things
that we have heard from afar have now drawn close to us. Therefore, and
according to the words of the prophet, I can see the sentence of divine
judgment looming over us, and I am compelled to rouse you from bodily
sleep. *Thus says the Lord God: One affliction, behold an affliction comes. The
end comes, the end comes, and it will keep watch against you. Behold, contrition
comes over you who live in the land. The time comes. The day of slaughter, not of
glory, is near.*[35] And again through the prophet Amos: *Thus says the Lord of
Hosts: In every street there shall be wailing, and in all places that are without, they
shall say: Woe! Woe! And they shall call the farmer to mourning and those who
are skilful in lamentation to lament.*[36] These are the words of the prophet
admonishing you.

Awake, I beg you! Awake from the sleep of the body and prepare
yourselves to conquer the anger of divine punishment. May the sleep fly

[34] Suggested, but undeveloped, by King, *Law and Society*, 170.
[35] Ez. 7:5–7.
[36] Amos 5:16

from your eyes, the torpor from your souls. May levity retreat, may joy flee. Let sadness alone possess your hearts, for behold, the fury of the wrath of God crashes upon us, for funebrial death now assaults our thresholds.

But perhaps, beseeching, we say: "Why should these judgments of God weigh upon us?" And you want to know why these evils should rage violently on us. Hear the prophet: *Because your land is full with the judgment of blood, your cities filled with iniquity, and because you accuse the stranger falsely.*[37] For these things the voices of all the prophets likewise accuse us. *Whereupon*, says the Lord, *I also have given you dullness of teeth in all your cities, and want of bread in all your places.*[38] Behold as, in the terror of sinners, we now hear the words of the prophets accusing us: *The joy of our hearts has ceased, our dancing is turned into mourning. The crown is fallen from our head. Woe to us, because we have sinned.*[39] What, I ask, can we now do to escape the ruin of so great a calamity, to appease God's anger? We take fright at diseases; let us request medicines. Pay attention, therefore, to the counsels of angels and seek out the remedies of the prophets. For the angel speaking to Tobit said: *Prayer is good with fasting and alms: for alms deliver from death and purge away sins and make to find everlasting life.*[40] Behold the counsel of angels, which frees from death the souls of the people. Attend, now, to what the counsels of prophets instruct for the cure of sins. For thus is it enjoined by the Lord through the prophet Jeremiah: *I will suddenly speak against a nation and against a kingdom, to root out, and to pull down, and to destroy it. If that nation against which I have spoken shall repent from its evil, I also will repent of the evil that I thought to do to it.*[41]

Behold I, unworthy minister of God's word, examine the angelic and prophetic counsels for you, and I see nothing better to persuade you than that we should change for the better, if we wish to alter the sentence of God. Let us come in tears to Him who, by frightening us, awaits our prayers. Before the blow is struck, let us anticipate Him who terrifies us completely with the deadly report, lest He strike; let us anticipate Him who mercifully waits for us to turn to Him, before He cuts us off by the judgment of His vengeance. Now, therefore, pour forth your confession of sins and do penance. I say to you, do penance; that is, make worthy fruits of penance, that each may drink the tears of his compunction just

[37] Cf. Ez. 7:23, 22:7
[38] Amos 4:6.
[39] Lament. 5:15–16.
[40] Tob. 12:8–9.
[41] Jer. 18:7–8.

as he remembers having been thirsty through guilt; and inasmuch as anyone sees that he has fallen on account of what is prohibited, so much the
more should he be eager to restrain himself from what is permitted. For
what is to do penance except to punish one's sins? For "penance" is so
called from "punishing." Therefore, dearest brothers, shed bitter tears if
you would prevail over the penalties of vengeance. Penance, beloved, cannot be made in satiety, but is effected through the virtue of continence.
Whatever the mind wickedly desires it is necessary to flee. Meanwhile, cast
deceit from your souls, quarrels from your minds, wickedness from your
hearts, knowing that you will in no way obtain that which you seek unless
you cast them out from your heart. Prayers that are poured out with love,
these are accepted by God. For prayer mixed with discord is a great blasphemy, and thus the prayer of such men obstructs the prayers of others,
because it is written: *One praying and another cursing. Whose voice does God
hear?*[42] For we do not deserve to be heard by God the Father if we are
waylaid by fraternal hatreds. For just as evil lands overwhelm those united
through love, likewise, from time to time, discordant people become the
ruin of their homeland. Therefore among other evils, hatred and discord,
which so divide quarrelers that they never make good supplicants, always
have more weight. And what can I say? Sinners' prayers are detestable to
God, even if they pray for something good. For so it is written: *Whoever
blocks his ears from hearing the law, his prayer shall be an abomination.*[43] Indeed
the law of God, that is the gospel of Christ, forbids hatred and urges charity. Thus it must be that the vow of him who resists this law will not be
received in prayer. For he who carries hatred of his brother in his breast,
he is himself called a murderer by voice of the apostle, as John says: *Whoso-
ever hates his brother is a murderer. And you know that no murderer has eternal
life abiding in him.*[44] And see what that same blessed apostle reveals from
that. For he says: *We know that we shall pass from death to life, if we love our
brother.*[45] But he who does not love remains in death. What we have said,
the blessed apostle offered: *Rooted, therefore, and fruitful in charity, which is
the fetter of perfection,*[46] let us lie upon foundations of penance. Let us make
crimes public by confession if we wish to temper the fury of the Lord that

[42] Eccl. 34:29.
[43] Prov. 28:9.
[44] 1 John 3:15.
[45] 1 John 3:14.
[46] Eph. 3:17.

is coming upon us. He gives us hope of forgiveness through the prophet, saying: *Declare your previous sins so that you are justified.*[47] For justification is quickly given to those in whom confession is called forth towards salvation. Therefore let the beginning of our righteousness be the confession of sins, which does not mix with the requirements of vanity, which has no truck with talkativeness, as it is written: *In the multitude of words there shall not want sin.*[48] Therefore restrain the tongue from useless words. Listen to the reader in silence. Attend to the Psalms. Attend not to chatter, but only pour forth your murmurs to God alone, with tears. Argue not, but attend to prayer. Your laughter is turned into mourning and your joy into sorrow. Set aside all care for this world and turn to almsgiving, purge your sins, attend to fasting. Offer to God a sacrifice of tears and together with us call out to the Lord with tears: *Lord, we have sinned against you. We have sinned and have acted unjustly, drawing away from you. Do not for the sake of your name, we beg, surrender us to disgrace.*[49] Remove now the plague from our borders. Let the disaster of the impending blow depart. Let the raging sword of pestilence fail against those it attacks and let it not, we beg you, come to us. Relieve now the wretched, succor the afflicted. Form in us what you would accept from us. Give to our hearts the disposition that can penetrate your hearing. Give us an overflowing of tears and the abundance of your sweetness, which is able to extinguish the anger announced against us. For we wretched ones have exhausted ourselves in tears, and saving remorse does not flow in us. But you, fountain of piety, reflect now upon the groaning of the contrite and take up the prayer of the groaners, so that we may not perish in evil days, but that we may bless you forever, because you will have *honor and glory,*[50] virtue and power forever and ever. Amen.

Conclusion

Behold, most beloved brothers, consumed by the message of a bloody death and disturbed by the terror of a threatening blow of anger, pour out the murmurs of your contrite hearts devoutly to the Lord, and all together cry out indulgence to God since we are pressed by the immense weight of our sins and flogged by the just judgment of God.

[47] Is. 43:26.
[48] Prov. 10:19.
[49] Cf. Jer. 14:7 and 20, Dan. 3:29 and 34.
[50] 1 Tim. 1:17.

Likewise a Sermon on the Catastrophe, to be Read
on the Second Day (Grégoire, *Les homéliaires*, 217–19)

Most beloved, yesterday we wept over the ills announced to us. Today
let us foster Christ by proclamations that are worthy of forgiveness. We
have confidence in the Lord, because a pious and devoted confession
in His presence does not go to waste. Believe the apostle's proclamation
when he says: *Be humbled under the strong hand of the Lord and he will exalt
you in time of trouble. Who has hoped in the Lord and been confounded? Who
has continued in His commandments and has been forsaken?*[51] In order, therefore, to nurture your faith in this, I will put before you something sweet
and memorable from exempla of evil men, that the words and deeds of
another time will lighten the calamity of your own time. I will expand on
what I have read for the comfort of sinners – not so that you lift the fear
of God from your hearts, but to instill in you the faith not to despair of
salvation.

Blessed Augustine in a sermon concerning the destruction of the City
reports that these things happened in the time of Emperor Arcadius.
He says: "A few years ago, in the time of the Emperor Arcadius, God
wished to terrify the city of Constantinople, and by doing so to amend,
convert, cleanse and change it. He came in a vision to a certain servant
of His, a soldier, and said that the city would be destroyed by a fire from
heaven. And He admonished him. When this was declared to the bishop,
the bishop did not despise the account, but told the people. The city
turned to penance, just as ancient Nineveh once did. However, so the
people did not think that the man who had spoken either was deceived
or had deceived by a fraud, the day came which God had threatened.
The people were tense and fearfully expected an army at nightfall. And
while the earth darkened, a fiery cloud was seen from the East, small at
first, but then gradually, so that it came towards the city, it grew terribly
large until it hung over the whole city. A horrible flame seemed to hang
down, nor was the odor of sulfur lacking. Everyone fled to the church,
and the place could not hold the crowds. Everyone begged baptism from
whomever could perform it. Not only in the church, but throughout the
houses, districts, and streets of the city, people demanded the salvation
of that sacrament by which anger (certainly not of the present, but of the
future) is driven away. But after that great tribulation when God proved
true to His words and fulfilled the vision of His servant, the cloud began

[51] James 4:10 and Eccl. 2:11–12.

to shrink just as it had grown. The people, gradually made safe again, heard that they must desert the city, because it would be destroyed the next Saturday. The entire city left with the emperor. No one stayed in his house or closed it up. The people, moving far away from the walls and seeing their sweet dwellings and houses left behind, miserably said goodbye to their homes. That whole multitude went forth some miles and gathered in one place to pour forth prayers to the Lord; they suddenly saw a great amount of smoke, and cried out loudly to the Lord. At last, when calm had been restored, they sent men out to report carefully what had happened after these words. After an hour had passed, when they reported that all the walls and dwellings stood sound, the people returned with great thanksgiving. No one lost anything from his house. Every man found everything just as he left it. What shall we say? Whether, in this, God's anger or mercy was the greater? Who would doubt that the most merciful Father wished to correct the people by terrifying them, not punish by destroying them, since the whole calamity harmed none of the people, houses or walls? Indeed, just as disasters are customarily raised up to strike, and when the one who was to be stricken is made contrite and called back by pity, so it happened to that city."[52]

These are the events of ancient times that the blessed Augustine recounts as happening. You should act likewise. Be frightened by divine terror and you will see the smiting persecution and pestilence wither away entirely. They, subject to divine terror and seeing destruction loom over their homeland, sought the church; you who are now within the church, quietly offer the Lord gifts of confession. With destruction threatening, they demanded baptism from whoever could perform it; you who are already baptized, let each of you who are able not close his inmost parts to mercy. There, leaving their city behind, they sought a place where they could lament the destruction of their falling homeland; you, living in the cities, judge rightly. They, when the Lord's fury abated, happily returned to the city; and you, if you listen to me, you too will happily maintain the liberty of your homeland. Yesterday you learned of the penance recommended by the counsel of angels and prophets; today you have learned this more fully by the examples of repentance. And you probably understand that the Lord Himself said in the gospel, rebuking evil men: *Unless you shall do penance, likewise you shall perish.*[53] And I, strengthened by the words of the Lord, say to you and to myself: Let us repent. Where? Where

[52] From Augustine's Sermon *de excidio urbis* (*PL* 40:715–24).
[53] Luke 13:3.

God can see. Where the bodily eye cannot perceive. *Let us rend our hearts and not our garments.*[54] Examining the ways of the Lord let us examine our hearts, and see if they are not fickle. Let us neither flatter ourselves, nor be gentle with ourselves, nor tender with our flesh, if we wish to avoid the punishment owed to flesh. Let us not mock God if we do not wish to anger Him by our actions and vices, if we want to be freed from both present and future punishments. But that Lord who saddens us by its report, would free us by the announcement of that scourge. He would both forgive our confessed sins and restore us who persevere to serve in fear of Him. And He would grant us both to enjoy the fruits of His sweetness here, and afterwards eternal blessedness with the angels, through the Lord Jesus, co-equal with Him and reigning co-eternal with Him and with the Holy Spirit forever and ever. Amen.

Conclusion

Behold, most beloved brothers, because of the example of the city of Constantinople, you know that people who were confident in God were saved and avoided the destruction of imminent ruin. Take on a similar disposition by confession, and publicly make bitterest lamentations to God. And let us all equally, with one heart and voice, seek indulgence from the Lord.

A Sermon on the Catastrophe, to be Read on the Third Day
(Grégoire, *Les homéliaires,* 219–21)

Most beloved, yesterday in the sermon I read everything written about the destruction of a city of ancient people, those people whom the terror of repentance so alarmed that they did not endure fearsome evils, and so happily returned to the city that they had sorrowfully left. Let that example indeed be enough for us, if the Lord orders the imminent blow to withdraw, and if that plague raging against should not come to pass. Otherwise, if it is the judgment of God to sweep us away by the scourge of such deaths, His will be done. By many counsels you ought to prolong providence to the future, lest unforeseen evils suddenly and horribly press upon an unexpecting people. Well advised, pay attention to me. Those about to die do not have many worries, such as what will kill them, but in dying they are compelled to go. Why do we so greatly fear that

54 Joel 2:13.

the groin disease should swallow us, as if varieties of other deaths were lacking to remove us from this life? One must be taken either by a fever or by a pestilence. Will we, even if this blow does not come, be able to have eternal life in this corruption? Or if it does come, has it cut short the predestined boundaries of human life, or does it snatch away anyone's life before the hour in which the preordained end comes to each? It is not fitting for us to doubt about this, because we have a very firm and solid proof from divine scripture: *The day of man is brief; the number of his months are with you. You have fixed his ends, which have not passed by.*[55]

If we carry on to the prescribed ends of our lives, what does the groin disease do to us? If it has duly attacked us, it will fulfill the hastening of death. However, it will not be able to cut short the years of our lives. Many perish by this disease, many by another, but no one dies before their prescribed end. Therefore, if this plague does not violate the preordained end of human life, why do the terrors of this disaster torture us? Why does this rumor disturb us, since we will not be able to avoid the preordained end of death whether the plague comes or not? If, God forbid, *what* we do not desire comes, then let no one murmur, no one be discouraged, no one despair and no one, God forbid, say despairingly: "What has penance profited us, since we have not avoided the plague?" May that blasphemy be absent from this Christian mouth. In everything that happens in our time, let the praise of God always be in our mouths. May His will be done for us and in us. *For if we have received good things at the hand of God, why should we not receive evil?*[56] He is the Father. Is He to be loved when He caresses, and refused when He rebukes? Is He not the Father both when promising life and when imparting discipline? But what should we say? You who take fright at this blow (not because you fear the uncertainty of slavery, but because you fear death, that is, you show yourselves to be terrified), oh that you would be able to change life into something better, and not only that you could not to be frightened by approaching death, but rather that you would desire to come to death. When we die, we are carried by death to immortality. Eternal life cannot approach unless one passes away from here. Death is not an end, but a transition from this temporary life to eternal life. Who would not hurry to go to better things? Who would not long to be changed more quickly and reformed

[55] Job 14:5.
[56] Job 2:10.

into the likeness of Christ and the dignity of celestial grace? Who would not long to cross over to rest, and see the face of his king, whom he had honored in life, in glory? And if Christ our king now summons us to see him, why do we not embrace death, through which we are carried to the eternal shrine? For unless we have made the passage through death, we cannot see the face of Christ our king. Or perhaps, God forbid, you think little of this vision and thus fear death? As to how unutterably this vision ought to be cherished, I shall draw a certain comparison from an earthly prince that should further your salvation.

Imagine that this earthly king has said to someone among you: "Behold, your house is full of all riches. Go into it. Be rich. Do whatever you wish, as you wish. Let no one oppose you in anger. Let all obey you when you govern. Let your will be done in all things. But I say only this to you, that you may not see my face." He says therefore: "Does a lover of this world, who desires most truly to gaze at the face of his king, not consider as dung all those things given to him? And would he not consider that this alone is punishment to him, that he is ignobly separated from the presence of his king?" Moreover, according to this analogy, make Christ say to you: "You do not wish to die. You fear to be made bitter. Behold, I neither bring in death nor send pestilence to you. Live as you wish in this life; only you may not see my face." Consider therefore from this analogy how impious that thought is and how it is oppressed by the darkness of eternal night. For whom is it sweeter to live in this life than to see Him who grants life, since no death is crueler or worse to the soul than not to see the face of God? Now with a balanced mind, with a very ready devotion, with strong faith and virtue, let us be prepared for every wish of God. And let us hasten with every desire of our hearts to see Him for whom we have struggled, and let us consider, with all fear of mortality being shut out, the immortality that follows. So that, when the day of our own calling comes, we go to the Lord swiftly and without delay, let us not dread death if we truly wish to come to life. But may the Lord Himself, who both conquered death and gave us life, by His fruitful tears, both prevent the death that you fear and grant the eternal life you seek.

Conclusion

Now, most beloved brothers, if by the Lord's inspiration we truly both despise death and love life, let us claim the voice that overthrows death. Now let us all in one, with sorrowful and contrite dispositions, seek indulgence from the Lord.

Likewise a Sermon on the Catastrophe
(Grégoire, *Les homéliaires*, 222–23).

Behold, most beloved brothers, the force of that stroke that we know rages among the people of God and has terrified the hidden places of our minds. For it terrifies us, this so tumultuous force of that blow to the groin, it terrifies us, this assault of unforeseen death. And yet what is there in this, brothers, what except that which we know to be fulfilled in us for our sins, that which we have moreover read was predicted by the prophet: *Who will stand before the face of the future blow, or who will withstand the rage of the Lord's anger? Because His indignation is poured out like fire and the earth quakes from His face.*[57] But why has it been proclaimed that these come for the casting out of our sins? What must we do, or what must all men do, except bewail the offences of our failings with tears and placate the rage of the Lord's anger with assiduous tears? For He is our maker, by whom we wish to be saved from these things, because we take fright at the Lord as our evils require. Let Him deign to give counsel on what it would be fit for us to do. He says: *Be converted to me from your whole heart in fasting and weeping and mourning. Rend your hearts and not your garments. For indeed if you were thus turned to me, I would heal your contritions.*[58] Behold, most beloved, this is the salvific voice of the doctor who does not wish us to perish under blows. Although there is vengeance for our offences, nevertheless a remedy from God is open to us through frequent lamentation. Pay attention, therefore, most beloved, pay attention to the prophetic predictions, pay attention to the prayers of my voice, if you wish to avoid the dangers of this pestilential death. He whom we know to abound in compassion and mercy indeed wishes to assist those who make tearful confessions. For so it is written, most beloved: *God is not mocked*[59] in tears, but must be sought from the heart. Let us groan here in prayers, therefore, sadly in lamentation, and with downcast expression let us display on our faces the mark of error. Behold our end, we already carry the torment of our groin blow. Will we not be able to bewail zealously? Brothers, therefore let us groan in order to destroy such an enormous danger of guilt, and let us conquer the ruin of the dire wound by continuing in lamentation. Pass the course of days in mourning and spend the spaces of nights in tears. Fill the hours by tearful waiting, and conquer the ruin of this blow through penance. We

[57] Nahum 1:6 and 5.
[58] Joel 2:12–13, cf. Hosea 14:5.
[59] Gal. 6:7.

have sinned greatly, let us weep greatly. Let vast veneration, borne upon
alms, be lively in the remedy of such an unforeseen wound. Be swift to
bewail and free-flowing to give mercies. And doing these things, let us
pour forth prayer with tears. Perhaps we will quickly sway the mercy of the
creator in order to remove the torment of this wound. For He, promising
His mercy to relieve penitents quickly has thus considered us worthy to
receive consolation through the prophet: *When you will have brought forth
conversion, then you shall be saved,*[60] and you will be able to avoid the evil
that threatens. And likewise He says: *I do not desire the death of him who dies,
says the Lord, so much as revere, and you may live.*[61] And Joel, prophet of the
same Lord, commanded piety to the same Lord with this warning: *Show
reverence to the Lord your God,* he says, *because He is merciful and holy and full
of compassion.*[62] And therefore seek Him in prayers, seek Him in all works.
For He is able to remove the wounds of the pestilence inflicted on us. He
is able to change the decision of vengeance into the antidote of salvation,
He who with God the Father and the Holy Spirit lives as one God.

[60] Is. 45:22.
[61] Ez. 18:32.
[62] Joel 2:13.

9

Plague in Seventh-Century England

John Maddicott

During the second half of the seventh century the English kingdoms, along with much of the rest of the British Isles, were affected by severe outbreaks of epidemic disease. They were described by contemporary writers in terms that varied from the briefly factual to the nearly apocalyptic. The most famous of those writers, Bede, recapitulating the events of his *Ecclesiastical History*, noted their onset in 664 with stark concision: 'And the pestilence came' (*et pestilentia venit*). In the body of his text, completed about 731, he had already provided a more elaborate and emotive record, speaking of 'a sudden pestilence raging far and wide with fierce destruction', that 'laid low a great multitude of men'. It was 'the mortality that ravaged Britain and Ireland with cruel devastation', 'the pestilence that carried off many throughout the length and breadth of Britain.'[1] Nor was Bede the earliest witness to its terrors. Adomnán, abbot of Iona and biographer of Columba, writing c. 697, close to the events that he recounts, alluded to 'the great mortality that twice in our time has ravaged a large part of the world'.[2] The anonymous Life of Cuthbert, composed between 698 and 705, drew upon the memories of a priest, Tydi, who recalled 'the mortality that depopulated many places';[3]

---

[1] Bede, *EH* 5.24, 3.27, 3.13, pp. 564–665, 310–12, 252–53; *Two Lives of St. Cuthbert*, 180–81. Bede's prose life of Cuthbert, the source here, was written c. 720: Bede, *Opera historica*, 1:cxlviii.

[2] Adomnán, *Adomnán's Life of Columba* xlii, pp. 178–79; idem, *Life of St Columba*, pp. 55, 203.

[3] *Two Lives of St. Cuthbert*, 118–19. Date of composition: Thacker, "Cult of St. Cuthbert," 115.

I am very grateful to John Blair and Paul Slack for their helpful comments on an earlier version of this essay. Reprinted with minor changes from *Past and Present: A Journal of Historical Studies*, no. 156 (August 1997): 7–54, by permission of the Past and Present Society.

while the biographer of Wilfrid, writing c. 715, spoke simply of 'the great mortality'.[4] All these authors had lived through the afflictions that they describe, and, as we shall see, they provide enough detail to substantiate their general recollections of what had clearly been, if they can be believed, a catastrophe. Without prejudging its nature, we shall henceforth call the agent of that catastrophe 'plague'.

Consideration of these plagues bears on some central topics in early Anglo-Saxon history: monasticism, rural settlement, and demography, for example. Yet their almost complete neglect by modern historians is perhaps less surprising than it may at first seem.[5] For our knowledge of the plague's effects, we are almost entirely dependent on literary sources of a special sort: ecclesiastical writers with a hagiographical bent, for whom plague was a helpful but incidental part of their story, used to illustrate the virtues of a king or the prophetic words of a saint or the miraculous powers of a vision.[6] The Anglo-Saxonist can only envy the Byzantine historian of plague, who can draw on epigraphy, numismatics, and administrative texts to control his comparable writers.[7] It goes without saying that we lack entirely both the manorial and church records that provide guidance on mortality during the plagues of the fourteenth century, and the statistics of prices and wages that allow us to chart the long-term effects of those plagues. Archaeology, more valuable for the seventh century than for the fourteenth, we do have; but archaeology offers no precise dates and therefore little sustainable correlation with historical events. Faced with all these difficulties in the assessment of plague, Anglo-Saxon historians have generally, and understandably, passed by on the other side.

Despite the inadequacies of our sources, it may nevertheless be worthwhile to set out what is known and what may be deduced about a series of disasters that were certainly fatal to many and probably traumatic for those who survived.

---

4 Eddius Stephanus, *Life of Bishop Wilfrid*, 40–41. Date of composition: Kirby, "Bede, Eddius Stephanus," 106–08.

5 For example, Stenton, *Anglo-Saxon England*, 130; Sawyer, *From Roman Britain to Norman England*, pp. 18, 85–86 (only on the sixth-century plagues). Loyn, *Anglo-Saxon England* appears to overlook the plague entirely. Russell, "Earlier Medieval Plague in the British Isles" does not fulfill the promise of its title.

6 For example, Bede, *EH* 4.14, pp. 376–78; *Two Lives of St. Cuthbert*, 246–49; Bede, *EH* 4.7, pp. 356–59.

7 Cf. Durliat, "La peste du VIe siècle," 107–12.

COURSE AND MORTALITY

The plague that first struck England in 664 fell within the cycle of plagues that affected western Europe and the Mediterranean lands from the mid-sixth to the mid-eighth centuries. Originating in Egypt, the plague spread to Constantinople in 541 or 542, where it is said to have caused many thousands of deaths.[8] Thence it quickly moved westward, presumably via seaborne commerce, reaching Italy, Gaul, Carthage, and Spain within a year and later extending far into the interior of Gaul, along the great river systems that were the arteries of inland trade. Through this whole region sporadic attacks continued until the 760s.[9] They appear to have been most frequent and destructive in the sixth century, but appearances may be deceptive here, for when Gregory of Tours ceased to write in 591 we lose our best-informed source for the history of plague in Gaul. In the notoriously unchronicled seventh century, outbreaks almost certainly went unrecorded. Fredegar, Gregory's feeble successor, mentions only one, although we know that there were others. It seems to be Bede alone, for example, who records the *pestilentia* in Rome, which carried off Wighard, the English candidate for the see of Canterbury, in 667 or 668.[10] That it was indeed bubonic plague whose course we can thus trace, rather than one of the other epidemic diseases current in this period, is proved by the three writers, Procopius, Gregory of Tours, and Paul the Deacon, who describe the characteristic plague buboes, the large hard swellings of the groin and other lymphatic glands, that marked out its victims. To Gregory the symptoms gave the plague its name: it was *lues inguinaria*, 'the groin plague'.[11]

The plague first arrived in the British Isles in 544 or 545, when it reached Ireland. 'The great mortality called "blefed,"' according to the Annals of Tigernach, it later became known as 'the first great plague' to distinguish it from the later and equally devastating plague of 664.[12] Although we lack the description of symptoms that would enable us to identify the disease as plague, there can be virtually no doubt as to its

[8] Procopius, *PW*, 1–557; Biraben and Le Goff, "La peste dans le haut moyen age," 1492.

[9] Biraben and Le Goff, "La peste dans le haut moyen age," 1492, 1494–95, 1497, 1499–1500.

[10] Fredegar, *Chronicle of Fredegar*, p. 12; Bede, *EH* 4.1, pp. 328–29; Biraben and Le Goff, "La peste dans le haut moyen age," 1496–97.

[11] Procopius, *PW* 2.22.16–17, pp. 457–59; Gregory of Tours, *The History of the Franks* 1:421–22, 2:119, 141; Paul the Deacon, *Historia Longobardorum* 2.4, p. 74.

[12] *Annals of Tigernach*, 137, 198; Adomnán, *Life of St Columba*, 348; MacArthur, "Identification of Some Pestilences," 172–73.

being that. In the geographical advance of what was certainly bubonic plague, northward transmission rather than the coincidental visitation of some other disease is likely to explain the Irish outbreak. The conclusions to be drawn from what is a chronological sequence – Constantinople, 541/2, western Mediterranean, 542/3, Ireland, 544/5 – gain added weight from our knowledge of Ireland's maritime connections with Gaul and the Mediterranean world. In the mid-sixth century those connections were numerous and extensive. Pottery came in on a large scale, more especially from Atlantic Gaul but also from the eastern Mediterranean; and there is more tentative evidence for the import of corn and cloth, traded commodities notorious for the mobility that they offered to the rats and fleas that were the source of bubonic plague infection.[13] Here, almost for certain, was the main route for the spread of plague, and one probably to be followed when plague moved into seventh-century England.

For some thirty years after the plague of the 540s, a variety of epidemic diseases affected Ireland, none of them clearly identifiable as bubonic plague and none recorded after the mid-570s. They almost certainly included smallpox, the 'yellow plague' (*buidhe chonaill*) recorded by the Ulster annals as bringing a 'great mortality' in 549, and a disease notorious for its virulence in societies previously unvisited.[14] Either this disease or, less probably, the earlier bubonic plague may well have spread to Britain, for the *Annales Cambriae* note the death of the Welsh ruler King Maelgwn of Gwynedd in the 'great mortality' of 547.[15] The reliability of this annal has been questioned.[16] Yet the close maritime contacts between

[13] Pottery: Thomas, *Provisional List of Imported Pottery*, 7, 11, 20–24, 27; James, "Ireland and Western Gaul," 381–83. Grain: ibid., 376–77. Cloth: Adomnan, *Life of St Columba*, 290. The grain trade from the Mediterranean to regions whose economies were mainly pastoral may have been extensive: note the seventh-century story of the ship's captain from Alexandria, his ship laden with a cargo of grain, who was blown off course toward a famine-stricken, south-west Britain. Was he steering for Ireland? The source is translated in Penhallurick, *Tin in Antiquity*, 245. For the importance of cloth and grain in the transmission of plague, see Slack, *Impact of Plague*, 12, and in this essay at nn. 108–10.

[14] For a list of Irish epidemics, see Bonser, *Medical Background of Anglo-Saxon England*, 59–60. MacArthur, "Identification of Some Pestilences," 173–75, argues that the "yellow plague" was relapsing fever, but the case made for smallpox by Shrewsbury, "Yellow Plague," 34–39, is more persuasive.

[15] "Mortalitas magna in qua pausat mailcun rex genedotae": Phillimore, "Annales Cambriae," 155. For Welsh references to this outbreak as the "yellow plague," see Lloyd, *Wales From the Earliest Times*, 1:131.

[16] Dumville, "Problems of Dating," 53–54.

western Britain and both Ireland and the Continent make the transmission of one or other disease seem entirely plausible. Whether it spread beyond Wales to lowland Britain we cannot know. Neither the silence of the exiguous sources nor the apparent (and perhaps illusory) separation of western Britons from midland and eastern English necessarily imply immunity;[17] and the seeming origins of many Anglo-Saxon kingdoms in the years after c. 550 – Bernicia, Deira, Essex, and Kent, for instance – could indicate a new start after a demographic and political hiatus.[18] But not much can be built on half a dozen words in a doubtful text.

As far as we can see, therefore, the plague was still sporadically active in continental Europe, extinct in Ireland, and either as yet unknown or at least long past, at the time of its simultaneous descent on both England and Ireland in the 66os. Before assessing its nature and effects in England, our first task must be to trace its course: an elementary prelude to any discussion, but one hitherto, and surprisingly, neglected.[19]

The history of the plague in England falls into two fairly well-defined phases: the first visitation of 664–c. 666, and the second of c. 684–c. 687, with other scattered outbreaks in the intervening years. The two visitations were also common to Ireland and were explicitly recognized for both countries by Adomnán, who wrote of the plague's ravaging 'twice in our time'.[20] The outbreaks recorded by Bede, our main source, conform to just this pattern. The plague first appeared in England during the summer of 664, shortly after an eclipse of the sun on May 1. It struck initially in the south, a starting place tentatively confirmed by the simultaneous deaths of Deusdedit, archbishop of Canterbury, and of Earconberht, king of Kent, on July 14.[21] In the south-east it also affected Essex, causing the reversion to paganism of the kingdom's joint ruler, King Sighere, and his subjects.[22] By the autumn of that year it had reached the north, killing Cedd, bishop of the East Saxons, in his Deiran monastery of Lastingham on October 23, and subsequently wiping out all Cedd's monks who had traveled north from their East Saxon monastery to dwell at their leader's

---

[17] *Pace* Morris, *Age of Arthur*, 222–23.

[18] Bassett, *Origins of Anglo-Saxons Kingdoms*, 645, 136, 219; Sawyer, *From Roman Britain to Norman England*, 85–86.

[19] The best account to date is provided in Plummer's notes to Bede's *Ecclesiastical History* 4.27 in Bede, *Opera historica*, 2:194–95.

[20] Adomnán, *Life of St Columba*, 203, 348–49.

[21] Bede, *EH* 3.27, iv.1, pp. 311–13; 328–29. For the date of the eclipse, see *Life of St Cuthbert*, 348–49.

[22] Bede, *EH* 3.30, pp. 322–23.

shrine. [23] About the same time it struck down Tuda, newly appointed after the Synod of Whitby as bishop for the Northumbrians, [24] and Boisil, prior of Melrose. Cuthbert, then a monk at Melrose, sickened but later recovered, living to succeed Boisil as prior and to reconvert those in the neighboring countryside who had apostasized during the plague. [25]

After 664 the plague declined but did not disappear. Bede refers to the frequency of Cuthbert's evangelizing journeys among the *errantes*, hinting at recurrent outbreaks. [26] One of these afflicted the Deiran monastery of Gilling (Bede's *Ingetlingum*), probably between 666 and 669, leading Tunberht, then abbot, Ceolfrith, later abbot of Jarrow, and other monks to withdraw to Ripon at Wilfrid's invitation. [27] It was during this intervening period too that plague returned to the south. At some point between 666 and 675 it struck the East Saxon double monastery of Barking, causing many deaths; [28] it carried off Bishop Chad and many of the monks at Lichfield in 672; [29] and about 680 it reached Ely, killing the first abbess, Æthelthryth, former wife of King Ecgfrith of Northumbria, and others. [30] As far as the very imperfect record indicates, therefore, this was not a period of remission but of more sporadic and scattered outbreaks affecting a spread of different regions.

After 684 these were overtaken and overshadowed by the more comprehensive return of the plague 'in many provinces of Britain'. Of the

[23] Ibid., 3.23, pp. 286–89. For the date of Cedd's death, possibly derived from a calendar, see John of Worcester, *Chronicle of John of Worcester*, 2:115, accepted by Grosjean, "La Date du Colloque de Whitby," 243.

[24] Bede, *EH* 3.27, pp. 310–13. See below, at n. 94.

[25] Bede, *EH* 4.27, pp. 432–33; *Two Lives of St. Cuthbert*, 181–87. That the plague that affected Cuthbert and killed Boisil was that of 664 and not some earlier outbreak, as used to be thought, is shown by Stancliffe, "Polarity between Pastor and Solitary," 30–31.

[26] *Two Lives of St. Cuthbert*, 184–87.

[27] *Historia Abbatum Auctore Anonymo*, in Bede, *Opera historica*, 1:388–89. Ceolfrith was ordained priest by Wilfrid at Ripon in 669 (ibid., 2:370). Wilfrid had returned from abroad in 666 (ibid., 317). This dates the plague at Gilling and Ceolfrith's departure for Ripon to between 666 and 669, and probably nearer 666 because it is clear from *Historia Abbatum Auctore Anonymo* (ibid., 1:389), that Ceolfrith was at Ripon for some time before his ordination.

[28] Bede, *EH* 4.7, 8, pp. 356–69. Barking was probably founded in 666 and the plague struck in the time of its first abbess, Æthelburh, whose successor, Hildelith, may have come into office in 675: Hart, *Charters of Eastern England*, 117; Bede, *EH* 4.10, pp. 362–63; John of Worcester, *Chronicle of John of Worcester*, 2:128–29; *Aldhelm*, 51.

[29] Bede, *EH*, 4.3, pp. 337–39; Bede, *Opera historica*, 2:208.

[30] Bede, *EH*, 4.19, pp. 390–97. Ely was probably founded in 673, according to John of Worcester and the Anglo-Saxon Chronicle, and Æthelthryth was abbess for seven years, according to Bede: John of Worcester, *Chronicle of John of Worcester*, 2:122–25; Bede, *EH*, 4.19, pp. 392–93; cf. Bede, *Opera historica*, 2:235–39. This would place her death in 680.

southern kingdoms, only Sussex, and specifically the monastery of Selsey, is known to have been affected,[31] but, as before, our information from Bede's Northumbria is much fuller. On Lindisfarne the plague lasted nearly a year, carrying off almost the whole congregation;[32] it struck equally hard at an unnamed monastery near Carlisle;[33] it killed Abbot Eosterwine and many of the monks at Wearmouth;[34] and at Jarrow all the choir monks died, leaving only Abbot Ceolfrith and a small boy to continue the offices.[35] Further south in the Northumbrian kingdom, the plague fell on Ripon.[36] Nor was it only the monasteries that were affected, for the epidemic left many rural settlements devastated and deserted, and in need of all the consolation that Cuthbert, traveling the country as bishop of Lindisfarne, could provide.[37] It lasted for some considerable time: Abbot Adomnán paid two visits to Northumbria, one in 685 or 686 and a second two years later, and on both occasions the plague was raging.[38] The first to write of the plague, about 697, Adomnán was the witness to what seems to have been its last assault; for after c. 687 we hear no more of it.

Even a summary will have brought out the scale of this disaster, in terms of both its geographical range and the number of its victims. If our sources can be believed, these were indeed national plagues, striking with exceptional virulence. The early plague almost certainly affected Kent, certainly reached Essex, and spread to some widely separated monasteries in

---

[31] Bede, *EH*, 4.14, pp. 376–81. Selsey was struck during the period of the kingdom's conversion by Wilfrid, 681 to 686, and probably late in that period, after the foundation of the monastery at Selsey: Bede, *Opera historica*, 2:319.

[32] *Two Lives of St. Cuthbert*, 244–49. The plague came to Lindisfarne during Cuthbert's own solitary residence on Farne, as he himself stated (ibid.); that is, between 676 and 685: Stancliffe, "Polarity between Pastor and Solitary," 33–35. I have assumed a late date in this period because most of the plague outbreaks in Northumbria were around 685, but the date could be earlier.

[33] *Two Lives of St. Cuthbert*, 242–45. The attack came shortly before King Ecgfrith's death at Nechtansmere on 20 May 685.

[34] *Historia Abbatum Auctore Baeda*, in Bede, *Opera historica*, 1:372–74. Eosterwine almost certainly died in 686: ibid., 2:362, 364.

[35] *Historia Abbatum Auctore Anonymo*, in ibid., 1:392–93. The episode cannot be precisely dated, but probably followed shortly after Eosterwine's death at Wearmouth, which it immediately follows in the text.

[36] Eddius Stephanus, *Life of Bishop Wilfrid*, 40–41. The plague struck at Ripon after Wilfrid's time as bishop there, 669–78, and because Wilfrid's biographer describes it as "the great mortality," it can be only the outbreak of c. 685.

[37] *Two Lives of St. Cuthbert*, 118–21, 259–61. Cuthbert was bishop from 685 to 687. For the plague and rural settlements, see the section on plague in the countryside in this essay.

[38] Adomnán, *Life of St Columba*, 46–47, 203–04, 351–52.

Northumbria: Lastingham, Gilling, and Melrose. Subsequently it touched Lichfield in Mercia, Ely in East Anglia, and Barking in Essex. When it returned in full force during the 680s it struck Selsey in Sussex, and a further group of monasteries in Northumbria: Lindisfarne, Wearmouth, Jarrow, Ripon, and the unknown monastery near Carlisle. Although there are many regions from which we have no information, there seems nothing implausible in Bede's claim that the 664 plague ravaged 'the length and breadth of Britain', or in Adomnán's that the later epidemic reached 'everywhere' in Ireland and Britain, save only the northern lands of the Picts and the Dalriadan Irish.[39]

Imprecise though they are, the mortality rates suggested by our sources provide other evidence for the destructiveness of these plagues. We know most about the monasteries, where death came to many, and, in some houses, to a majority: to all save one small boy among the thirty or so monks who traveled to Lastingham to reside near the body of their bishop, Cedd; to almost all the monks of Lindisfarne; to the abbot and 'no small company' of monks at Wearmouth; to all but the abbot and a boy at Jarrow. The bishops provide us with a slightly sharper statistical picture. Of the eight active in 664 – Deusdedit of Canterbury, Damian of Rochester, Wini of the West Saxons (Winchester), Cedd of the East Saxons, Boniface of the East Angles, Jaruman of the Mercians, Chad of York, and Tuda of the Northumbrians – two, Tuda and Cedd, certainly died of the plague, and two others very probably did. The death of Deusdedit, recorded by Bede almost immediately after his notice of the coming of plague in 664, occurred on the same day as that of King Earconberht of Kent, suggesting that both were the sudden victims of plague; and Damian of Rochester ·may well have died shortly before his metropolitan.[40] Eight bishops hardly provide a large or representative sample of the English population. Even so, a death rate of 25–50% is strikingly high, and considerably higher than that among the episcopate in 1348–1349, when the sole plague death among the seventeen bishops was that of Thomas Bradwardine, archbishop of Canterbury (although the preceding archbishop-elect had also died in the same way).[41]

39 *Two Lives of St. Cuthbert*, 180–81; Adomnán, *Life of St. Columba*, 203.
40 Bede, *EH* 4.1, pp. 328–29; Bede, *Opera historica*, 2:195, 207. Both Grosjean, "La Date du Colloque de Whitby," 246, and Brooks, *History of the Church of Canterbury*, 68, see Deusdedit (and in the case of Grosjean, Damian too) as a victim of the plague. I have omitted Wilfrid (York?) from the reckoning because he was probably overseas for his consecration when the plague struck.
41 Ramsay, *Genesis of Lancaster*, 1:361.

Among the more numerous bishops of the 680s, no deaths are known to have been due to plague, but the succession to a number of sees (Dunwich, Elmham, Lichfield, Lindsey, Rochester, and Selsey) is so uncertain that no reliable conclusion is possible. In this second wave of plague, monasteries appear to have been more at risk than bishops, to an extent that again suggests some surprising comparisons with the fourteenth century. Then, some houses escaped very lightly (only four deaths at the large community of Christ Church, Canterbury), while others were virtually extinguished;[42] but the impression given by Bede of a wide and almost wholesale devastation of monastic communities is not generally replicated for the later epidemic.

The only other seventh-century group open to examination is that of kings. Here there were two probable victims of the plague: Earconberht of Kent (whose fate hangs on the same arguments as that of Deusdedit) and Alhfrith, son of King Oswy of Northumbria, and his father's co-ruler.[43] Wilfrid's friend and patron, Alhfrith disappears from history after his despatch of Wilfrid for consecration in 664; Wilfrid would hardly have submissively retired to Ripon on his return two years later had his champion still been active.[44] It is often said that Alhfrith rebelled against his father in the mid-660s, bringing about his death or exile.[45] But the coincidence of his disappearance with the onset of the plague, and the complete silence, not only of Bede but also of Wilfrid's biographer 'Eddius', the two writers with an interest in Alhfrith's fortunes, may point to a different explanation: an unrecorded death in illness and obscurity, perhaps on some upcountry royal estate, rather than one brought about by a rebellion that could hardly have been anything other than public and publicized.

BEDE AS WITNESS

A survey of the evidence suggests, then, that the plague of 664–c. 687 had a lethal effect on those communities and individuals whom it touched. Even in advance of our discussing the nature of the disease, this seems inherently plausible. Any epidemic disease striking what epidemiologists call a 'virgin population' would cause very high mortality, and it is safe to assume that the English peoples were indeed 'virgin'. Even had there

---

[42] Knowles, *Religious Orders in England*, 2:10–11.
[43] For Alhfrith's position, see Eddius Stephanus, *Life of Bishop Wilfrid*, 14–15.
[44] Ibid., 30–31; Bede, *EH* 3.28, 5.19, pp. 314–17, 520–23.
[45] For example, Bede, *Opera historica*, 2:198; Mayr-Harting, *Coming of Christianity*, 108.

been an epidemic of plague (rather than the marginally more likely small-pox) around 550, nothing suggests that a single episode (and at best only a possible one) had led to endemic infection; and without that there could be no established biological immunity. The examples of Ireland, struck in the 540s and again in the 660s, and later of Iceland, devastated in 1402–1404 and again in 1494–1495, show that no security was conferred by a first plague separated by a long interval from a second.[46] Bede's silence on the subject prior to 664, and his laconic notice in his chronological summary for that year, *et pestilentia venit*, both point to a new scourge that may have cut down the unprotected English, lacking biological resistance, just as smallpox cut down the unprotected natives of eastern America in the seventeenth century.[47] Prima facie, therefore, we can argue that Bede may not have exaggerated what he had to say about the plague's victims.

Do we have internal grounds for thinking that he is a reliable witness? Unlike the Byzantine historians of the sixth-century plague, who looked back to Thucydides' account of the Athenian plague and who wrote accounts that themselves became stereotyped,[48] Bede had no model for the plague episodes he described. Although he knew Gregory of Tours' *Historia Francorum*, which provided the fullest survey of the ravages of the plague in the west, he probably came by Gregory's work only after completing his *Ecclesiastical History*,[49] and his own comments owed nothing to Gregory. Unlike Gregory, for example, he gives neither a specific name to the plague, beyond the general *pestilentia*, nor any explicit description of the plague's symptoms. What he wrote thus drew, not upon precedents and conventions, but presumably upon the oral testimony that underlay much of his work, upon a few earlier texts that mentioned plague, such as the anonymous *Life of Cuthbert*, and, more unusually, upon personal experience. He may not have been the 'young boy' who, as he recounts, was the only survivor besides the abbot when the plague struck Jarrow in the 680s, for it has been plausibly argued that his own monastery was Wearmouth.[50] But there he would have been a novice, aged about fifteen, when the plague cut down Abbot Eosterwine and many of the monks in

[46] Karlsson, "Plague Without Rats," 266–67, 270.
[47] Bede, *EH* 5.24, pp. 564–65; Shrewsbury, "Yellow Plague," 35–38.
[48] Durliat, "La peste du VIe siècle," 116.
[49] Levison, "Bede as Historian," 132.
[50] As argued by J. McClure and R. Collins in their trans. of Bede's *Ecclesiastical History* (New York, 1994), xiii. But for a contrary view, see Wood, *Most Holy Abbot Ceolfrid*, 34, n. 207.

the Black Death, which made landfall at the Dorset port of Melcombe, and probably in Bristol too, in June or July 1348.[70]

The seasonality of these epidemics suggests their occasional identity with a disease still more terrifying than bubonic plague: that is, plague in its pneumonic form. Pneumonic plague is usually contracted via infected sputum spread through coughing, or sometimes via the breathing in of infected flea feces. Because of its airborne transmission, it is far more infectious than bubonic plague, which can be caught only from the bite of an infected flea. Pneumonic plague differs in one other significant way from its bubonic cousin in that it lasts through the winter; bubonic plague can survive the winter in warm climates, but in cold weather infected fleas will often die and certainly cease to breed.[71] Now one feature of the plague that Bede describes is its sporadic occurrence during the winter months. At Lindisfarne in the 680s the plague broke out at Christmas, lasting for almost a year, and at Wearmouth, Abbot Eosterwine died of it on March 7.[72] The possibility that the plague in its early medieval cycle was at least in part pneumonic has hardly been considered.[73] Yet the English evidence points in that direction. It is drawn from the cold northeast, where bubonic plague would hardly be active during the winter, and from a newly invaded area, of the sort said to be more prone to pneumonic plague than other regions where plague has become well established and endemic.[74] If the disease did take on a pneumonic form from time to time, then its remarkable virulence and its ability to obliterate whole communities would be all the easier to comprehend: a point to which we shall return when we consider the plague's incidence and mortality in the countryside.[75]

Beyond the factors of place and season, any firm identification of Bede's *pestilentia* with plague must hang on the presence in England of the black rat. The rat is the main agent in the spread of plague, acting as host for the bacillus *Yersinia pestis*, whose transmission via the rat flea is the main route to human infection. Although infected fleas may themselves be carried long distances without the transport provided by rats, to infect

---

[70] Horrox *Black Death*, 10, 62–64.
[71] Ibid., 6–7; Morris, "Plague in Britain," 39.
[72] *Two Lives of St. Cuthbert*, 244–49; *Historia Abbatum Auctore Baeda*, in Bede, *Opera historica*, 1:372–74.
[73] But see Riché, "Problèmes de démographie historique," 47; Charles-Edwards, *Irish and Welsh Kinship*, 473.
[74] Twigg, *Black Death: A Biological Reappraisal*, 161–62.
[75] See in this essay at nn. 111–28.

their human hosts, 'it is likely that rodent infection was the necessary foundation for a major epidemic'.[76] If bubonic passed into pneumonic plague, this may have been less true, for the latter could then take off and acquire a momentum of its own, dependent on human transmission but independent of rats and fleas.[77] Yet, whatever the case for secondary pneumonic infection in seventh-century England, the buboes indicated in the cases of Cuthbert and Æthelthryth are peculiar to bubonic plague, pointing to flea bites as the source of infection and ultimately to the existence of the rats on which fleas were parasitic. Were there then rats in Bede's England?

Unfortunately this is a question to which there is no certain answer. Rats were not a late, post-Conquest introduction into Britain, as was once thought. Archaeology has shown that they were active in Roman towns – at York, Lincoln, London and, as late as the fifth century, at Wroxeter – and they had re-established themselves at York and Lincoln, and probably elsewhere, by the ninth century.[78] But for the intervening period there appears to be virtually no evidence anywhere for the presence of rats. Dependent as they were on centers of population and their food stores, they may have died out with the death of Roman town life and have been reintroduced from abroad at a time of renewed urban growth under the Vikings.[79] With the exception of one rat bone from the seventh-century Anglian village of West Stow (Suffolk), apparently – and frustratingly – lacking a firm context, no rat bones have been recovered from any early Anglo-Saxon site.[80] None appears to have been found in excavations at the *wics*, the great trading ports of early and middle Saxon England: neither at *Lundenwic* nor *Eoforwic* (York), nor Hamwic (Saxon Southampton), where the Melbourne Street excavations alone have produced nearly 50,000 identified bones.[81] Nor have the Northumbrian monasteries of Hartlepool and Jarrow produced any.[82] If rats were active

[76] Slack, *Impact of Plague*, 7–12.

[77] Cf. Karlsson, "Plague Without Rats," esp. 276–84.

[78] Armitage, West, and Steedman, "New Evidence of Black Rat in Roman London," 375, 380–82; O'Connor, *Bones from 46–54 Fishergate*, 257; idem, *Bones from the General Accident Site*, 105, 108.

[79] O'Connor, *Bones from Anglo-Scandinavian Levels*, 189; idem, *Animal Bones from Flaxengate*, 40; idem, "On the Lack of Bones," 318–20.

[80] West, *West Stow*, 1:86.

[81] Rackham, *Environment and Economy*, 128; O'Connor, *Bones From 46–54 Fishergate*, 257–58; Holdsworth, *Excavations at Melbourne Street*, 79, 114.

[82] Daniels, "Monastery at Church Close," 197; Noddle, *Animal Bones*, 6.

in early Anglo-Saxon England, their post-mortem disposal seems to have been extraordinarily inconspicuous.

These negative arguments are, however, much less than conclusive. The intermittent visitations of what was indubitably bubonic plague in sixth- and seventh-century Gaul must signify the presence of rats there; and indeed Gregory of Tours once comments on the multitude of rats in the Paris of the 580s.[83] The almost equally indubitable bubonic plague in Ireland of the 540s suggests their shipboard transport from the Continent. If rats were present across the Channel, there is nothing inherently improbable, given the volume of maritime contacts between England and the Continent, about their passage to England. Nor is the absence of skeletal remains at all decisive. We are considering what is, in archaeological terms, a very narrow slice of time: the period of some twenty-three years from 664 to c. 687. After that time rats may have disappeared, just as they had disappeared from late Roman Britain, until their arrival once again, but now plague-free, in the towns of the ninth century: a process of extinction and reintroduction characteristic of rat populations.[84] If this was the sequence of events, there may be nothing significant in the absence of rats from Hamwic, which was not founded until the early eighth century, or from Anglian York, where the excavated area (and perhaps the whole site) dates only from the very end of the seventh century or the beginning of the eighth.[85] Rats may have come and gone again before these places got going. Other *wics* were indeed thriving in the second half of the seventh century: notably London, whose commercial importance dates from at least the 670s.[86] But they have been excavated so incompletely and patchily that little weight can be attached to their yielding no rat bones. In general, too few sites occupied during the plague's comparatively short reign have been excavated for much importance to be attached to what is admittedly an almost entirely negative record.

There can, therefore, be no absolute certainty about the nature of the late seventh-century plague. But the known presence of plague on the Continent, Bede's two crucial descriptions of symptoms, and the epidemic's advent in 664, at a time and place characteristic of bubonic plague's arrival, should weigh more heavily than the lack of hard evidence

[83] Gregory of Tours, *The History of the Franks*, 2:358; Morris, "Plague in Britain," 44.

[84] Davis, "Scarcity of Rats," 458–60.

[85] Morton, *Excavations at Hamwic*, 26–28; O'Connor, *Bones From 46–54 Fishergate*, 211–12; Hall, "York, 700–1050," 127–29.

[86] Lobel, *City of London*, 25.

for the presence of rats, to suggest that Bede's *pestilentia* was indeed this disease.

TRANSMISSION AND SPREAD

It was not only their lack of prior experience that made the population of late seventh-century England vulnerable to disease. Other circumstances were more favorable to its transmission than at any time since the first Anglo-Saxon settlements. Since the Roman occupation of the fourth century there had probably been no larger concentrations of population than those found in the new coastal trading ports and in the new monasteries. We know nothing about the effects of plague on the few *wics* already in existence. But in the case of the monasteries we can go beyond Bede's demonstration of their mortal exposure in the face of disease to identify the conditions that left them so exposed. The number and contiguity of their residents was perhaps the most significant. Some houses were already quite large. If thirty or so monks traveled from Cedd's East Saxon monastery in 664 to dwell near his body,[87] how much more numerous than thirty was their home community? If twenty-two brothers (or seventeen according to Bede) migrated from Wearmouth to the new foundation at Jarrow in 682, how many more than twenty-two resided at Wearmouth before their departure?[88] The common life of the monks, emphasized, for example, by the common refectory and dormitory at Wearmouth, as well as the normal practices of monastic life, created ideal conditions for the spread of infection, particularly when the very concept of infection was quite unrecognized.[89] If the Northumbrian monks shared in the common view of the ancient and medieval world, which was also Bede's view, namely, that epidemics were the products of aerial miasmata, they would have had no reason to avoid contacts during times of plague.[90] Those contacts might be of the most intimate kind. There could hardly have been a more innocently lethal act of charity than

[87] Bede, *EH* 3.23, pp. 286–89.
[88] *Historia Abbatum Auctore Anonymo*, in Bede, *Opera historica*, 1:391; *Historia Abbatum Auctore Baeda*, in ibid., 370. If the discrepancy in numbers is due to a manuscript confusion between "xvii" and "xxii," as Plummer thought (ibid, 2:361), the larger figure of the Anonymous is likely to be right because he states that the twenty-two comprised ten tonsured and twelve untonsured brethren.
[89] *Historia Abbatum Auctore Baeda*, in ibid., 372.
[90] For the absence of any notion of contagion before the sixteenth century (except in the notable case of Thucydides), see Holladay and Poole, "Thucydides and the Plague of Athens," 296–97. I am very grateful to Barbara Harvey for this reference.

the kiss of peace given by Abbot Eosterwine to each of the Wearmouth monks as he lay dying of *pestilentia* in March 686.[91] Alhough Wearmouth and Jarrow were each struck hard by the plague, their exceptional stone buildings may have made them a degree less vulnerable than, say, Lindisfarne or such lesser houses as Hartlepool, where timber construction was extensively used; for if rats were the agents of disease, stone gave them less 'access and leeway' than walls of wood and wattle.[92] It is salutary to remember (and we shall find later evidence to confirm this) that, hard hit though the greatest and wealthiest of the Northumbrian monasteries were by the plague, their country cousins among the smaller monasteries, about whose fortunes we know much less, may have been hit still harder.

In Gaul, it was the great towns and particularly the ports that were the bases and launching points for the spread of plague: Narbonne, Albi, Avignon, Lyons, and especially Marseilles are the names scattered through Gregory of Tours' desultory chronicle of its progress.[93] In seventh-century England there were no comparable surviving Roman towns, but the new monasteries in some ways resembled them, as communities, centers of population, and points of convergence that brought together food supplies, buildings, and human hosts in an environment favorable to the parasites that were the agents of infection. Like the Gaulish towns too, the monasteries did more than just provide a passive stage for the plague's most obviously destructive visitations. They also played a more active role in its dissemination, as the sites for its initial reception and, as we shall argue later, for its onward transmission to the countryside.

The problem of the plague's reception and of the monasteries' part in it is best approached by considering the speed of its spread. One of the most remarkable features of the first plague of 664 is the apparent rapidity of that spread. After striking first in the south, probably in June or July, it had reached the north by the autumn, to judge by Cedd's death at Lastingham on October 23. The absence of anything but a mere record for the episcopate of Tuda, appointed to the Northumbrian see after the Synod of Whitby in the first half of 664, bishop for 'a very short time' (*permodico tempore*), and an early victim of the plague, again argues

[91] *Historia Abbatum Auctore Baeda*, in Bede, *Opera historica*, 1:372.

[92] For the buildings of Wearmouth and Jarrow, see Cramp, "Monkweathmouth and Jarrow," esp. 10–11, 13–16. For Lindisfarne: Bede, *EH* 3.25, pp. 294–95. For Hartlepool: Daniels, "Monastery at Church Close," 203–4; Daniels, "Hartlepool," 273. Benedictow, *Plague in Late Medieval Nordic Countries*, 136–38, emphasizes the role of stone buildings in reducing the risk of plague infection; cf. Slack, *Impact of Plague*, 322.

[93] Gregory of Tours, *The History of the Franks*, 2:264, 394–96, 459, 461.

for a rapid onset in the north.[94] This was a much swifter progress than that of the later Black Death, which came to southern England in June or July 1348, but did not reach York until May 1349, the Lincolnshire Wolds until July, and Meaux Abbey, in the East Riding, until August.[95] It was also considerably faster than the speed at which plague generally spread in the late medieval and early modern period, for which recent calculations suggest a rate of progress rarely in excess of 1.5 kilometers a day. If we reckon the period between the plague's arrival in the south and in the north to be some thirteen weeks or ninety-one days (say, July 15 to October 15), and the distance between, say, Dover and Lastingham to be some 385 kilometers as the crow flies, we are left with a rate of progress of about 4.2 kilometers per day, considerably faster than almost any record for the later period; and plague will hardly have traveled with a crow's notional directness.[96]

This comparative evidence argues strongly against the overland transmission of plague, from south to north, in 664 and in favor of an alternative – the disease's spontaneous and near simultaneous introduction to the north via maritime contacts either with the south coast or, perhaps more plausibly, with the Continent. The concurrent arrival of plague in Ireland on August 1, 664 seems to fall into this pattern of multiple introductions. It is entirely possible that the plague was borne overseas via rats carried in the ships from some Frankish port such as Quentovic (where Archbishop Theodore embarked for England in 669), to strike independently in all these parts of Britain.[97] Such an advance on several fronts characterized the spread of plague in 1348–1349, both in England, where the plague seems to have made separate landfalls in Dorset, Bristol, and possibly London, and in Norway, where it arrived both at Bergen on the west coast and around Oslo in the south-east.[98] In both periods, multiple entry points would do more to explain plague's national and catastrophic effects than any thesis of transmission from a single source.

The monasteries are likely to have provided those entry points, at least in the north of England. Much recent work has emphasized the coastal and estuarine situation of the early Northumbrian monasteries, their

---

94 Bede, *EH* 3.26–27, pp. 308–13.
95 Horrox, *Black Death*, 10.
96 Benedictow, *Plague in Late Medieval Nordic Countries*, 79–81, brings together much useful material on the rate of spread of plague. The calculations discussed earlier are based on his figures.
97 Bede, *EH* 4.1, pp. 332–33.
98 Horrox, *Black Death*, 10; Benedictow, *Plague in Late Medieval Nordic Countries*, 75–94.

being well placed for sea communication, and their role as trading centers, confirmed, for example, by the large number of sceatta coins found at Whitby.[99] Whitby, Hartlepool, and Lindisfarne, the latter possessing 'a fine natural harbour and a strategic anchorage', were all flourishing monastic houses in 664 and all coastally located.[100] Other Northumbrian seaboard monasteries – Coldingham and Tynemouth – were founded at unknown dates in the seventh century,[101] and others again – Wearmouth and Jarrow – post-dated the first plague. Of non-monastic places with access to the sea, only the Anglian port of York is likely to have been of any consequence, but we have already noted that there was probably little or no economic activity there before c. 700.[102] If the plague came by sea to Northumbria, it is far more likely to have arrived at a monastic port than anywhere else. Nor need this have been true of Northumbria alone. Tilbury in Essex, with its estuarine site, early monastery, and numerous sceatta finds, may provide a parallel case further south.[103] We may be witnessing what would emerge again more visibly in the early modern period: the development of distinct 'maritime epidemics', initiated by ship, growing from coastal centers, and spreading widely through the single maritime region that the small British landmass constituted.[104]

PLAGUE IN THE COUNTRYSIDE

The monasteries are thus likely to have played a crucial part in the history of the seventh-century plague, both as communities in some ways like towns, whose size and close-quarter living made them peculiarly susceptible to the disease, and as probable entry points for the seaborne rats that were the agents of plague. Their prominence in Bede's references to the plague reflects not only Bede's own monastic sources and interests but also the monasteries' preeminent vulnerability to infection. The majority of the population, however, did not live in monasteries but in a countryside whose social and economic contours have become much

[99] Cramp, "Northumberland and Ireland," 192; Campbell, "Background to the Life of St. Cuthbert," 17–18; Blair, "Ecclesiastical Organization and Pastoral Care," 201; Hill and Metcalf, *Sceattas*, 265. For other sceatta finds at Jarrow see ibid., 253.
[100] Rollason, "Why was St. Cuthbert so Popular?" 17.
[101] *Two Lives of St. Cuthbert*, 80–81; Bede, *EH* 4.19, 5.6, pp. 391–93, 464–65.
[102] See at nn. 83–86 in this essay.
[103] Hamerow, *Excavations at Mucking*, 2:86–89.
[104] For later "maritime epidemics," see Eckert, *Structure of Plagues*, 67–73.

clearer over the past two decades. It was one of small and scattered settlements, where houses shifted within settlements in a constant process
of abandonment and rebuilding, and where settlements themselves were
sometimes mobile features in the landscape, lacking the fixed and permanent anchorages later provided by church and manor. Such fixed points
as existed were provided by the monasteries, which may already have
begun to function as markets, by the local churches occasionally served
by monastic priests, and by the royal vills that were the stopping places
for itinerant kings and the collection points for food rents and tribute.
Even these might be impermanent, as the mid-seventh-century abandonment of the Northumbrian *villa regia* at Yeavering shows. Settlement was
thus extensive rather than intensive, and lacking in the market towns and
orderly nucleated villages that would begin to focus the landscape from
the tenth century onward.[105]

The impact of plague on this loosely structured countryside and its
thin spread of people is an important question. No matter how high the
death rate in the monasteries, if they were virtually the sole communities
affected it would be hard to argue that plague was of great general significance. A priori, it might seem that in our period rural society – there was
hardly any other – could not possibly have been so endangered by plague
as its fourteenth-century counterpart. By that time a densely populated
landscape of villages, markets, and small towns, bound together by trade
and exchange, lay mortally exposed in the face of plague; so that, for
example, the large Worcestershire village of Halesowen, with an adult
population of some 680, saw nearly 43% of those adults die between May
and August 1349.[106] But in Bede's England there were no Halesowens.

These differences might easily reinforce the commonsense assumption that the rural Northumbria of King Oswy and King Ecgfrith was
relatively less vulnerable to plague than the rural England of Edward III.
We may be less inclined to accept that assumption, however, if we consider the plague's impact, in a later age, on two countries that were in
some ways comparable to Bede's England: fourteenth-century Norway
and fifteenth-century Iceland. The late medieval Norwegian plague fell
on a countryside more like that of seventh- than of fourteenth-century
England. It was a land of poor communications, divided by mountains,

---

[105] A composite picture chiefly derived from Taylor, *Village and Farmstead*, 109–24; Blair,
       "Minster Churches"; Hamerow, "Rural Settlements and Settlement Patterns"; Welch,
       Anglo-Saxon England, 29–53. The case of Yeavering is discussed next.
[106] Razi, *Life, Marriage and Death*, 25, 31, 103–04.

fiords, and forests, virtually without inland towns and with few villages, but scattered instead with the small hamlets of the more prosperous peasantry and the single holdings of the poor, which lay on their outskirts.[107] Yet Norway's population, contrary to all natural expectations, seems to have fallen by about the same proportion as that of England during the Black Death and subsequent outbreaks of plague.[108] How such a scattered and often isolated people may have succumbed to plague has been provisionally worked out by Ole Jørgen Benedictow. Central to the process was the transport of infected fleas, either by humans or by rats, and here two mechanisms were especially important: the flight of flea-bearing refugees from plague-stricken areas to others as yet unstricken; and the carriage of grain, and with it not just rats but also fleas apparently able to subsist independently on grain and grain debris, between settlements. Grain-borne infection might be accomplished in several ways, notably through the exchange of grain for animal produce between arable lowlands and pastoral uplands, and through grain payments made to laborers in return for services. Other forms of trade, especially perhaps in salt, might promote other adventitious contacts.[109] Once established by these means in a settlement, infection was spread via the normal practices of religion and local society: the attendance on the sick and dying of family friends and priests, whose movements between households made them active disseminators of infection; the holding of funeral feasts, which brought together the dead, the sick and the living in flea-ridden households; and the distribution of the flea-harboring clothes and bedding of the dead.[110] These forms of interdependence, both commercial and social, ensured almost paradoxically that isolation favored infection rather than immunity. It is true that this reconstruction contains much hypothesis and that the means of contact between peoples and settlements are easier to detect than the precise links between contact and infection. But it is difficult to posit other ways in which plague's devastation of a widely scattered population could have occurred.

The experience of Iceland, discussed by Gunnar Karlsson, both resembled and differed from that of Norway.[111] The two Icelandic plague epidemics of 1402–1404 and 1494–1495 afflicted a countryside where

---

[107] Benedictow, *Plague in Late Medieval Nordic Countries*, 109, 192.

[108] Ibid., 104–09, 113–15, 193–205. A shade of doubt remains about Benedictow's calculations, however, because he does not make them available in his text.

[109] Ibid., 185–89.

[110] Ibid., 182–85.

[111] Karlsson, "Plague Without Rats," esp. 265, 267, 270, 281–84.

'practically everyone lived on individual farms; there were hardly any villages and certainly no towns'. Yet by Karlsson's reckoning the death rate
may have been as high as 50–60% in the first epidemic and 30–50% in
the second. It certainly brought a wide and general desertion of home-
steads. How then did plague spread, and to such mortal effect, in this
other land of isolated settlements? Not by rats, as Benedictow argues
(wrongly in Karlsson's view) for Norway: there is no sign of their presence in Iceland; the climate was too cold for their survival, let alone
for that of their parasitic plague-bearing fleas, and even had it not been,
there was virtually no overland movement of grain to provide the means of
flea-transmission proposed for Norway. Because both Icelandic epidemics
continued through the winter, the evidence favors not bubonic but pneumonic plague, spread presumably by human contacts and through some
of the same means prevailing in Norway: the flight of the fearful, the
pastoral travels of priests, the journeys occasioned by funerals. Although
pneumonic plague must take its distant origins from a flea bite, the Icelandic epidemics provide the best available evidence for plague's further
diffusion without the agency of rats.

To the investigator of the seventh-century English plagues, both these
models have their uses, for they suggest ways in which plague could ravage
a population dispersed across a rural landscape of small-scale settlements.
In the case of England, where we have argued for the same combination
of bubonic and pneumonic plague as was to occur again at the time of
the Black Death, each of the mechanisms invoked by Benedictow and
by Karlsson to explain the spread of plague in their respective countries
may have come into play.[112] Perhaps the closest parallel between possible routes to infection in late medieval Norway and in early Anglo-Saxon
England lies in the transport of grain. Benedictow's stress on the primacy
of grain movements and on the symbiotic economies of highland and
lowland, which often occasioned such movements, immediately brings
to mind both the transport of the king's food rent (*feorm*) from dependent settlements to the central places marked by royal vills, and also the
location of those vills. The only surviving statement of what a king could
draw from his estate in *feorm*, contained in a grant made by Offa to the
church of Worcester between 793 and 796, mentions, among other foodstuffs, thirty 'ambers' of unground corn and four 'ambers' of meal, to be
delivered to the royal vill (*ad regalem vicum*). The best known royal vill,
at Yeavering, lay at the junction of highland and lowland zones, on the

---

[112] Lindley and Ormrod, *Black Death in England*, 24–25.

edge of both the pastoral Cheviots and of the grain-producing area of the coastal plain and the Tweed valley.[113] Although Yeavering had British origins, its siting may partly be explained in terms of its convenience for the exchange of grain and stock, and for the delivery of these complementary products for the king's use. Behind these links between agriculture and royal power we can thus dimly discern contacts similar to those that may later have spread infection in rural Norway.

Other parallels were more directly and unambivalently related to plague. One common reaction to plague, in England and Ireland as in Norway and Iceland, was flight, with the attendant likelihood of the onward transmission of disease.[114] In England, as in Norway and Iceland, priests were expected to visit the sick, even those sick with plague. Theodore's Penitential, quoting the opinion of 'the Greeks and the Romans', lays down that 'in case of plague ... the sick ought to be visited, as [are] other sick persons': a ruling that, despite its foreign origins, was presumably thought to have some relevance to the English situation.[115] In England, as in Norway, the trade in salt served to link different regions.[116] Other contacts were probably more sporadic and unregulated. Luxury goods found on rural sites – a cowrie shell at Puddlehill in Bedfordshire, north French pottery at Chalton in Hampshire – suggest wealth, exchange, and more than subsistence agriculture;[117] sceatta finds at hillforts point to the marketing of livestock;[118] the warriors who traveled in search of ring-giving kings are likely to have moved from one royal vill or high-status site to another;[119] bishops, if they did their duty, took the Gospel into remote countryside;[120] a traveling Briton, passing through a settlement, could join the locals in a feast.[121] There were a dozen forms of mobility to provide the putative means of transport for the infected fleas of bubonic plague and to link separated settlements via the infected humans of pneumonic plague. If, in seventh-century England, isolation fostered economic interdependence, as in Norway, these other sorts of

[113] *Cartularium Saxonicum*, 1: no. 273; *English Historical Documents*, 1: no. 78; Hope-Taylor, *Yeavering*, 12, 17–23.
[114] Below, at nn. 172–75, 184; Karlsson, "Plague Without Rats," 277–78.
[115] *Theodore's Penitential* 8.6, in *Medieval Handbooks of Penance*, 206.
[116] Blair, *Anglo-Saxon Oxfordshire*, 84–87.
[117] Hinton, *Archaeology, Economy and Society*, 26; Champion, "Chalton," 369.
[118] Metcalf, "Sceattas Found at the Iron-Age Hill Fort," 1–2.
[119] Bede, *EH* 3.14, pp. 256–59, for the ability of King Oswin of Deira to attract "noblemen from almost every kingdom."
[120] *Two Lives of St. Cuthbert*, 208–09, 256–61.
[121] Bede, *EH* 3.10, pp. 244–45.

contact, 'political' and religious, owed more to the particularities of time and place.

This was especially true with regard to the monasteries, whose pastoral functions bred contacts that had no exact parallel in the Europe of the later Middle Ages. At this time the monasteries were anything but enclosed communities. Not only did monks and their attendant priests have a pastoral role to play in the countryside, but also the monasteries themselves drew in the faithful. On Sundays, Bede says, monastic churches were the venue for popular devotions;[122] both Bede's own homilies and the pictures on Biblical themes displayed around the churches at Wearmouth and Jarrow suggest the occasional presence in those churches of the unlettered laity, some of them probably extramural laborers on the monastic estates and all of them there to be instructed.[123] Grander visitors at the monasteries included kings and their thegns;[124] and women and children as well as men, presumably some of them laymen, were buried in monastic cemeteries.[125] This close integration of the monasteries into the religious life of their neighborhoods was fostered by other contacts of a less distinctively religious kind. Some monasteries almost certainly functioned as markets, both for imports brought by sea to places whose coastal location has already been noted, and also for the surplus produce of monastic estates. Whitby and Jarrow, with their sceatta coins and craft products, may be cases in point.[126] At others, the reputation of a saint's shrine such as Cuthbert's might be expected to draw in 'fugitives and guilty men', probably more intent on sanctuary than religious experience.[127] Of course, not all regions were thickly planted with monasteries and not all monasteries filled all these functions. Nevertheless many monasteries, like the royal vills, were in effect central places, and often designedly so.[128] If, during the plague, they became reservoirs of infection, the exchange between center and periphery, monastery and locality, salvational in purpose, may have become lethal by result.

So far we have done no more than to scout the superficially plausible view that the plague was largely confined to monasteries; to use evidence

---

[122] Ibid., 3.26, pp. 310–11.
[123] Thacker, "Monks, Preaching and Pastoral Care," 140–41; Meyvaert, "Church Paintings at Wearmouth-Jarrow," 69.
[124] Bede, *EH* 3.26, pp. 310–11.
[125] Thacker, "Monks, Preaching and Pastoral Care," 140.
[126] Campbell, *Anglo-Saxon History*, 141; Cramp, "Monkwearmouth and Jarrow," 8, 14.
[127] *Two Lives of St. Cuthbert*, 278–79.
[128] Cf. Blair, "Ecclesiastical Organization and Pastoral Care," 201.

from other times and other countries to suggest that dispersed rural settlements were not necessarily immune from its visitations; and to propose ways in which it may have spread, sometimes via the monasteries, to and between those settlements. But this begs the question of plague's actual impact on the English countryside. In attempting an answer we go first to the continental sources.

Rather more informative than the English sources, they suggest that plague was by no means restricted to large centers of population. Gregory of Tours, for all the close association he establishes between towns and plague, also makes it clear that plague was not confined to towns. The first Gaulish plague of the 540s, he says, 'raged ... in divers regions'; that of 571, the Auvergne (hardly the most urbanized part of Gaul) and 'all that region', with such ferocity that 'the legions of men who fell there might not even be numbered', and the dead were buried in common pits; and that of 584, 'various regions'.[129] Much more vivid and precise is Paul the Deacon's record of the plague of the 560s in rural north Italy – the best account of any Dark-Age plague in the West, and worth quoting in full:

A very great pestilence broke out particularly in the province of Liguria. For suddenly there appeared certain marks among the dwellings, doors, utensils and clothes, which, if anyone wished to wash away, became more and more apparent. After the lapse of a year indeed there began to appear in the groins of men and in other rather delicate places a swelling of the glands, after the manner of a nut or date, presently followed by an unbearable fever, so that upon the third day the man died. But if anyone should pass over the third day he had a hope of living. Everywhere there was grief and everywhere tears. For as common report had it that those who fled would avoid the plague, the dwellings were left deserted by their inhabitants, and the dogs alone kept house. The flocks remained alone in the pastures with no shepherd at hand. You might see villages (*villas*) or fortified places lately filled with crowds of men, and on the next day all had departed and everything was in utter silence. Some fled, leaving the corpses of their parents unburied; parents forgetful of their duty abandoned their children in raging fever. If by chance long-standing affection constrained anyone to bury his near relative, he remained himself unburied, and while he was performing funeral rites he perished; while he offered obsequies to the dead, his own corpse remained without obsequies. You might see the world brought back to its ancient silence; no voice in the field; no whistling of shepherds; no lying in wait of wild beasts among the cattle; no harm to domestic fowls. The crops, outliving the time of the harvest, awaited the reaper untouched; the vineyard with its fallen leaves and its shining grapes remained undisturbed while winter came on; a trumpet as of warriors resounded through the day and night; something like the murmur of an

[129] Gregory of Tours, *The History of the Franks*, 2:119, 140–41, 264.

army was heard by many; there were no footsteps of passers by, no murderer was
seen, yet the corpses of the dead were more than the eye could discern; pastoral
places had been turned into a desert, and human habitations had become places
of refuge for wild beasts.[130]

Paul the Deacon's words are of special value. They portray a catastrophe. They clearly identify its cause as bubonic plague by describing
the plague buboes; they reveal the reaction of potential victims – terror,
flight, the abandonment of the most binding obligations; and, most significantly for us, they show how plague left a countryside void of people.
It is a picture to keep in mind as we move back to the less well-evidenced
terrain of seventh-century England. Were such scenes replicated here?
Were there no longer whistling shepherds on the hills of Northumbria?

Although our accounts have most to say about the effects of plague on
the monasteries, their remarks about its impact 'throughout the length
and breadth of Britain' and 'everywhere in Britain and Ireland' suggest
that its sickle cut a much wider path.[131] Peoples and provinces were not
immune, as the apostasy of the East Saxons during the first plague of 664
suggests.[132] More valuable, however, because more specifically related
to rural conditions, are Bede's descriptions of Cuthbert's Northumbrian
activities during the two plagues of 664 and c. 685. As in Essex, the 664
plague brought lapses from the faith, and it was to the apostates in the
hill country around Melrose that Cuthbert went out to preach.[133] Writing
of the effects of the later plague, Bede is fuller and more helpfully precise. He paints Paul the Deacon's picture in miniature. 'A most grievous
pestilence ... brought with it destruction so severe that in some large
villages and estates (*in magnis ... villis ac possessionibus*) once crowded
with inhabitants, only a small and scattered remnant, and sometimes
none at all, remained'. It was to these 'poor few' survivors that Cuthbert
ministered.[134] Bede here builds upon the earlier account of the same
episode in the anonymous Life of Cuthbert, which speaks of the plague
depopulating many regions (*plures depopulavit regiones*) and of Cuthbert
again preaching to the survivors in a certain village (*villa, vicus*), which

[130] Paul the Deacon, *Historia Longobardorum* 2.4, p. 74. Though Paul the Deacon wrote
c. 790, his account does not draw on any known source. With its careful account of
the plague symptoms, which at that date are unlikely to have been known to Paul from
firsthand experience, it may well draw on the evidence of an eyewitness.
[131] As seen in the opening paragraph of this essay.
[132] Bede, *EH* 3.30, pp. 322–23.
[133] *Two Lives of St. Cuthbert*, 184–87.
[134] Ibid., 258–61.

Bede later calls a *viculus*.[135] Adomnán too, an eye-witness traveling to the Northumbrian court, speaks of this second plague as devastating many villages (*multos . . . vicos*).[136]

Here is some unequivocal evidence, generally neglected, of the plague's effects on the Northumbrian countryside: of depopulation, the shrinkage of some settlements, and the abandonment of others. We can do something to define the nature of those settlements. The words used by Bede and Adomnán to describe places – *villa, vicus, viculus* – signify, in a general way, small villages; although 'village' conveys an anachronistic sense of concentration, density, and order. *Villa, vicus* and *possessiones* may additionally have stood for royal estate centers and their dependent settlements.[137] Our textual evidence does not extend beyond Northumbria. But if we can trust it – and we are drawing here on three authors – a variety of rural places proved vulnerable to the plague's depredations.

To go further than this we must turn from texts to archaeology. Leading on as it does from the textual record just discussed, our most useful corpus of material here is provided by the rural settlements that excavation has shown to have been both occupied and abandoned between c. 600 and c. 700. Few in number, they nevertheless constitute a large proportion of those settlements known for the early and middle Saxon period. Although their history is very difficult to reconstruct, against our written sources, all from Northumbria, they have one advantage: They are widely distributed over the country, from Northumberland south to Hampshire, and from Suffolk and Essex across to Bedfordshire and Oxfordshire. Here we attend particularly to their size and period of occupation because it is these factors that bear most strongly on the possible reasons for their desertion.[138]

Moving clockwise, south from Northumbria, the sites and their chief characteristics are these:

1. Thirlings (Northumberland): some twelve buildings, mainly constructed in the late- fifth and sixth centuries, with the start of the latest building having a *terminus post quem*, obtained by radiocarbon

---

[135] Ibid., 118–21.
[136] Adomnán, *Adomnán's Life of Columba*, 178–79; Adomnán, *Life of St Columba*, 203.
[137] Campbell, *Anglo-Saxon History*, 108–12.
[138] In what follows I have omitted (except for Raunds) those very few sites thought either to have been deserted before c. 600 (e.g., Bishopstone, Sussex) or to have continued after c. 700 (e.g., Catholme, Staffs). For these sites, see Welch, *Anglo-Saxon England*, 32–34, 39.

dating, of 604–681; all were abandoned, after systematic demolition of the six major buildings, at an unknown date.[139]

2. Yeavering (Northumberland): a royal vill, founded in the late-sixth century at an earlier British center, probably visited intermittently by the kings of Bernicia and later of Northumbria, but not permanently occupied, and abandoned some time after 633, probably between c. 655 and c. 685.[140]

3. West Stow (Suffolk): a small settlement, founded during the mid-fifth century, containing some four 'farm complexes', reduced to two by c. 650, and entirely abandoned at some later date.[141]

4. Mucking (Essex): a large settlement with a possible population of around 100 at any one time, occupied from the first half of the fifth century until the beginning of the eighth.[142]

5. Cowdery's Down (Hampshire): like Yeavering, probably a high-status site rather than a normal village, occupied from the late-sixth century and through the seventh; in its final and most extensive phase it may have had a population of sixty or more, before the whole settlement was destroyed by fire and not rebuilt.[143]

6. Chalton (Hampshire): a small settlement, founded in the late-sixth or early seventh century; at its most thriving in the seventh century, it may have lasted into the early eighth, to judge by finds of north French pottery, possibly imported through Hamwic; at no time is it likely to have consisted of more than 'three to four fenced farm units'.[144]

7. New Wintles Farm (Oxfordshire): one or two farms, occupied from the end of the sixth century until the late-seventh or early eighth century.[145]

8. Puddlehill (Bedfordshire): a small settlement of nine buildings, 'perhaps one family and its dependents', probably occupied from early to late in the seventh century.[146]

---

[139] Miket and O'Brien, "Settlement of Thirlings," 57, 60–61, 88.

[140] Hope-Taylor, *Yeavering*, 277; Welch, *Anglo-Saxon England*, 44, 46.

[141] West, *West Stow*, 167–70; Welch, *Anglo-Saxon England*, 30–31.

[142] Hamerow, *Excavations at Mucking*, 2:90; Hamerow, "Rural Settlements and Settlement Patterns," 3–8; Welch, *Anglo-Saxon England*, 31–32.

[143] S. James and Millett, "Excavations at Cowdery's Down," 197–200, 212, 218, 222, 249; Welch, *Anglo-Saxon England*, 17–18, 29–30.

[144] Champion, "Chalton," 367; Welch, *Anglo-Saxon England*, 30.

[145] Briggs, Cook, and Rowley, *Archaeology of the Oxford Region*, 83–84.

[146] Matthews and Hawkes, "Settlements and Burials on Puddlehill," 59, 61, 101–02.

9. Raunds (Northamptonshire): beginning as a large, scattered settlement in the sixth century, Raunds continued into the tenth century, unlike the other sites listed above; but at some point between c. 650 and c. 750 there occurred an important change: extensive settlement was abandoned and reduced to four principal buildings placed within a ditched enclosure.[147]

The peculiar pattern of desertion revealed by these sites has long been recognized, although its seeming focus on the years around 700 has been noticed less often. It has been accounted for in various ways, but two explanations hold the field. The first, that of C. J. Arnold and P. Wardle, sees the process of abandonment as an extended one, spread through the seventh and eighth centuries, and representing the relinquishment of marginal land in favor of something better.[148] The second, that of H. F. Hamerow, sees that process as merely another phase in the constant dynamic of settlement mobility that characterized the early and middle Saxon countryside. By Hamerow's reckoning, many settlements simply relocated to neighboring sites, as yet undiscovered, and indeed very difficult to discover because of the dearth of eighth-century artifacts. With the disappearance of both grave goods and apparently of datable pottery, settlements sink into virtual invisibility.[149] Divergent though these views are, their authors share a belief in the mobility of the rural population rather than its decline. Only one historian, Christopher Taylor, has suggested a bolder 'catastrophe' thesis. The 'considerable abandonment of settlement', he writes, 'may be explained only by a large decrease in the population of England'. This he tentatively attributes, among other reasons, to epidemic disease, although mainly to the supposed epidemics of the fifth century.[150]

The evidential value of these deserted sites is thus qualified by the lack of agreement on what their desertion signifies. This in turn results largely from the difficulty of fixing even approximate dates for their desertion; for dating purposes, the few artifacts they yield are blunt rather than precision implements. Yet although closely defined limits cannot be ascertained, it is surely significant that in all cases abandonment fell within the seventh or early eighth centuries, and predominantly around 700.

[147] Report on the Raunds Area project in *Current Archaeology* 96 (1987): 325.
[148] Arnold and Wardle, "Settlement Patterns in England," 145–48. Cf. Aston, Austin, and Dyer, *Rural Settlements of Medieval England*, 278–80.
[149] Hamerow, "Rural Settlements and Settlement Patterns," 11–17.
[150] Taylor, *Village and Farmstead*, 121.

The majority of sites had long been occupied: in the cases of Yeavering, Thirlings, West Stow, Chalton and perhaps New Wintles, probably for a century or more. After such continuous occupation it is curious that all should have been abandoned within a space of fifty years or so. If settlement shift provides the explanation, it might have been expected to be as prevalent in the sixth century as in the seventh, resulting in a more extended sequence of desertions. There are sixth-century desertions (e.g. Bishopstone, Sussex), but they are rare by comparison with those that spread around the end of the next century.[151] Earlier desertions may to some extent be more difficult to spot because the buildings that denominate sites were often smaller and less substantial in the sixth century than in the seventh. Yet identified sixth-century sites, although fewer than their seventh-century successors, are not uncommon: the tally of A. Marshall and G. Marshall notes nine sites containing twenty-three buildings for the sixth century, as against thirteen sites containing eighty-seven buildings for the seventh.[152] Had there been any general pattern of desertions and relocations prior to our period, it is unlikely to have gone undiscovered.

It should remain an open possibility, therefore, that the abandonment of sites long occupied does not provide a mere optical illusion of rural depopulation. It may instead mark a real decline, although one whose nature and duration remain to be considered. Given what our literary sources have to say about such depopulation – evidence ignored by the archaeologists – it is hard to doubt that plague had at least some part to play in the story.

Two examples may strengthen the case by bringing the textual and the archaeological evidence rather more closely together: Yeavering and Mucking. In decay during its mid-seventh-century final phase, Yeavering comprised a mere four buildings, their erection dated to the early 650s by their excavator.[153] One of them, a probable barn with an unloading bay and winnowing doors, points both to Yeavering's continuing function as a center for the delivery of food rents in grain and to the possible hospitality that it might thus offer to rats.[154] The crucial witness to the settlement's occupation at this time, a Flemish coin minted in the 630s or 640s and

[151] Welch, *Anglo-Saxon England*, 32–34.
[152] Marshall and Marshall, "Change and Continuity in Anglo-Saxon Buildings," 376, 378.
[153] Hope-Taylor, *Yeavering*, 166–68, 277.
[154] The suggestion of Alcock, *Forts of the North Britons*, 26. Alcock's further suggestion, in *Neighbours of the Picts*, 26, that Yeavering was finally deserted in the year after King Edwin's death in 633, seems very unlikely in view of the 630 to 650 date of the coin.

found in the remains of the hall, does not preclude, and may support, a date for desertion during the period of the plague; for the coin must have circulated for some time before its loss.[155] When Cuthbert was ministering to the plague-stricken around Melrose in 664 and again, as bishop, to those dependent upon Lindisfarne in the 680s, it is unlikely that the men and women of the Yeavering area, some twenty-three miles from Melrose and fourteen from Lindisfarne, remained sublimely unaffected by these disasters. After all, the estates that made up the core of the see of Lindisfarne came almost to Yeavering's doorstep.[156] A sharp reduction in the numbers of those who looked to Yeavering as an estate center may have contributed to, or even caused, the final redundancy of the villa. Mucking is less susceptible to such finely balanced arguments. But when the plague struck Essex about 664, causing King Sighere and his people to apostasize, and when it returned some years later to devastate the monastery at Barking, it is again unlikely that it exempted this large rural settlement, within the kingdom, and only some fifteen miles from Barking.

We would expect some sites to be especially vulnerable to demographic disaster: that is to say, small settlements, more hamlets than villages, perhaps *viculi* rather than *vici* in Bede's terminology, and often located on marginal land, long recognized as prejudicial by those who see marginality as a step along the road to desertion.[157] Puddlehill, with its few settlers living high on the Chilterns and exposed to the westerly gales, was one such settlement; West Stow, its dwindling band of mid-seventh-century inhabitants residing on a low, infertile sandy bluff above the river Lark, was another.[158] Many other rural sites seem, like these, to have been small;[159] and some, like both West Stow and Yeavering, with their shrunken clusters of buildings, were clearly ailing before the advent of the plague. If such settlements were struck by disease, their antecedent decline, small size, and marginal location would immediately place them in jeopardy, sapping their vitality and population to a point where the survivors (if survivors there were) could no longer support a life of pastoral and arable husbandry, and so migrated. It was just such small settlements, with some

[155] Hope-Taylor, *Yeavering*, 57, 182–83, 277.
[156] Ibid., 277; compare the map in Rollason, *Cuthbert, Saint and Patron*, 15–16, with that in Hope-Taylor, *Yeavering*, 2.
[157] Cf. Campbell, *Anglo-Saxon History*, 108, 111.
[158] Matthews and Hawkes, "Settlements and Burials on Puddlehill," 59–60; West, *West Stow*, 1:9–10, 105, 108.
[159] Cf. Blair, *Anglo-Saxon Oxfordshire*, 22–25.

pre-existing weakness of economy or location, that were most vulnerable to shrinkage, decay, and sometimes extinction after the plagues of the fourteenth century.[160] Larger villages would have had a greater chance of survival; Mucking, with its population of 100 or so, and its continuity into the eighth century, may be an example. But to judge by what has been excavated, robust and populous settlements of the Mucking sort were the exception in the early Anglo-Saxon period. That by the later Middle Ages they had become the rule, at least in lowland England, perhaps explains why epidemic disease may have been more disruptive to settlement patterns in earlier times than in later.

If we look for more direct and conclusive archaeological evidence for the possible impact of plague, we shall be disappointed. Archaeology cannot tell us much about the progress of epidemic disease in any period. If we relied on it alone, we would hardly be able to detect the Black Death: a warning of what may lie concealed in this much earlier period, when the written sources record so much less than those of the fourteenth century. Some possible indicators of plague are worth a mention. There are, for example, a few burial sites that may indicate the hasty disposal of its victims: an adult woman with a child in her arms, accompanied by a tall man lying supine and with head bent up, both buried carelessly, at Kintbury (Berkshire); pits containing carelessly buried bodies, including a large rectangular pit holding several bodies, at Saffron Walden (Essex); the unlaid-out skeletons found in shallow irregular graves at Marina Drive, Totternhoe (Bedfordshire).[161] Most suggestive of all are the two cemeteries at Camerton (Somersetshire) and Winnall (Hampshire). From Camerton came 115 skeletons, including 40 children, buried hurriedly in the positions in which they died. Here, in a cemetery firmly datable to the seventh century, the excavator himself was inclined to see the burial of plague victims. At Winnall, where the cemetery can be more closely dated to the second half of the seventh century, some bodies had been buried in rigor mortis and in shoddily dug and sometimes very shallow graves.[162]

---

[160] C. Taylor, *Village and Farmstead*, 171. For a particular example, consider Tusmore, Oxon, *Victoria County History, Oxfordshire*, 6:337; Allison, Beresford, and Hirst, *Deserted Villages of Oxfordshire*, 26, 45. But for a different view, see Aston, Austin, and Dyer, *Rural Settlements of Medieval England*, 57.

[161] Meaney, *Early Anglo-Saxon Burial Sites*, 48, 88, 41; Meaney and Hawkes, *Two Anglo-Saxon Cemeteries*, 29–30. See Meaney, *Early Anglo-Saxon Burial Sites*, 145, 287–88, for other possible examples.

[162] Meaney, *Early Anglo-Saxon Burial Sites*, 218. Meaney and Hawkes, *Two Anglo-Saxon Cemeteries*, 29–30, 46–49.

Such 'disorderly' cemeteries point us back to what our texts have to say about the disposal of plague victims: to the burials in a common pit, ten or more at a time, recorded by Gregory of Tours for the Auvergne, and to the corpses left unburied by fleeing survivors remarked on by Paul the Deacon for Liguria.[163] They cannot be diagnostic; but they put us in mind of possibilities.

Our conclusion must be that the effects of plague on the countryside remain certain but unquantifiable. It is highly unlikely that the deserted settlements spoken of by Bede and our other sources for Northumbria were not also found elsewhere, in regions unprovided with historians and hagiographers. They may well be visible in at least some of the shrunken and abandoned sites laid bare by archaeology. Yet the archaeological evidence is too imprecise to be interpreted solely, or even in any particular instance, as the product of plague. Even in the landscape of small and scattered settlements revealed by the spade, plague could spread quickly, as the evidence from the comparable societies of Norway and Iceland suggests. All that was needed was a degree of human mobility to provide the means to epidemic infection. In England such mechanisms as the complementary economies of arable and pastoral agriculture, and the force of royal power, visible in the travels of warriors and of countrymen delivering food rents, were there to induce that mobility. Under the onslaught of the resulting epidemics the population of rural England declined; that decline may conceivably have been on the scale of the Black Death; the evidence tentatively points in this maximal direction. But the unsatisfactory truth is that the plague of 664 to c. 687 cannot with confidence be placed at any particular point on the ascending scale between minimum and maximum.

AFTERMATH AND CONSEQUENCES

What were the long-term effects of the seventh-century plague? In all probability they were small, chiefly for the reason that plague ceased completely after about 687. After that, no source records anything resembling an epidemic in England until the ninth century.[164] Nor, on a more local level, does plague figure in any of the numerous miracles of healing associated in 687 and afterward with the dead Cuthbert and the living

---

[163] Gregory of Tours, *The History of the Franks*, 2:140–41; Paul the Deacon, *Historia Langobardorum* 2.4, p. 74.

[164] Bonser, *Medical Background of Anglo-Saxon England*, 61–62.

John of Beverley, and recorded by Cuthbert's anonymous biographer and by Bede. Generalized illness – *languor, morbus, infirmitas, aegritudo* – is much in evidence in their narratives; *pestilentia*, never.[165] In confirming once again that these authors could distinguish perfectly well between plague and other ailments, the evidence separates the lethal but exceptional from the troublesome but routine. Here the English experience of declining mortality tallies with that of Ireland and the Continent. In Ireland there were three years of famine and pestilence around 700, an unidentifiable epidemic around 709, and then an apparent respite from all epidemics until 743; although the accounts in the annals suggest that these were all minor disturbances compared with the great mortalities of the 660s and 680s. In the rest of western Europe, recorded plagues after the 680s are confined to an outbreak around Narbonne in 694 and a final visitation in southern Italy in 767.[166] Although the termination of plague in England was possibly more clearcut than plague's decline elsewhere, it thus fitted into a common European pattern. That the failing cycle of European infection, in which England participated, was indeed one of bubonic plague strengthens still further the case for identifying Bede's *pestilentia* with that same disease.

It also points to a sharp contrast with the late medieval experience of plague. Then, the Black Death was only the first, if also the most severe, of many plagues and other epidemics whose recurrence worked to prevent any recovery in population for some 150 years. The plagues of the seventh century, on the other hand, constituted a well-defined episode lasting some twenty-three years. Their cessation after c. 687 is likely to have allowed the population to recover fairly rapidly, perhaps partly through the mechanism of more and earlier marriages that characterized the years following the plagues of 1348–1349 and of 1361–1362. In the later Middle Ages that process was soon checked by high rates of infant mortality in the plagues following the Black Death;[167] but no such check would have operated in the late seventh and early eighth centuries. However virulent the early plagues may have been, they did not become endemic or project cycles of high mortality far into the future. In the years following

---

[165] *Two Lives of St. Cuthbert*, 133–39, 289–91, 297, 307; Bede, *EH* 4.31, 32, 5.2 pp. 444–49, 456–69.

[166] Bonser, *Medical Background of Anglo-Saxon England*, 61–62; MacArthur, "Identification of Some Pestilences," 181, 185–86; Biraben and Le Goff, "La peste dans le haut moyen age," 1497.

[167] Hatcher, *Plague, Population and the English Economy*, 16–20, 55–62; Razi, *Life, Marriage and Death*, 131–38.

their disappearance there is every probability (although no certainty) that fertility outstripped mortality as the main determinant of demographic change.

That probability has some bearing on the history of the only two sorts of community about whose post-plague fortunes we can even speculate: the monasteries of Northumbria and the settlements of the country-side. At first glance, any maximal view of the plague's effects seems to be resoundingly gainsaid by the cultural achievement of the Northum-brian monasteries in the years around 700. Hardly needing rehearsal, that achievement comprehended not only the writings of Bede and of the lesser figures who provided lives of Cuthbert, Wilfrid, and the abbots of Wearmouth and Jarrow, but also the making of the Lindisfarne Gospels, the Echternach Gospels, the Durham Gospels (the latter two probably also the products of the Lindisfarne scriptorium), and the Codex Amiat-inus, as well as Cuthbert's coffin and its treasures.[168] Cultural and artistic enterprise on this scale depended on the availability of wealth and – more importantly for our subject – of manpower. The two years or more needed to complete the Lindisfarne Gospels, the nine scribes who worked on the Codex Amiatinus, and the trained craftsmanship of those who carved the figures on Cuthbert's coffin, all suggest religious com-munities well enough supplied with men to do more than provide for the liturgical offices that were the foundation of monastic life.[169] This deduction is confirmed by Bede's much quoted remark that when Abbot Ceolfrith departed for Rome in 716 he left behind him 'around six hun-dred brethren' at Wearmouth and Jarrow. Even if we allow that a pro-portion of those 600 may have been estate workers rather than monks *sensu stricto,* these were clearly large and thriving houses.[170] Yet in the 680s, only a generation earlier, it had been just those houses at the cen-ter of Northumbria's cultural achievement, Lindisfarne, Wearmouth, and Jarrow, which, if Bede is to be believed, had been almost overwhelmed by the plague. The contrast is striking and has been surprisingly ignored. Should it make us revise our earlier view of the plague's virulence?

To answer that question we need to take into account more than just the plague's abrupt ending and the possibly rapid growth of population

---

[168] Backhouse and Webster, *Anglo-Saxon Art and Culture,* nos. 80–82, 88, 98–99.

[169] Backhouse, *Lindisfarne Gospels,* 14; Parkes, *Scriptorium of Wearmouth-Jarrow,* 3.

[170] *Historia Abbatum Auctore Baeda,* in Bede, *Opera historica,* 1:382. The anonymous Life of Ceolfrith says that there were "more than six hundred": *Historia Abbatum Auctore Anonymo,* in ibid., 400. For monks and estate workers, see Thacker, "Monks, Preaching and Pastoral Care," 141.

thereafter. These remain, however, central considerations. Those born in the decade following the plague's disappearance, and later intending to follow a monastic life, might have been expected to enter the noviciate in the first two decades of the eighth century. If population was rising quickly from a low base, there would have been no obvious hindrances to a healthy level of monastic recruitment. Nor need that process have been entirely a natural one, for external forces may have contributed to it. Æthelwulf, the early-ninth-century author of the poem *De Abbatibus*, for example, writes of how some Northumbrians were driven to take the tonsure in monasteries during the reign of the tyrannical King Osred (c. 706–16), presumably by way of refuge: a reminder that political disturbances are not incompatible with cultural growth and that quite adventitious factors may have increased the numbers of monks.[171]

There is another possibility that may help to explain the Northumbrian monastic boom of the post-plague decades: that is, the abandonment of smaller houses during the plague and the concentration of both their surviving members and of potential future members in the larger (and better known) houses. The evidence for this course of events is sparse but suggestive, and comes in part from Ireland. There, the plague precipitated the flight of monks from their churches and sometimes the abandonment of the churches themselves. In the first great plague of 664, Bede tells us, the monks of Rathmelsigi (Clonmelsh, Co. Carlow) were almost all carried off by the disease 'or scattered about in various places' *(vel per alia essent loca dispersi)*.[172] The double process of mortality and flight described here might lead to total desertion. *Tírechán*, the late-seventh-century account of St. Patrick's churches, speaks of churches being taken over by the monastic community at Clonmacnoise, apparently after their abandonment during the plague.[173] In England, migration is more in evidence than permanent desertion. At Gilling around 666, for example, the abbot Tunberht, his kinsman Ceolfrith, and many of the monks withdrew from their plague-stricken community to Ripon, at Wilfrid's invitation. It would be tempting to assume from the subsequent silence of the sources that the house ceased to exist, but the later topographical and archaeological record (a round churchyard, Anglo-Scandinavian sculpture, Gilling as a mother church with detached chapelries) counsels

[171] Æthelwulf, *De Abbatibus*, 6.
[172] Bede, *EH* 3.27, pp. 312–13. For Rathmelsigi, see Adomnán, *Life of St Columba*, 349.
[173] *Patrician Texts in the Book of Armagh*, 143. I am very grateful to Richard Sharpe for this reference.

against this view.[174] The earlier part of this process, by which the plague allowed a 'receiving' house to draw upon new blood from outside, was not peculiar to Gilling and Ripon. After the plague had devastated Jarrow in the 680s, Ceolfrith and his diminished band of inexpert choristers continued with the liturgy (according to Ceolfrith's biographer) until the abbot had been able to train 'or gather from elsewhere' *(vel aliunde colligeret)* competent replacements for the monks.[175] The clear implication is that those coming from 'elsewhere' were not new recruits but seasoned monks: perhaps the nucleus of the large community that Ceolfrith left behind him at his departure in 716.

If such a shift was at all general, the 'losing' houses were probably mainly to be found among the very small monasteries, least known from our sources. Small in size because they were small in resources, there may have been many of them, all peculiarly vulnerable to plague's attacks.[176] The difference between extinction and survival may have been the difference between Abbess Hild's first and unnamed monastic house, on the north bank of the Wear, and, say, Wearmouth: the first, where Hild dwelt with a very few companions *(cum perpaucis sociis)*, endowed with only a hide of land, the second with seventy hides.[177] So it was in the plagues of the fourteenth century. The major houses, such as Westminster and St Albans, the Jarrows and Wearmouths of their day, were initially hard hit by the plague, but recovered and flourished, while at some of the smaller houses the religious life was temporarily and sometimes permanently extinguished, leading to annexation by a more powerful neighbor.[178] For this process the plague in Bede's England may have provided precedents.

If these various surmises are right, we could explain the flowering of Northumbrian monasticism in terms that do not demand any modification of our earlier views on the plague's severity. A steady recovery of population, the attractions of the monastic life for such unfortunates as political refugees, and a possible concentration of survivors and recruits

[174] *Historia Abbatum Auctore Anonymo*, in Bede *Opera historica*, 1:388–89. I am very grateful to John Blair for drawing my attention to the later history of Gilling. Note also Kirby's view that Bede may have drawn on information from Gilling: "Bede's Native Sources," 347–48, 351.

[175] *Historia Abbatum Auctore Anonymo*, in Bede, *Opera historica*, 1:393.

[176] Cf. Campbell, *Anglo-Saxon History*, 51.

[177] Bede, *EH* 4.21, pp. 406–07; *Historia Abbatum Auctore Baeda*, in Bede, *Opera historica*, 1:367–68.

[178] Knowles, *Religious Orders in England*, 2:10–11; Power, *Medieval English Nunneries*, 180.

in the larger houses may all have helped to provide the intellectual energy and human resources underlying the Northumbrian renaissance. But to some extent these assets were independent of plague and its consequences. They derived from the substantial endowments in land that reflected the territorial power of the Northumbrian kings and, more particularly, from the wealth of Benedict Biscop, the virtual creator of the buildings and libraries of Wearmouth and Jarrow. By about 652, when he retired from the secular life of a royal thegn and the profitable warfare with which it was no doubt filled, Biscop is likely to have accumulated sufficient treasure to finance his six subsequent journeys to Gaul and Rome, and the purchase of 'countless valuable gifts', notably the books that provided the foundations for Bede's learning.[179] Deeply stricken though the major Northumbrian monasteries were by the plague, their wealth partly predated the plague's coming and was immune from its attack. In that sense Northumbrian monastic culture stood entirely beyond the range of the plague's effects and does not have to be explained in terms that take account of that disaster.

When we turn from monastic life to the countryside, our sources take us from shadow toward darkness. The long-term effects of plague on rural settlements can hardly be charted with even the tentative caution applicable to the monasteries. As Hamerow has noted, the archaeological record for eighth-century settlements, if not entirely blank, is nevertheless very thin. Taking the eighth and ninth centuries together, only fourteen sites, containing a total of fourty-four structures, have been identified, compared with our thirteen sites and eighty-seven structures from the seventh century alone. The degree to which this reduction represents a real decline cannot be ascertained because the scarcity of eighth-century artifacts makes it impossible to distinguish between non-existence and mere invisibility.[180] On this slippery ground even the most intrepid may find it difficult to get a footing.

Some pointers there are, however, and in the decades around 700 change is what they seem to indicate. Those small and often run-down sites that were deserted about that time were not reoccupied, to judge by the absence from them of the one class of artifact that is both new and conspicuously plentiful in the early eighth century. That artifact is

[179] *Historia Abbatum Auctore Baeda*, in Bede, *Opera historica*, 1:364–65, 373; Campbell, "Impact of the Sutton Hoo Discovery," 90.

[180] Hamerow, "Rural Settlements and Settlement Patterns," 13; Marshall and Marshall, "Change and Continuity in Anglo-Saxon Buildings," 378–79.

the sceatta, the commonest of all Anglo-Saxon coins. Yet only at Mucking have sceattas been found, to provide firm evidence of continuity beyond the c. 700 watershed; and Mucking, as we have seen, was a large settlement and one therefore probably more resistant to demographic disaster than the isolated farmsteads of Puddlehill or Chalton.[181] Slightly more determinative perhaps is the change in housebuilding styles that separates the seventh century from the eighth. In the first period, Anglo-Saxon houses generally conformed to the pattern of the 'two-square module'; that is, a rectangular longhouse, consisting of two square units usually separated by opposing doors. But in the next century 'conformity had vanished, two-square plans no longer dominated, and a wide variety of plans was used as the established tradition was apparently abandoned'. Its investigators tentatively interpreted the 'breakdown in the coherent building tradition', surviving from the fifth century, as evidence for unspecified 'instability and change'.[182] Irish developments may throw some light on this, for in Ireland something more dramatic seems to have happened, with a virtually complete break in building, detectable through dendrochronology, following the late-seventh-century plagues.[183] If such a break occurred in England – and how, lacking the precise evidence of dendrochronology, would one detect it? – the change in building styles would be the more comprehensible.

Can we reconcile, however provisionally, the various factors bearing on rural settlement after the plague: the epidemic's end, the likely rise in population thereafter, the permanent desertion of some smaller places, the rupture in building styles, the eighth-century decline, real or illusory, in the number of occupied sites? One model that would take in most of these developments is that already invoked as a partial explanation of the monastic recovery: that is to say, initial high mortality in small communities, migration, the community's immediate extinction or reduction to an unsustainably low level, and the reconcentration of the emigrants in surviving larger communities. Of course, for the rural *viculi* this remains little more than a working hypothesis, and one predicated upon the plague's devastation of the countryside to an extent that cannot be proved. It is nevertheless a plausible scenario, having for its foundation what we know to have been the first reaction to plague almost everywhere

[181] Blackburn and Grierson, *Medieval European Coinage*, 168; Hamerow, *Excavations at Mucking*, 2:86.
[182] Marshall and Marshall, "Change and Continuity in Anglo-Saxon Buildings," 397–98, 400.
[183] Baillie, "Marker Dates," 154–55.

and at all times. That reaction was flight: as characteristic a response in the Gaul of Gregory of Tours and the Liguria of Paul the Deacon as in the Florence of Bocaccio or fifteenth-century Iceland or sixteenth- and seventeenth-century Bristol.[184] Although the anonymous *Life of Ceolfrith* shows us something of monastic flight, in tracing the departure of the monks of Gilling to Ripon, the scanty textual evidence for plague in the countryside reveals depopulation without distinguishing between death and flight as its causes. Yet it is unlikely that late seventh-century England was exempt from so universal a response to plague.

If there were migrants, we can know nothing about their destinations. But we should note, for instance, the suggestion, based on pottery finds, that the modern villages of Chalton and Catherington, adjacent to the early settlement of Chalton, were already occupied during the lifetime of the early village, whose desertion they must have survived. We should note, too, the further possibility that Maelmin, the royal vill that took Yeavering's place, was already an occupied site at the time of the vill's re-establishment there – or so its British place-name and the large-scale settlement denoted by about forty huts may imply.[185] These examples barely constitute even straws in the wind. But the process they perhaps point toward may have more in common with Arnold and Wardle's model of a purposeful relocation of settlement than with Hamerow's picture of settlements shifting and changing in something like a constant game of musical chairs across an open landscape. One consequence of plague may have been a degree of premature settlement nucleation.

CONCLUSION: PLAGUE AND POPULATION

In a larger context than that of England alone, the problem of the plague's long-term effects has not been widely addressed, and the few answers ventured have been insubstantial, hesitant, diverse, and justifiably full of uncertainties. In Europe as a whole, we are told, plague mortality was 'probably great', but there is no evidence that its demographic effects were as severe as those of the Black Death.[186] The presence of plague in southern Europe and its absence in the north (an unfounded contrast) may explain the movement of power from the Mediterranean

---

[184] Gregory of Tours, *The History of the Franks*, 2:264, 396; above at n. 114; Horrox, *Black Death*, 29–30; Karlsson, "Plague Without Rats," 277–78; Slack, *Impact of Plague*, 124–25.

[185] Cunliffe, "Saxon and Medieval Settlement-Pattern," 4–5; Champion, "Chalton," 369; Hope-Taylor, *Yeavering*, 281; Gates and O'Brien, "Cropmarks at Milfield," 1–9.

[186] Pounds, *Economic History of Medieval Europe*, 144.

Basin to the Carolingian realms.[187] In the cities of the Byzantine Empire, plague brought a population decline that was no more than temporary: 'the Black Death, this plague and its successors were not'. In rural Italy the population may or may not have declined.[188] In Ireland, the plagues of the 540s and of the late seventh century are likely to have been 'major demographic disasters', but 'the population was resilient and recovered quickly'.[189] As their authors admit, none of these statements, once they move beyond the obvious link between plague and mortality, offers more than a hypothesis. In the absence of statistics, with little more than the uncertain and sporadic record of the literary sources, and with many parts of Europe lacking even that, how could they offer more?

The English evidence has been insouciantly dismissed by those who have written most fully on the continental plagues, largely because it does not provably testify to bubonic infection.[190] Yet not only can the English epidemics be reasonably identified with bubonic, and perhaps pneumonic, plague, but the English sources also provide a narrower and more microcosmic view of plague's effects, and for that reason a more sharply focused one, than any comparable evidence from the Continent. Bede's stage is smaller than that of Gregory of Tours, his time-scale more limited, his interest greater in just those sorts of communities – monasteries in his case – that were most susceptible to plague. The same applies to those other, lesser writers who worked in his shadow and whose writings have been drawn on here. Unlike the Irish annalists, all told their story in some detail, and unlike the story told by Gregory of Tours, it is one with a precise beginning and an almost equally precise end. The contained and circumscribed nature of the English plague, already emphasized, makes it easier to judge plague's effects in England than in Ireland or in continental Europe. In those parts, epidemic outbreaks (though not of plague alone) were often localized and recurrent over a long period, reducing, it must be assumed, any rising curve of population to a fluctuating and undulant line. In England, there is reason to think that the plague's immediate impact was probably countrywide in its range and cataclysmic in its consequences for peoples lacking any acquired immunity and any

---

[187] Biraben and Le Goff, "La Peste dans le Haut Moyen Age," 1508.

[188] Wickham, *Land and Power*, 110.

[189] Charles-Edwards, *Irish and Welsh Kinship*, 473; cf. Cróinín, *Early Medieval Ireland*, 108, 160.

[190] "Enfin, l'epidémie décrite par Bède le Vénérable, et qui frappe les Îles Brittaniques en 664, ne peut pas être la peste": Biraben and Le Goff, "La Peste dans le haut moyen age," 1494.

knowledge of the principles of infection. Here the evidence of archaeology and of the written sources can be cautiously brought into alignment, in a complementary relationship difficult to achieve for continental countries. The changes to which archaeology bears witness – the desertion of settlements, the break in building styles, and, in Ireland, the interruption of building itself – seem to coincide with the period of plague and its immediate aftermath and may be among its more long-lasting effects. But little else falls into that same category. With the cessation of epidemics from c. 687, the likelihood is that the population made an unimpeded and rapid recovery, one free from further national disasters and to the advantage of the monasteries that had earlier been the foyers of infection.

If the population history of Anglo-Saxon England is ever written, therefore, the plagues of the seventh century, horrific though they were for those who lived through them, are likely to be seen as a brief and temporary intermission in an upward trend. This conclusion has necessarily to be couched in tentative terms. But one man's tentativeness is another's incaution; and it would be imprudent to say more.

10

The Plague and Its Consequences in Ireland

Ann Dooley

Analyses of plague visitations in medieval Ireland, including the epidemic of 544, were first advanced in some detail by William P. MacArthur in 1949.[1] Apart from the discussion by J. R. Maddicott of the plague in seventh-century England, which also uses Irish evidence, there has been no subsequent analysis of the Irish material in any detailed way.[2] It may be useful then, in fleshing out the trajectory and consequences of the Justinianic Plague outbreaks in Europe generally, to consider the evidence from Ireland, where a contemporary annalistic record survives. The witness afforded by these early Irish records remains sketchy, however, and

---

[1] MacArthur, "Identification of Some Pestilences," 169–88.

[2] See chapter 9. Maddicott himself, while using the Irish data very effectively, is not primarily concerned with Ireland, and although he did look again at what the Irish annalistic sources and what Adomnán had to say about the plague of 664, he took much of what MacArthur proposed at face value. Most important for him is the time of the plague's arrival in Ireland – August 1, 664, pinpointed so carefully by the Irish annalists – which fills in an expected westward progress from Bede's date for the first English casualties on July 14. Again, he differs from MacArthur on the nature of the epidemic termed *buide chonaill* by the Irish annalists and accepts Shrewsbury's diagnosis of small-pox rather than MacArthur's relapsing fever for this term. What was especially attractive about MacArthur's work was its genealogy as a sociomedical discourse. He consciously set it in the tradition of the great nineteenth-century Irish medical practitioners (Graves, Corrigan, and Sir William Wilde – whom he does not cite for his ground-breaking statistical study of Irish famine), whose research into epidemics arose out of the shadows of the great Irish Famine of 1846–1848. MacArthur reminds his reader constantly that he knows of what he speaks – plague and all – first-hand. Thus, the assumption of a close relationship and a human sympathy, even an unbroken historical one, between medical investigator and suffering poor, gives his work a very particular kind of authority within an Irish historiographical tradition.

thus part of the purpose of this essay, besides assessing the outbreaks themselves and their immediate historical consequences, is to map something of the cultural form that evolved from the impact of these events; plague visitations provide an insight into the formation of a particular crisis-management mentality in Ireland and Irish-influenced European zones.

The arrival of a plague in Ireland in 544 would seem to concur with the westward trajectory of the outbreak of Justinianic Plague at this time; it had arrived in central Gaul by 543.[3] The exact mode of ingress is not clear, but one possible way was the one that ran through the western route from Narbonne to the Garonne and thence past Brittany to western Britain.[4] Such a route extends to southern Ireland also and does not necessarily make landfall in Britain. There is no record of a British outbreak at this time. However, the comments of Gildas, vague though they are, on the contemporary tribulations of the Britons, equivalent to the plagues of Egypt, may have a germ of reality behind their prevailing biblical language.

A sudden climate change can be observed from a dendrochronology study of Irish trees, beginning in 538 and continuing through the next decade; Irish climate was especially slow to recover, and reduced food harvests, noted already in the Annals for 538, might have had a significant impact on the heightened ability of a plague to wreak devastation on a weakened population.[5] McCarthy has noted the implications of this discovery for dating issues in the Irish Annals.[6]

Only one Irish personage is registered as having died in 544, Mobhí Clárinech: *mortalitas magna quae blefed dicitur in qua moBí Clairineach cui nomen est Berchan brecano poeta periit.*[7] This individual, named in later hagiographical tradition as one of the twelve apostles of Ireland, a disciple of St. Finnian of Clonard, and of the Leinster tribal group of the Fothairt, is associated with Glas Noenden (Glasnevin) in the Corpus of Irish saints' genealogies. He is also noted as tutor to Colum Cille;[8] he is associated with the latter in the traditions about the hymn, *Noli pater indulgere,* recorded

[3] See Michel Rouche in Fossier, *History of the Middle Ages,* 1:475–77.

[4] There is no record of actual Irish contacts with Gaul before Columbanus arrived there in the late sixth century, but the pottery record in Britain and Ireland indicates continuous imports from Gaul from the period of conversion on. See Bowen, *Saints, Seaways, and Settlements,* 14–17, 24–26.

[5] See the dendrochronological chart in Baillie, "Patrick, Comets, and Christianity," 70.

[6] McCarthy, "Chronology of Colum Cille."

[7] *Annals of Tigernach,* sub anno 544. I use these annals rather than any other version of the early Irish annals because they are closest to the original "Annals of Iona" prototype.

[8] *Corpus Genealogiarum,* 44, 51, 62, 92, 136, 172.

in the Middle Irish notes to the *Liber Hymnorum*.[9] McCarthy suggests that it was Colum Cille himself who recorded his death in the annals as a tribute to his former teacher. This does not, however, mean that the entire entry, although in Latin, is original to Colm Cille.

In 550, another epidemic struck Ireland, described as the *cróin Chonaill* (redness of C) or the *buidhe Chonaill* (yellowness of C), and here a list of saints who died is recorded: *Findia mac hui Tellduib 7 Colum mac Crimthaind 7 Colam Indse Cealtra 7 Sineall mac Cenandain ab Cilli Achaidh Drumfhada 7 Mac Tail Chilli Cuilind qui nominatur Eogan mac Corcrain.*[10] The geographical distribution of these names suggests a fairly widespread outbreak with a focus on the Shannon area: Findia from Clonard; Colum mac Crimthaind from Terryglass; Colam from Inis Cealtra in the Shannon; Sin[ch]eall from Killeigh, Co. Offaly, Mac Táil of Kilcullen, Co. Kildare. The focus also seems to be monastic rather than episcopal at a time when the great establishment period of Irish monasticism is just beginning. In none of the sites, however, is there any evidence that the monastery was crippled by the fatalities. There is one possible citation of a secular fatality recorded for this year, *Duach Tenga Uma mac Fergasa,* king of Connacht, but this is a badly garbled entry.[11] The relative sparseness of the Irish Annals for the first half of the sixth century sets severe limits on the degree to which they can be used to present a reliable social picture. The one political figure who dominates the mid-century is Diarmait mac Cerbaill (+565) of the dynasty of Síl nÁedo Sláine, and king of Tara during the period.[12] His predecessor in the kingship, Tuathal Máelgarb of another dynastic line, was assassinated in 544; Diarmait is considered by later legend as the ruler whose misdeeds provoked the ire of St. Ruadhan, whose curse, in turn, caused the definitive abandonment of Tara as a royal site and possibly the end of the celebration of the royal ritual Feast of Tara.[13] In local political terms, a weakness perceived in one segment of the descendants of Níall, founder of the Uí Néill dynasty, and acted upon opportunistically by another in this

---

9 *Irish Liber Hymnorum,* 87. In the *Annals of Clonmacnoise* he is equated with Merlin! This is probably for no better reason than his association with prophecy.

10 *Annals of Tigernach,* sub anno 550.

11 *The Annals of Ulster* retool this entry as the obituary of an abbot of Armagh (548). The name has Connacht associations, and this is the dynasty that will be known in Irish history as the Uí Briúin Seóla; but the annalistic records for the west are even more sporadic than those of other regions in this period, and the doubling of an ancestor's name for a great-grandson, as here, is most suspect.

12 See Byrne, *Irish Kings,* 87–105.

13 Ibid., 105. The title "king of Tara" continued in use, however, long after the site was abandoned.

year of the plague may possibly be significant but not unusual in Irish dynastic segments' power relationships with each other.

Generally, it has been claimed that it is in this period that older gentilic tribal nomenclatures of the *moccu* kind are replaced by the more "dynastic," or more properly parentelic, nomenclature, *Uí*, "grandson/descendant of," and that plague disturbance may lie at the root of this superseding of tribal by dynastic interests.[14] It might also be queried whether the abandonment of royal centers such as Tara, and perhaps the Leinster complex at Dún Ailinne, at this time was not partly a result of some naturally occurring catastrophe such as the plague.

One other factor needs to be clarified. The plague of 544 is called *blefed* by the Irish annalists, and the British *Annales Cambriae* also seem to waver between their records for this outbreak and the subsequent one.[15] The Welsh annals variously refer to these occurrences as *pestis flava, lues flava*, in Welsh, *y fad felen, lallwelen*. MacArthur and other scholars after him, including Maddicott, are intent on differentiating between the two sixth-century outbreaks by keeping the graphic "yellow" as a distinctive diagnostic marker for the latter 554 one; they also discount the use of the Irish "yellow" terms for the outbreak of plague in the century following.[16] The etymology of *blefed* in the Irish annals for 544 has not been established. The annalists obviously saw it as a distinctive name in the sequential taxonomy of epidemics, but we do not know if it is a term that came with the plague. From all its variants (*blefed, belfeth belefeth*), it is clear the word caused some problems of transcription. I suggest a tentative solution to the lexical problem by treating the word as a compound made up of *blá-* and *-féth*. *Blá* seems to be a term for "yellow," though not well attested outside a learned glossary context;[17] it is obviously related to its related Latin *flavus* (possibly **bh_l -uo-s > *bhleuos* with variation of **bhl-a/bhl-e*, e.g. Irish *gel, glan*). *-Fed* has variants *-feth*, and it seems reasonable to assume that this is for *féth*, "appearance of health or the reverse," with compounds such as *drocféth, féth galair*, "ill appearance, appearance of disease."[18] This yields a yellow color-coding for all the epidemics. If this

[14] Byrne, "Tribes and Tribalism," 149–53; Etchingham, "Irish History," 129–30; Jaski, *Irish Kingship*, 201–02. I am not sure the inference is justified. A good example of an old *moccu* name misunderstood as *mac hui* occurs in the 550 citation noted earlier.

[15] *Mortalitas magna in qua pausat mailcun rex genedotae* (the great plague in which Maelgwn, king of Gwynedd, perished); Phillimore, "Annales Cambriae," 155.

[16] MacArthur notes that the references to the term *crón Chonaill, buide Chonaill* is the work of the fifteenth-century scribe of the *Annals of Ulster*, but this does not necessarily invalidate his usage as genuine for the earlier periods.

[17] *Dictionary of the Irish Language*, blá, 2, 110

[18] Ibid., *féth* 5, 103.

explanation of the term is correct, then it would at least have the virtue of simplifying the picture, for the two distinct epidemics of the mid-sixth century could now be considered as a single, "natural" plague cycle.

David Woods has recently drawn attention to a misunderstood entry in the Irish Annals for 576 on an outbreak of leprosy and an abundance of mast (*scintille lebre et habundantiam nucum inaudita*). He shows convincingly that the original entry must have read *magna pestis glandularia* and hence be a direct reference to bubonic plague.[19]

Information is much more varied for the next major outbreak of plague in Britain and Ireland in 664. Here, as Maddicott has shown, there is symptomatic evidence from Bede that it really is an outbreak of bubonic plague that is in question, and it is clear from a comparison of Bede and the Irish sources that they are speaking of the same epidemic.[20] Both Bede and the Irish Annals concur in noting also a solar eclipse in May of that year, but the Irish timing of the eclipse is accurate, whereas Bede's is not, and this may actually indicate that he is relying on an indirectly transmitted Irish source. The Irish evidence that it struck in Ireland on August 1 is compatible with Bede's information on a July commencement in Britain. The mortality record from this second outbreak in Ireland is much more extensive than the first and seems to have lasted longer – five years or so according to *The Annals of Ulster*. It is clearly tagged in the Irish Annals as an epochal occasion, linked by chronological calculation, both with the first outbreak and the death of St. Patrick. This may attest to some kind of editorial scrutiny of part of the earliest annalistic stratum somewhat similar to the retroactive regularization of the later *buide Chonaill* notational tag. It should be noted, moreover, that the Irish historical record of the seventh century is much more reliable and copious than that of the century before. On the annalists' evidence, both monasteries and the secular elite were hit hard this time. With notable exceptions, the core of Irish Annals information from this period still comes from a posited "Iona Chronicle," so it follows that, from all the major provincial dynasties, the main emphasis will be on the dynastic family of Colum Cille and the subsequent abbots of Iona, the Uí Néill. The main secular fatalities noted are the joint kings of Tara, the brothers Diarmait and Blathmac, sons of Áed Sláine, founder of the midlands dynastic line of the Uí Néill that bore his name. We have no

---

[19] Woods, "Acorns, the Plague and the 'Iona Chronicle'." I am grateful to the author for allowing me to read his article before publication. The regular term for plague in Irish sources is *mortalitas*, but *pestis* is used for outbreaks in 554.

[20] See the essay by Maddicott at notes 64 and 65.

means of knowing what, in effect, a joint-kingship actually signified. It is possible too that Diarmait's son, Cernach Sotail, who died in 668 (664 in *The Annals of Ulster*), may also have been a plague casualty, as the outbreak continued through that year.

Is the date given for the outbreak, August 1, 664, significant for Ireland? By this time, the most public ritual associated with the kingship of Tara – it was the prerogative of the king of Tara to call it – was the fair of Tailtiu, celebrated annually on this date, that is, the feast of Lugnasad. If so, then it might have proved to be a triggering situation, as it would have attracted to it not just a local and regional public, but possibly also overseas mercantile representation.[21] The principal vassal group with special links to the kingship of Tara and the Uí Néill at this time were the Airghialla group of peoples. Of these, the closest segment geographically and almost certainly present for a feast of Tailtiu would have been the Mugdorna of Breg segment. The king of Mugdorna, Máel Bresail, son of Máel Dúin, is listed by *The Annals of Ulster* as having died in the same year as Blathmac. Among these Airgialla associates of the Uí Néill were other casualties: Cellach son of Guaire (+666), Fergus son of Muiccid (+668), and Mael Fothartaig son of Suibne (+669). In the west, Dub Innrecht son of Dunchad, king of the Ui Briuin Aí, died (666).[22] In the south, the king of Munster from the ruling dynastic branch of the Eóghanacht Glendamnach, Cú Cen Máthair, succumbed. Also named as a casualty in this list is an "Óengus Ulaidh," founder of the Cenél nÓengusa, the son of Máel Cobo (+647) of the Dál Fíatach, king of Ulster and brother of another Ulster ruler, Blathmac, who died in 670. Other Ulster notables are Eochaid Iarlaithe, king of Cruithne from the Dál nAiride, and Máel Cáich of the Dál Fíatach. Other Uí Néill fatalities of the year 666 include Máel Dúin, king of the Cenél Coirpri, and Ailill Flann Esa of the Cenél Conaill.[23]

---

[21] See MacNeill, *Festival of Lughnasa*, 311–38; Charles-Edwards, *Early Christian Ireland*, 476–80, 556–59. Later poems on the Fair of Tailtiu do not mention overseas merchants, but the poem on the fair of Carmun in Leinster does. It may also be of interest that the first outbreak of plague seems to have been associated with a curious story concerning Saint Cíarán of Clonmacnoise cursing a certain man at the feast of Tailtiu who swore a false oath; he then developed a suppurating sore (*aillse*) on his neck (*Annals of Tigernach*, sub anno 543).

[22] Neither Byrne nor Charles-Edwards lists this individual; he is either a misplaced entry for Indrechtach, son of Dunchad Muirisci (+683) of the Ui Fiachrach (+707), or else the king-lists' tradition is in error at this point.

[23] This is how the *Annals of Ulster* describes him. Charles-Edwards gives him as son of Suibne from another family line in the group; Charles-Edwards, *Early Christian Ireland*, 607.

All annals except *The Annals of Ulster* give the deathdate of Fáelán mac Colmáin, king of Leinster, as 666, a possible victim; but Byrne has shown that he must have died more than a decade earlier and that this date is merely a calculated guess extrapolated from the Irish regnal lists.[24]

It would seem that there are, surprisingly, no mortalities listed for the Leinster elites, and this raises an interesting question. As we have seen, one of the as-yet-unsolved mysteries is the annalists' term for the plague, *buide Chonaill* (the yellowness of Conall). It is just possible that there is a Leinster candidate for this personal name associated with the outbreak, at least for its second occurrence. Fáelán's son, Conall, was never king of Leinster, although the latter's son Bran Mut (+693) was so named. In a note in the *Félire Óengusso* on a certain Saint Emene, head of foundations in south Wexford and Kildare, it is said that he died of the yellow plague after Bran mac Conaill and his fifty saints and Bran king of Leinster with his fifty kings.[25] Conall's deathdate is not listed in the annals, but to suppose he was a plague victim would help to tie in some of this floating plague lore about his family.[26]

All ecclesiastical centers seem to have been hard hit (bishops – two named – abbots, kings, and innumerable others died: *Tigernach*, 665),[27] none more so than Bangor in the territory of Dál Fiatach, in which four abbots died of plague in this time: Berach (feast day April 21), Cuimíne, Colum, and Áedán.[28] Other houses were also visited: Clonmacnoise lost two abbots in one year, Colmán Cas and Cuiméne. Other casualties included Ultán grandson of Cunga (feast day December 29) and Ailerán na hecna, abbot and lector of Clonard, respectively; Manchán

---

[24] Byrne, *Irish Kings*, 151.

[25] *Félire Óengusso*, 260. A tradition of association between this dynasty and a major grouping of Leinster saints began with Fáelán, not his grandson Bran, and also a special patronage of Brigid's monastery of Kildare (Byrne, *Irish Kings*, 151–53); indeed the dynasty count Murchad (+1042) as the fiftieth and last of his family to hold the kingship of Leinster.

[26] In the *Fragmentary Annals*, for example, the death of Blathmac son of Áed Sláine at Calatruim is immediately followed by a legend of Diarmait (either his grandfather or his brother?) who died in the same place and was buried stretched against a cross facing the Leinster hosts who had come to kill him (see *Three Fragments of Irish Annals*). This amalgamation of death motifs illustrates well the slippage of historical fact into legend, and one might view the Leinster evidence in much the same way.

[27] *Annals of Tigernach*, sub anno 665.

[28] Can those with feast days – i.e., death dates – for the earlier part of the year be considered plague victims of 664? This again points to the confusion in the annals as to who is listed as dying in which year between 664 and 668.

of Liath Mancháin (Offaly, taken over by Clonmacnoise at a later date); and Fechín, abbot of Fore (Westmeath).[29]

Maddicott has raised the interesting question about the effect of the plague on monasticism in Northumbria and incidentally in Ireland, and its role in the absorption of smaller houses and their property by larger foundations. He has noted the express role given to the plague in Tírechán's complaint in his biography of St. Patrick about the takeover by Clonmacnoise of the outlying Patrician foundations across the Shannon; he also notes the devastation of Rath Maelsige in the south, reported by Bede's *Ecclesiastical History*.[30] It may be that the plague caused a major disruption of this latter house as a major center for Anglo-Saxon monastic studies when Ireland was receiving migrating groups, probably in reaction to the Synod of Whitby, as well as a group from the Island of Skye.

Perhaps the more intriguing question to ask is the effect of the plague on Irish secular polity, and here it does seem as if some clear trends are immediately discernible. Among the Uí Néill, the early part of the seventh century sees the rivalry between the midlands dynastic branch of Síl nÁedo Sláine and the northern branches of Cenél Conaill and Cenél nEogain for the kingship of Tara. After the plague, the family of Diarmait son of Áed Sláine, who also lost his son Cernach Sotail at this time, loses its drive for a while, and the successful claimants to the kingship come rather from his brothers' kindred. His family misfortune is limited, however; from his son Cernach descends a powerful subgroup based at Lagore in Meath and known as kings of southern Brega thereafter. In Munster, the traditional alternation of regional kingship between the different branches of the dominant Eóganacht dynasty complicates the picture somewhat for this region: Máenach (Eóganacht of Cashel) was succeeded in 662 by Cú Cen Máthair (Eóganacht Glendamnacht), who died in the plague; after him comes an Eóganacht of Cashel dynast, Colgu; then Cú Cen Máthair's sons reign in succession. In the genealogical poems on Cú Cen Máthair and his friendly co-dynasts ascribed to the seventh-century poet Luccreth moccu Chérai, there is one poem to Eóganan of the Uí Fidgeinti of west Limerick, who may also be a plague casualty

---

[29] Dáibhí Ó Cróinín gives the amusing, if in somewhat poor taste, anecdote from the Latin Life of St. Gerard of Mayo, which accuses these saints of having fasted against God to bring down a plague in the interests of a population cull. According to the *Vita*, they rather got their just desserts by dying themselves (Ó Cróinín, *Early Medieval Ireland*, 101–2); MacLean, "Scribe as Artist."

[30] See chapter 9 at n. 173.

(+667).[31] There is no mention of the Eóganacht Caisil in the earliest form of the collection, so it would seem that in this instance there is a significant but by no means mortal blow to the fortunes of a particular provincial ruling line and its allies. In Connacht, the dominant figure of the mid-century is Guaire Aidne of the line of Uí Fiacrach Aidni, who died in 663. His son Cellach, however, died in 666, and another son, Muircertach Nár (whom only one annal, the *Chronicon Scotorum*, lists as king of Connacht), died in 668. There is a brief interruption of immediate family succession with the intrusion of Cenn Fáelad of the Uí Briúin Seóla (+682) before the return of Guaire's grandson, Fergal Aidne (696). Thereafter, however, it is the line of Uí Briúin Aí that supplies the great majority of Connacht provincial kings. Guaire became the material of legend as the archetypal generous ruler, but in his lifetime his political influence and ambitions extended into Munster.[32] After him, Connacht retreated into something of a backwater until the twelfth century, so one might say that in an indirect way the plague redirected the course of Irish provincial history even if the leader in question, Guaire, was not himself a victim.

The general conclusion one may draw here is that the influence of the plague on religious and secular institutions in Ireland was not necessarily catastrophic. Given the Irish succession system, which eschews primogeniture in favor of a succession among eligible male members of the extended family, and the frequent marriages of high-status males, political recovery could and did occur quickly if other factors were favorable.

Thus far, I have been using the annalistic sources in a straightforward way as items in a discursive system whose function it is to provide more-or-less reliable reportage. In handling sources in this way, one is, of course, making large assumptions as to their historical transparency. The dossier of textual responses to the plague in Ireland is fuller and more complex, however, than simply the sum of historically oriented texts. There exists also another textual way of referencing and absorbing the impact of the plague, and it is to these materials that I now turn. This group of texts brings us closer to what one might call a plague-response mentality, and it affords some insights into the way in which such a disaster is incorporated into a functional belief system on a number of levels.

---

[31] Meyer, "Laud Geneaologies," 292–338. The poems are discussed by Byrne, *Irish Kings*, 179.

[32] Byrne, *Irish Kings*, 239–46.

THE PLAGUE AND ITS REDRESS

The first group is the cluster of legal and para-legal texts that took shape in the years between 664 and the 680s, that is, between the two related plague outbreaks of the seventh century. Of these, the most significant is the early Old Irish *Speculum Principis* text, *Audacht Morainn* (The Testament of Morann).[33] In a passage that the editor considers as one of the oldest sections of the text, in the first of a series of alliterative statements beginning with the phrase "It is by the truth of the ruler," there occurs the following: "Say to him, it is by the truth of the ruler that plagues, great hostings and great lightnings are kept from the people."[34] The series itself describes the truth of the ruler as one of the royal virtues that maintains a society free of natural disasters, law-abiding, and naturally prosperous. The Old Irish law text, *Crith Gablach,* written toward the end of of the seventh century, describes the special crisis conditions under which a king may assert special powers as including plague time. The list includes specific historical references to events of 684, and I am inclined to think the plague reference refers to recent events also.[35] *Corus Béscnai,* which forms the concluding tract in the first third of the great *Senchas Már* collection of Irish legal texts, formulates the principle thus:

There are three occasions when the world is in disorder: a sudden onset of plague, the flood of war, when verbal contracts are dissolved. There are three things that cure them: tithes, first fruits and alms prevent a sudden onset of the plague, the enforcement of treaty by king and *túath* prevents the flood of war, the binding of each in his advantageous and disadvantageous contracts prevents the dissolution of the world.[36]

Of all the medieval Irish discussions of the role of the king, it is this insistence on his *fír*, his truth – a value that reaches cosmic proportions – that

---

33 *Audacht Morainn.*
34 *Is tre fhír flathemon mortlithi mórslóg no márlóchet di doíninb dingbatar.* Irish *mortlith* < *mortalitas,* is one of the very few Latin loanwords in this text, as its editor notes, p. 26 and Introduction, xvii. It invariably means "plague" in Irish contexts. In the Old Irish glosses to Sanctán's hymn, *mortlaid* is glossed as *quando plurimi pereunt uno morbo, .i. luath écai .i. anaichnide* (*Thesaurus Palaeohibernicus,* 2:352); also glossed *mortluath . . . luath .i. bás* ("when many die in one infection, that is, swift death, that is unusual [death]. *Mortluath . . .* early, that is death").
35 *Crith Gablach,* ch. 38, p. 20.
36 The triadic structure and the vices/remedies argument would seem to be characteristically Irish. There is a striking resemblance between this statement and the letter of Pepin to Bishop Lull in 765. Here, after a difficult year with a threat of famine, there had been a very good harvest. The king orders that litanies be said in thanks to God, that alms be given to the poor, and that each one pay tithes. *Die Briefe des heiligen Bonifatius,* No. 118, p. 254. I am very grateful to Prof. Alain Stoclet for this reference.

is the most striking feature. Conversely, it is his *góe*, his falsehood and lack of judgment, that brings down ruin. Plague, then, at a particular historical moment close to the composition of these texts, sits beside famine and frequently replaces it as the most far-reaching cosmic effect of the king's personal virtue, or lack thereof; it forms with the other two – war and lawlessness – a triad that might be said to have distinct shades of Indo-European tripartite social stratification.

The idea reappears in a number of ways in early Irish texts from the Old Irish through to the Middle Irish period. The following anecdote from the notes to the early ninth-century *Félire Óengusso* has no particular historical value; the king cited, Diarmait mac Cerbaill, came to power in 544 but is not otherwise associated with a memory of plague, and the saint, Ultán of Louth, is also misplaced.[37] It rather shows that the ministry to the plague-stricken on the part of holy men could supersede other aspects of the disaster triad (natural disaster, invasion, and abdication of legal responsibility) as this related to the work of a king:

[Ultan] used to be called 'the cleric of the children,' for after the plague called Buide Chonnaill every babe without maintenance was brought to Ultan, so that often fifty, or a hundred and fifty, of them were with him at the same time, and he himself used to feed them, i.e., the children of the women whom the Buide Chonnaill had killed. This is what Ultan used to do, to cut off the cows' teats... and pour milk into them, and the babes a-playing around him. Thus then he used to wend, with his gospel on his back, without any strap on it! At that time Diarmait son of Cerball was king of Ireland. There happened to come a vast seafleet which filled most of Ireland's estuaries. Great fear affects Diarmait, and then he said: 'Yon cleric of the children who wends with his gospel on his back and no strap on it, in him lets us put our trust that the plague may be taken from us.' So envoys were sent from Diarmait to Ultan. Then was Ultan feeding the children when the messengers arrived, and they tell him their errands. 'That is a shame,' says Ultan, 'that you do not leave me alone till my right hand was free. My hand that is free, i.e., the left hand, I will raise against these ships. But if it were my right hand no foreigner would ever invade Ireland.' So that that hence is 'the proverb' 'Ultan's left hand against the evil!'[38]

Thus, hand in hand with the idea that the ruler is responsible for the cosmic well-being of his kingdom goes the Christian belief that the prayers of saints are a powerful factor in protecting their clients from harms such

[37] There is an Ultán who died in 665, an abbot of Clonfert. The present figure is given in the Irish sources as the brother of St. Fursey of Peronne. This foundation became the conduit to this area of the continent of a number of Irish saints' cults, including that of St. Colum Cille.
[38] *Félire Óengusso*, 198–203.

as the plague. The anecdote is also precious as a witness to the social disasters that plague leaves in its wake and for showing the ability of an Irish tradition of sainthood to pick up on the social responsibilities for children left without any legal standing in a stricken community where normal family law has broken down.

The help of the saint is expressed in a triumphalist way by Adomnán in the *Vita Columbae* from the last decade of the seventh century but containing some earlier strata. One passage concerns the role played by the great patron in protecting his monasteries and the regions under his influence from the plague's ravages.[39] Perhaps the chapter is deliberately cautious, however, for while Adomnán speaks of his own plague experience, at no time does he cite a specific instance where Colum Cille's help is invoked by or for a victim with miraculous results. This is in sharp contrast to a chapter preceding the plague account where a specific rain-making ritual procession is devised, using Colum Cille's own monastic habit and his books, which successfully wards off the imminent disaster of total crop failure.

Many early Irish devotional hymns and prayers contain in themselves certain performative passages where the speaker confidently asks God's favor for having just composed or recited the piece in question. One of the first of the Old Irish vernacular hymn's, "Sanctán's Hymn," contains such a formula against fearsome kinds of death: "May mercy come to me on earth, from Christ, invoked in public song/May not death nor wailing come to me, may neither plague nor epidemic come to me."[40]

In such prayer performance, speech and effective performative act coincide. In other contexts, however, one can begin to see a supplemental ritual act added to the prayer performance in the interests of greater efficacy. In the second of the Litanies of the Irish Saints, a separate "Litany of the Seven Bishops" is inserted with the following instructions:[41] "Sing this over water against the *bolgach*, and against yellow disease (glossed *arin plaidh*, against plague), and against every destruction by a seizure and put the water on the sick person and he will be completely healed."[42] In a series of charms written into a St. Gall manuscript (probably early ninth century), there is evidence of magical formulae that would

---

[39] Adomnán, *Life of St Columba* 2.46, pp. 203–4.

[40] *Dommair trócaire tolam. ó Chríst nád cétla celar/ nímthairle éc ná amor. nímthair mortlaid ná galar. Thesaurus*, 352.

[41] *Irish Litanies*, 74–75.

[42] MacArthur takes *bolgach* as small-pox on the evidence of the *Annals of Clonmacnoise* entry for 675.

seem to include plague protection where no Christian element is at all evident:

I save the sick unto death: against mutilation, against spear-thong, against sudden tumor [plague buboes?], against bleeding from weapons, against what fire burns, against *ub*[?] that a dog eats. May *acuhrú* [?] that withers, three nuts that tremble,[43] three sinews that weave. I strike its disease, I vanquish blood... may it not be a tumor. May what it goes on be whole. I put my trust in the salve that Diancecht left with his family that it may be whole whereon it goes. This [an ointment or the charm in written form?] is always put in your palm full of water when washing, and you put it in your mouth and you put the two fingers nearest the little-finger into your mouth, one at each side.

There is one aspect of divine protection and saintly intercession that seems to have had a long history both in Ireland and on the Continent in areas of Irish influence, about which Jean-Michel Picard has collected a rich folkloric dossier.[44] To understand its popularity and its mechanisms, one must return to the basics of information about the seventh-century plague. I refer to the use of St. Colum Cille's hymn, *Noli Pater*, traditionally sung as a protection against lightning. On the Continent, such a tradition has crossed over into the cult of St. Gertrude of Nivelles in the fifteenth century and is strongly present in the folklore of the "ghost" saint Kakukilla, whom Picard demonstrates convincingly is originally Colum Cille. The writing of verses, invoking Colum Cille (Gertrude/Kakukilla) against lightning and also against rats and mice, and the leaving of them in the four corners of a room, is widespread in early modern northwestern Europe: In the Dunkirk area in the seventeenth century, Colum Cille is also invoked against the plague. This tradition, as Picard shows, goes back in Ireland at least to the plague fears of 1095 – indeed the word *uridine* in the opening verse of the *Noli Pater* is understood by the eleventh-century glossator of the *Irish Liber Hymnorum* as referring both to lightning and to plague. The Irish annalist, then, who observed lurid skies and storms in the late summer of 664, was placing two natural forces of terrifying power together – one of which, lightning, was already part of Columban protective tradition – in a conjunction that made cosmic sense to him, though not in the modern scientific way that some would read the evidence today. It was, moreover, a conjunction that long endured in popular belief. Both kings and saints bore responsibility for averting these dangers from their communities. Let us recall again the words of the *Audacht Moraind* cited

---

[43] *Crethaid*, trembles?
[44] Picard, "Adomnán's *Vita Columbae*," 17–21.

above: "It is through the truth of the ruler that plagues, hostings and great lightnings are kept from the people." This triadic formula may have a more precisely dated context than its editor realized.[45] The text bears every sign of being composed in the second half of the seventh century and was part of an early collection of Northern saga materials, *Cín Droma Snechta*.[46] Perhaps the kind of collaboration between southern and northern Columban scholars that gave us the *Collectio Canonum Hibernensis* with its wealth of material on the duties of kings lies behind the *Audacht Moraind* also.[47] It may point to a Columban sphere of influence not only for this early important text but also for a whole complex of devotional materials relating to plague protection.

[45] Kelly, the editor of *Audacht Morainn*, considers *mórslóg* (hosts) as a later gloss, but a triadic formula without connective would be more appropriate to the context. In any event, it is the linking of plague and lightning that is of interest here.

[46] *Audacht Morainn*, xxv.

[47] *Die irische Kanonensammlung.* See also Breatnach, "Canon Law and Secular Law."

V

THE CHALLENGE OF EPIDEMIOLOGY
AND MOLECULAR BIOLOGY

11

Ecology, Evolution, and Epidemiology of Plague

Robert Sallares

Many of the essays in this volume focus on the Justinianic Plague in relation to particular geographical areas.[1] This essay sets out to complement the various regional perspectives by offering a general overview of the ecology, evolution, and epidemiology of plague.[2] It is argued here, in opposition to recent heretical views, that the most important plague epidemics recorded by historical sources, such as the Justinianic Plague and the Black Death, were indeed caused by the species of non-motile, gram-negative bacteria called *Yersinia pestis*, commonly known as

---

[1] Most important previous works on the Plague of Justinian: Allen, "'Justinianic' Plague"; Biraben and Le Goff, "La peste dans le haut moyen age"; Bratton, "Identity of the Plague of Justinian"; Bray, *Armies of Pestilence*, 19–47; Conrad, "Die Pest und ihr soziales Umfeld im Nahen Osten," "Epidemic Disease in Central Syria," "Epidemic Disease," "Plague in Bilād-Shām," "Biblical Tradition for the Plague," "*Tāūn* and *Wabā*," and "Arabic Plague Chronologies and Treatises"; Crawfurd, *Plague and Pestilence*, 76–99; Dols, "Plague in Early Islamic History"; Durliat, "La peste du VIᵉ siècle"; Harrison, "Plague, Settlement and Structural Change"; Keys, *Catastrophe*; Kislinger and Stathakopouloss, "Pest und Perserkriege bei Prokop"; Leven, "Die 'Justinianische' Pest"; Maddicott, "Plague in Seventh-Century England"; McCormick, "Bateaux de vie, bateaux de mort"; Rijkels, *Agnosis en Diagnosis*; Russell, *Control of Late Ancient and Medieval Population*, 111–38; Seibel, *Die grosse Pest*; Stoclet, "Entre Esculape et Marie." Stathakopoulo's "Die Terminologie der Pest" is the best review of the literature.

[2] Standard reference works on *Yersinia pestis*: Hirst, *Conquest of Plague*; Jennings, *Manual of Plague*; Teh, *Treatise on Pneumonic Plague*; Perry and Fetherston, "*Yersinia pestis*"; Pollitzer, *Plague*; Wilcocks and Manson-Bahr, *Manson's Tropical Diseases*, 458–77.

This essay is dedicated to the memory of M. D. Grmek (1924–2000).

plague.[3] However, the author does have some sympathy with the theory, advocated by Shrewsbury in his *magnum opus* on plague in the British Isles and later applied to Renaissance Italy by Carmichael, that some of the lesser "plague" epidemics recorded in historical sources might have been caused by other pathogens, particularly typhus and meningitis.[4]

There are three possible ways of trying to identify the pathogen that was responsible for the Justinianic Plague. First, a retrospective diagnosis can be made by studying the descriptions of the symptoms of the disease in early medieval authors. Second, the techniques of the molecular biology laboratory can be applied to the past to investigate ancient biomolecules (DNA, RNA, proteins, and lipids) extracted from human skeletal remains. Third, the behavior of the pathogen in question can be characterized by examining its epidemiology. Clearly, the strongest possible interpretation would unite the evidence yielded by all three approaches, and it is argued here that all three approaches do yield the same conclusion with regard to the identity of the pathogen responsible for the most important historical "plague" epidemics. The state of play with the first method, using literary sources, is briefly summarized. The results of recent research on plague using ancient DNA were presented at the Rome conference on the Justinianic Plague and have been published elsewhere, but a few comments are made about the problems encountered in this field of research and about the evolution and early history of *Y. pestis*. After that, the main and original focus of this essay is on the third approach, the epidemiology of plague. I argue that historical plague epidemics do exhibit numerous features also found in other diseases transmitted by arthropods, such as typhus and malaria. These parallels strongly support the conclusion that the major historical plague epidemics were indeed caused by an

---

[3] A selection from the vast literature on the Black Death and the succeeding epidemics: Arrizabalaga, "Facing the Black Death"; Bazin-Tacchella, "Rupture et continuité"; Benedictow, *Plague in the Late Medieval Nordic Countries*; Biraben, *Les Hommes et la peste*; Bleukx, "Was the Black Death a Real Plague Epidemic?"; Cantor, *In the Wake of the Plague*; Carmichael, *Plague and the Poor*; Carpentier, *Une ville devant la peste*; del Panta, *Le epidemie*; Dols, *Black Death in the Middle East*; Eckert, *Structure of Plagues*; Ell, "Interhuman Transmission"; Gottfried, *Black Death: Natural and Human Disaster*; Herlihy, *Black Death and the Transformation of the West*; Horrox *Black Death*; *La peste nera*; McNeill, *Plagues and Peoples*; Morpurgo, "La peste"; Panzac, *La peste dans l'Empire ottoman*; Shrewsbury, *History of Bubonic Plague*; Twigg, *Black Death: A Biological Reappraisal*; Ziegler, *Black Death*.

[4] Carmichael, *Plague and the Poor*. Shrewsbury, *History of Bubonic Plague*, 124–25, reckoned that murine typhus was transmitted from rats to humans before being transmitted from person to person by the body louse. Cantlie, "Signs and Symptoms," 1230, stated that "a few cases in every extensive epidemic of plague exhibit a rash almost identical with that in malignant typhus."

arthropod-borne pathogen such as *Y. pestis*. I argue also that the comparative history of diseases is an interesting exercise and that it is illuminating to keep diseases such as typhus and malaria constantly in mind when considering the evidence for historical plague epidemics.[5] The main focus of this essay (apart from the next paragraph) is on the biological process of disease, not the social construction of disease (for which see Hays in this volume).

PLAGUE AS DESCRIBED BY ANCIENT AUTHORS

When the Justinianic Plague reached Constantinople in about April 542 AD from Egypt, Procopius states that some doctors did attempt to investigate the pathology of the new disease rationally, in the spirit of the ancient Hippocratic tradition, by performing autopsies and dissecting buboes,[6] inflammations of lymphatic glands most commonly found in the groin, armpits, neck, or by the ears, because *Y. pestis* has a tropism for lymphatic tissues.[7] The explanation of diseases in terms of "bad air" arising from marshes, based on the ancient experience of malaria but frequently transferred to other diseases as well, could be applied only with great difficulty to the initial wave of the Justinianic Plague, which occurred at all times of the year.[8] The disaster was ascribed to bad luck by some people because Agathias states that Persian astrologers described

---

[5] As an inspiration for this exercise the long forgotten but still interesting work of Gill, *Genesis of Epidemics*, should be mentioned. In his long book he discussed the epidemiology of plague and malaria and noted many parallels between them.

[6] Procopius, *BP* 2.22.17, 29, pp. 252, 254; Kislinger and Stathakopoulos, "Pest und Perserkriege bei Prokop" on the chronology of the beginning of the Plague of Justinian, and Conrad, "Arabic Plague Chronologies and Treatises," 54, for the anecdote about the Abbasids that marked its end.

[7] In the epidemics at Mahajanga in Madagascar from 1995 to 1998 inguinal buboes represented about 80% of all cases in adults, but the frequency of axillary and cervical buboes was significantly higher in children (Boisier et al. "Epidemiologic Features"; cf. Pollitzer, *Plague*, 420–23). In many of the plague epidemics in the Orient from 1894 onward, almost all cases were bubonic in character, but in some outbreaks a third of all cases were non-bubonic (Cantlie, "Signs and Symptoms").

[8] Procopius, *BP* 2.22.5, p. 250 and Evagrius, *Ecclesiastical History* 4.29, pp. 177–79 on the lack of seasonality of the Plague of Justinian; Sallares, *Malaria and Rome*, 122–23, on the transfer of the idea of "bad air" from malaria to other diseases; Horrox, *Black Death*, 160–61 and 173–77, and Ducos, "L'air corrompu," on the role of "bad air" in some tractates written after the Black Death. See Stathakopoulos in this volume and Congourdeau and Melhaoui, "La perception de la peste," for the interesting evidence of the *Miracles of St. Demetrius* and Anastasius of Sinai, indicating popular reactions against rational explanations.

the period as unlucky and bad.[9] Others took an agnostic view. However, our main sources all suggest that most people at the time regarded the Justinianic Plague as a calamity sent by God in anger at the sin of the people, a calamity often personified as a demon. Even if Procopius was simply biased in locating the arch-demon inside the Emperor Justinian in the *Secret History*, there is no doubt that in this period not only plague but also other diseases were regularly attributed to demons.[10] There is archaeological evidence at the late Roman infant cemetery near Lugnano in Teverina in Umbria in central Italy, dating to the fifth century AD, that magical rituals were used to combat the demons thought to cause the intermittent fevers of malaria.[11] The lives of the late antique saints are full of references to healing miracles involving the exorcism of demons. Today, infectious diseases are attributed to specific pathogenic micro-organisms rather than demons. Nevertheless, even for a doctor today, it can be very difficult to diagnose plague caused by *Y. pestis*, especially in the early stages of the disease and particularly if modern laboratory techniques are not immediately available.

For example, when plague reappeared in India in 1994 after an absence of twenty-seven years, there was some controversy about the identification of the disease until it was eventually decided, using the techniques of molecular biology, that the pathogen in question was indeed *Y. pestis*.[12] A second example: In 1997, in the highlands of Madagascar, a patient with high fever came to the attention of medical staff. They diagnosed the illness as malaria, which is indeed common in Madagascar, and prescribed antimalarial drugs, which had no effect. It was not until three days later, when the patient developed an inguinal bubo, that the doctors realized that they were not dealing with malaria, but with

---

[9] Agathias, *Historiae* 5.10.5, pp. 175–76.

[10] Procopius, *BP* 2.22.1 (ἐξ οὐρανοῦ) and 10–13, pp. 249, 251–52; Agathias, *Historiae* 5.10.6, pp. 175–76; numerous references to God's wrath and demons in John of Ephesus in Pseudo-Dionysius of Tel-Mahrē, *Chronicle, passim*; Evagrius, *Ecclesiastical History* 4.29, pp. 177–79; *Life of St. Symeon Stylite the Younger*, ch. 69 and pp. 126–29; John of Naples, *Gesta Episcoporum Neapolitanorum* 42.16.2, p. 425: *irato Deo* (for the dating of this, the last episode of the Plague of Justinian in the western Mediterranean, see McCormick in this volume); Procopius, *SH* 18.36–37, pp. 222–25.

[11] Sallares, *Malaria and Rome*, 231–32.

[12] E.g., Dar et al. "India: Is it Plague?"; John, "India: Is it Plague?"; Mavalankar, "Indian 'Plague' Epidemic"; and other articles too numerous to list here. See also Wills, *Yellow Fever Black Goddess*, 90–102 and Garrett, *Betrayal of Trust*, 15–49. Shivaji et al., "Identification of *Yersinia pestis*," settled the controversy, using 16S rRNA gene sequencing and RAPD analysis.

bubonic plague. Further study of the bacteria isolated from this patient revealed that this was the first known case of a multidrug-resistant strain of *Y. pestis*, resistant to all the antibiotics generally used to treat plague. It had obtained this property by the horizontal transfer of a plasmid, a movable group of genes, from another species of bacteria, probably one of the intestinal enterobacteria to which *Y. pestis* is closely related.[13] The first important result provided by molecular biology is that the appearance on Madagascar of new strains of *Y. pestis*, which only reached the island during the third pandemic, demonstrates that *Y. pestis* can undergo noticeable evolution in less than a hundred years.[14]

This case in Madagascar illustrates the difficulty of identifying plague in its early stages. All acute infectious diseases produce a high fever. Fever is probably a non-specific immune response by the human body, an attempt, crudely speaking, to make it too hot for pathogens to thrive (in some cases), or alternatively, a mechanism for enhancing the human immune response.[15] Cases of the septicemic form of plague, in which there is no externally visible bubo, would have been very difficult to diagnose in the past simply by looking at a patient, particularly an isolated case, and even today could be confused with other gram-negative septicemias. Septicemic plague causing sudden heart failure is the best explanation for observed cases of people dying suddenly with a paucity of symptoms, as recorded by Agathias who described the epidemic of 558 AD.[16] Black or purple spots or patches, caused by disseminated intravascular coagulation, and leading to death within twenty-four hours according to Procopius, are perhaps the most obvious symptom of septicemic plague.[17] They are recorded as a symptom in a minority of cases in plague epidemics throughout history, for example by John VI Cantacuzenus in his account of the Black Death at Constantinople, as well as in the epidemic at

---

[13] Galimand et al., "Multidrug Resistance in *Yersinia pestis*"; Pollitzer, *Plague*, 450–51, considered the differential diagnosis of plague and malaria; Jennings, *Manual of Plague*, 91 noted that co-infections of plague and malaria have been observed; cf. Sallares, "Pathocoenoses."

[14] Guiyoule et al., "Recent Emergence of New Variants of *Yersinia pestis*" reported that three new ribotypes of *Y. pestis* first appeared in 1982–1984 on Madagascar.

[15] Hasday et al., "Role of Fever."

[16] Agathias, *Historiae* 5.10.4, cf. 5.10.3, pp. 175–76, for people dying as if attacked suddenly by apoplexy; Hirst, *Conquest of Plague*, 31; Pollitzer, *Plague*, 413 and 439–40.

[17] Procopius, *BP* 2.22.30, p. 254: τισί τε φλυκταίναις μελαίναις ὅσον φακοῦ μέγεθος ἐξήνθει τὸ σῶμα, οἳ οὐδὲ μίαν ἐπεβίων ἡμέραν, ἀλλ᾿ εὐθυωρὸν ἅπαντες ἔθνησκον; John of Ephesus in Pseudo-Dionysios of Tel-Mahrē, *Chronicle*, 88; Evagrius, *Ecclesiastical History* 4.29, pp. 177–78: καὶ ἄνθρακες δὲ ἐξαλλόμενοι τοὺς ἀνθρώπους ἠφάνιζον.

Marseilles in 1720.[18] Plague can indeed present similarities to many other diseases besides malaria; one account lists a total of eighteen other diseases that plague can mimic.[19] Major infectious diseases such as typhoid fever and typhus inevitably figure in any such list, besides malaria, as well as rarer zoonotic diseases like tularaemia, and such diseases may well be active at the same time of the year as plague. For example, in Upper Egypt during plague outbreaks in the early twentieth century, typhus and relapsing fever were active at the same time of the year as plague.[20] Nevertheless, the case from Madagascar also shows that once the bubo appeared, there was no longer any real doubt about the diagnosis, which was confirmed by microbiology. It is only in plague epidemics that buboes appear in a *large* proportion of cases. This was already realized in the late medieval period by writers such as Bernhard of Frankfurt.[21] Pollitzer wrote that "a clinical prima-facie diagnosis of well-developed 'typical' bubonic plague is easy because, as has been described earlier, the symptoms and signs present in such cases, particularly the manifestations in the primarily affected lymphnodes, are rather characteristic,"[22] also adding that "the general appearance of severely affected plague patients is often so characteristic that, at least during an outbreak, the presence of the disease may be suspected at a glance."[23]

---

[18] John Cantacuzenus, *Historiae* 4.8, in *PG* 154:57–62: μέλαιναι φλυκτίδες στίγματα μέλανα. Miller, "Plague in John VI Cantacuzenus" and Schoten, "Joannes VI Cantacuzenus over de pest" discussed this text. In the 1967 epidemic in Nepal, 2 of the 17 fatal cases had multiple black spots scattered over the body before death (Laforce et al., "Clinical and Epidemiological Observations").

[19] Gregg, *Plague! The Shocking Story*, 264.

[20] Petrie and Todd, "Report on Plague Investigations," 146, cf. Crawfurd, *Plague and Pestilence*, 32–33.

[21] Bernhard of Frankfurt, cited by Sudhoff, "Ein Pestkonsilium," 247: *"facit etiam in initio morbus iste, ut dicit, et febris communis non multum differunt, nisi quia tumor iste putridus per anhelitum et spiramen frigidioris et humidioris est causatus et recollectus circa venas pulmonis et cordis et maturatus in venis lateralibus et inguinalibus et capitalibus. . . ."*

[22] Pollitzer, *Plague*, 448. Cohn, "Black Death: End of a Paradigm," 711, claimed that buboes can occur in numerous other diseases – relapsing fever, malaria, typhoid, typhus, glandular fever, tularaemia, lymphogranuloma inguinale, and filariasis. However, it is very striking that Cohn was not able to cite a single instance of *a major epidemic* of any of these diseases in which *a large proportion of all acute cases presented with buboes*, the defining feature of a bubonic plague epidemic (chronic diseases such as glandular fever and filariasis could hardly be confused at the population level with acute bubonic plague under any circumstances.) It is curious that Cohn relied so heavily on the summary description in *Manson's Tropical Diseases* while paying little attention to the much more detailed accounts in books specifically devoted to plague such as Pollitzer's.

[23] Pollitzer, *Plague*, 412.

Twigg, in his book, *The Black Death: A Biological Reappraisal*, a major challenge to the conventional identification of the pathogen responsible for historical plague epidemics, claimed that similar swellings can occur also in smallpox and anthrax.[24] Although carbuncles resembling the skin lesions of cutaneous anthrax did occur in the Bombay plague epidemics in India, their frequency was very low, only about 3% of all cases.[25] Moreover, the skin lesions of anthrax and smallpox are not confined to the specific parts of the body in which the buboes of plague occur. That is why the Greek word ἕλκους, applied by Thucydides to the skin lesions all over the bodies of victims of the so-called "plague of Athens" in 430 BC, cannot be a reference to bubonic plague.[26] When the constant references to buboes in all our sources for the Justinianic Plague are added to all the other symptoms mentioned that are also features of bubonic plague, even if individually of much less utility for diagnostic purposes, such as the continuous acute fever with sudden onset, hallucinations, headache, delirium or coma,[27] diarrhea,[28] the length of the illness, increased chance

---

[24] Shrewsbury, *History of the Bubonic Plague*, 13, claimed that "bubonous ulcers can occur in the groins in fatal cases of confluent smallpox." According to the standard modern reference book on smallpox (Fenner et al., *Smallpox and Its Eradication*, 1297, with the photographs on pp. 1298–99), significant lymph-node enlargement, sometimes only in the groin and neck but frequently more generalized, is a prominent symptom of human monkeypox (a rare zoonotic viral disease from Africa that has recently spread to the United States) but does not occur in smallpox. The presence of gross lymphadenopathy is the most distinctive clinical symptom distinguishing human monkeypox from smallpox. Consequently, it is extremely improbable that smallpox could have caused historical plague epidemics in Europe in which buboes were mentioned as a symptom.

[25] Pollitzer, *Plague*, 424–27, described cutaneous symptoms of plague.

[26] Thucydides, *Peloponnesian War* 2.49.5, in vol. 1:344–45; *pace* Hooker, "Buboes in Thucydides?"

[27] According to Pollitzer, *Plague*, 415–16, following Simpson, "next to the local manifestations of plague the most characteristic symptoms of plague are those connected with the nervous system."

[28] Procopius does not mention diarrhea, but it was reported as a symptom in 7.1% of the cases in the plague epidemics at Mahajanga in Madagascar (Boisier et al., "Epidemiologic Features," cf. Pollitzer, *Plague*, 416–17.) Diarrhea has also been a prominent symptom in recent cases in the United States of primary pneumonic plague in humans transmitted from cats (Doll et al., "Cat-Transmitted Plague"; Gage et al., "Cases of Cat-Associated Human Plague.") Consequently Evagrius, *Ecclesiastical History* 4.29, pp. 177–79, was right to report it as a symptom (ἄλλοις ῥύσις γαστρὸς ἐγίγνετο), cf. John of Ephesus (as emphasized by Morony in this volume). Evagrius was a more critical and careful observer than Procopius. Crawfurd, *Plague and Pestilence*, 85, rightly characterized Evagrius' account as follows: "the description that Evagrius gives of the symptoms of the disease, though brief, is wonderfully comprehensive. It shows that he was cognizant of the tonsillar, the bubonic, and the carbuncular or pustular types at least, and the rapidity of the issue in a proportion of the cases suggests that pneumonic and septicaemic forms were also

of survival in the case of suppuration of the bubo,[29] and the long-term aftereffects on survivors such as withered thighs and tongues, there is no doubt that *Y. pestis* caused the Justinianic Plague.[30]

Even the skeptics are sometimes forced to admit the strength of the case for *Y. pestis*. Twigg wrote as follows about Procopius' description of the Justinianic Plague: "Clearly, there is much in this account that leads us to think that bubonic plague was present although there may also have been other diseases."[31] The idea that the most important plague epidemics were a mixture of different diseases in fact has nothing to recommend it. It is explicitly rejected by some historical sources, for example John Cantacuzenus on the Black Death at Constantinople.[32] Twigg himself suggested that the Black Death was anthrax. The weakness of this idea is clearly shown by the acts of bioterrorism in 2001 in the United States involving anthrax. Anthrax cannot be transmitted directly from person to person and has no vector to transmit it from person to person. Even when someone is deliberately trying to spread it, it is not causing a major epidemic anywhere in the world, although a few people have unfortunately died. Anthrax is not an ideal biological weapon, and it is extremely unlikely that it played a significant role in the Justinianic Plague or the Black Death.[33] In contrast, plague caused by *Y. pestis* does have a long history as a biological weapon, starting with its use by the Tartars besieging the Genoese in Caffa in the Crimea in 1348, as described

rife." Crawfurd's interpretation that Evagrius was describing the various manifestations of a single disease, plague, is much more plausible than the suggestion of Shrewsbury, *History of Bubonic Plague,* 18, that Evagrius is referring to simultaneous epidemics of plague, diphtheria, influenza, bacillary dysentery or cholera, not to mention smallpox!

[29] Pollitzer, *Plague,* 423.

[30] The mean incubation period was 3 days and the mean duration of illness in fatal bubonic plague cases in the Bombay epidemics was $5^{1}/_{2}$ days (*Reports,* XXII: "Epidemiological Observations Made by the Commission," 765). This clearly matches the five-day length of illness recorded by Agathias, *Historiae* 5.10.3, pp. 175–76, describing the epidemic of 558 AD, cf. Evagrius, *Ecclesiastical History* 4.29, pp. 177–78, Gregory of Tours, *Historia Francorum* 4.31, pp, 166–68, and Paul the Deacon, *Historia Longobardorum* 2.4, p. 74 for death in 2 or 3 days after the appearance of the bubo. Allen, "'Justinianic' Plague" and Bratton, "Identity of the Plague of Justinian," discussed the symptoms of the Justinianic Plague in detail.

[31] Twigg, *Black Death: A Biological Reappraisal,* 33.

[32] John Cantacuzenus, *Historiae* 4.8 in *PG* 154:57–62: ἄνοσον μὲν γὰρ ἦν ἐκεῖνο τὸ ἔτος παντάπασιν εἰς τὰς ἄλλας ἀσθενείας, cf. Thucydides, *Peloponnesian War* 2.49.1, in vol. 1:344 on the "plague of Athens."

[33] Carmichael, *Plague and the Poor,* 14, suggested that small-scale anthrax epidemics might have been quite common in the past in localities with a significant textile industry. This is plausible, but it is irrelevant to plague pandemics.

by Gabriele de' Mussis. More recently the Japanese army used it in China during the Second World War.[34]

A small epidemic in Nepal in 1967 is an instructive example of how plague may masquerade as anthrax.[35] Both humans and cattle were affected during an outbreak of disease in a village in Nepal. That fact, together with the presence of carbuncles on the skin resembling the symptoms of cutaneous anthrax in three of the human cases, suggested an initial diagnosis of anthrax.[36] However, further investigation revealed that the human cases had plague, but the cattle were suffering from rinderpest, a completely different disease caused by a virus related to measles. Just as human populations were regularly hit by epidemics of many different infectious diseases in the past, similarly animal populations were regularly attacked by epidemics of their own specific diseases. An epidemic of a specifically human disease must have not infrequently coincided with an epidemic of an unrelated animal disease, without any causal connection whatsoever between them, as in Nepal in 1967.[37] Consequently, when, for example, John of Ephesus mentions the effects of the Justinianic Plague on domesticated animals, or Nicephoros Gregoras states that dogs and horses and birds died during the Black Death at Constantinople, or Thucydides says that animals that normally eat human corpses became ill if they did so during the so-called "plague of Athens" in 430 BC, all these statements should be dismissed as coincidences. It is a mistake to attach any great significance to them in attempts to identify the pathogens responsible for epidemics among humans in the past, even though plague can infect domestic animals such as cats and a wide variety of other animals as well, besides its normal rodent hosts (more than 200 mammalian species are susceptible to plague).[38] The only animal we

---

[34] Horrox, *Black Death*, 14–26, translated Gabriele de' Mussis, the primary source for the origin of the Black Death; Derbes, "De Mussis and the Great Plague"; Inglesby et al., "Plague as a Biological Weapon."

[35] Laforce et al. "Clinical and Epidemiological Observations."

[36] Pollitzer, *Plague*, 425–27, noted that primary plague carbuncles are quite often situated on the wrists or ankles, while secondary plague carbuncles may occur all over the body. Jennings, *Manual of Plague*, 87–89, observed that petechiae can occur in any position, while pustules up to an inch in diameter are common on the trunks and limbs. Consequently the medieval accounts that mention such symptoms are plausible (*pace* Cohn, "Black Death: End of a Paradigm," 715–16).

[37] Biraben, "Rapport," 124, also expressed this opinion.

[38] John of Ephesus in Pseudo-Dionysios of Tel-Mahrē, *Chronicle*, 87; Nicephorus Gregoras, *Historiae Byzantinae* 16.1, in *PG* 74:517–18, cited by Bartsocas, "Two Fourteenth-Century Greek Descriptions of the Black Death"; Thucydides, *Peloponnesian War* 2.50.1–2, in vol. 1:345–49; Miracles of St. Demetrius 3, in Lemerle, *Les plus anciens recueils*, 1:32,

need to consider in descriptions of historical plague epidemics is the rat, which is discussed later, in the final section.

The only real point of uncertainty about the symptoms of the Justinianic Plague as described by historical sources is not its attribution to *Y. pestis*, but the relative importance of the bubonic, pneumonic, and septicemic forms of the disease. The pneumonic form of plague arises initially from secondary pneumonic involvement in bubonic cases after hematogenous spread of plague bacilli to the lungs, or from pneumonic involvement in certain other animals such as cats, before direct person-to-person transmission by the respiratory route commences. The inhalation of large droplets leads to tonsillar plague, while small droplets pass on down to the lungs and cause pneumonic plague. Sylvatic plague among wild rodents is frequently pneumonic, but rats rarely develop pneumonic plague. Consequently, human infection directly arising from rats usually takes the bubonic form.[39] Cohn drew attention to late medieval accounts of plague epidemics that give the impression that the neck was the commonest site for buboes, followed by the armpits, with the groin in third place. This evidence is indeed very important, and Cohn was right to emphasize it, but he did not appreciate its real significance.[40] Buboes under the ears are linked to tonsillar plague, since the bacilli migrate to the nearest lymphatic glands. As Pollitzer stated: "As proved by observations on 'tonsillar' plague, the fact that oral infection of man with *Y. pestis* led as a rule not to primary pneumonic plague but to bubonic plague – often followed by secondary lung-involvement – also deserved great attention."[41] Tonsillar plague normally manifests itself in a bubonic form, with cervical buboes. Nevertheless, it is the result of infection by the respiratory route (like pneumonic plague). This is the crucial point that Cohn did not consider. Consequently, there would have been no need whatsoever for fleas to jump several feet off the ground and bite people on their necks to create cervical buboes, as Cohn's discussion implies. Instead,

---

on the epidemic at Thessalonica in 586 AD; Agnellus, *Liber pontificalis* 94, p. 337: *"anno quinto Iustini II imperatoris pestilentia bovum et interitus ubique fuit"*; on the epidemic of 571 AD, the diary of the Emperor Jahangir in India described a historical case of cat plague leading to human plague in Agra in the Punjab in 1619: Jahangir, *Tūzūk-I-Jahāngīrī*, 2:66.

[39] Hirst, *Conquest of Plague*, 206–7.
[40] Cohn, "Black Death: End of a Paradigm," 716–17.
[41] Pollitzer, *Plague*, 504, cf. p. 421: "cervical buboes are apt to be frequent *pari passu* with a frequent occurrence of an entry of the infection through the faucial mucous membranes leading to tonsillar plague." Tonsillar plague can also be contracted by eating contaminated meat – D. F. Rijkels personal communication; Arbaji et al., "12-Case Outbreak."

the late medieval sources for the frequency of cervical buboes cited by Cohn actually provide evidence that plague transmission *by the respiratory route* played a significant role in the Black Death and succeeding plague epidemics, and it is a reasonable suggestion that this was also the case during the Justinianic Plague. That is why the sources for late medieval plague not infrequently give the impression that the pathogen behaved like an airborne disease transmitted directly from person to person, as Cohn observed, a point to which we return in the final section.[42]

Without any palpable lymphadenopathies or skin lesions, pneumonic plague has fewer distinctive symptoms than bubonic plague. These symptoms are mostly concentrated in the respiratory system and can be confused with other pulmonary diseases.[43] Pneumonic plague has occurred widely but sporadically in modern plague epidemics; for example in Manchuria in 1910–1911 and Shensi in 1920–1921 in China, in Senegal in 1914–1915, in East Anglia in England in 1906–1918, in the Girga and Qena provinces of Upper Egypt, in the 1994 epidemic at Seurat in India, and in the highlands of Madagascar where plague epidemics are still in progress.[44] It seems to arise quite readily but not to generate large epidemics, at least under modern conditions in which the cause of plague is known and appropriate countermeasures are taken.[45] It is sometimes asserted that pneumonic plague *requires* cold weather, as in Madagascar, but this does not appear to be always true because there were small-scale but nevertheless frequent outbreaks of pneumonic plague under hot

[42] Cohn, "Black Death: End of a Paradigm," 712; Pollitzer, *Plague*, 103, rightly thought that "pneumonic plague was rampant during the Black Death."

[43] Pollitzer, *Plague*, 440–46. The only photograph of a pneumonic plague case in the color atlas of Peters and Gilles, *Colour Atlas of Tropical Medicine*, 37 plate 51, for example, is simply an x-ray of the patient's chest and lungs; cf. Pollitzer, *Plague*, 452.

[44] Wu, *Treatise on Pneumonic Plague*; van Zwanenberg, "Last Epidemic of Plague"; Black, "Plague in East Suffolk"; Boisier et al., "Epidemiologic Features"; Petrie and Todd, "Report on Plague Investigations," critically discussed by Gill, *Genesis of Epidemics*, 358–61. Scott and Duncan, *Biology of Plagues*, 341, accepted that pneumonic plague was probably important in the 1720 Marseilles epidemic. If so, it is inconsistent for them to deny that it could have played an important role in other historical plague epidemics as well (Scott and Duncan, *Biology of Plagues*, 68–70.)

[45] It is worth noting that pneumonic plague is less frequent on Madagascar now than it used to be because of treatment with antibiotics cutting short the natural course of bubonic cases and preventing late secondary pneumonic involvement (Chanteau et al., "Current Epidemiology of Human Plague.") This point needs to be kept in mind when very recent statistics for plague are being considered. According to Pollitzer, *Plague*, 415 and 424, "involvement of the respiratory tract is not peculiar to the primary pneumonic type but is almost invariably present in severely affected patients suffering from any form of plague."

conditions during the third pandemic in Upper Egypt.[46] The evidence
from Upper Egypt emphasized in this essay is particularly interesting as
an indication of the possibilities for the Justinianic Plague because it is
so much closer to the Mediterranean world than China, India, or Madagascar. These possibilities are considered at the end of this essay.

Historically, pneumonic plague characterized by a highly infectious
spitting of blood and death within three days played an important role
in the first two months of the Black Death, as indicated by Guy de
Chauliac's account; direct person-to-person transmission of pneumonic
plague explains the very rapid development of the epidemic in its initial
stages.[47] The extremely fast spread of the Black Death at Genoa is one of
the objections that has been made to bubonic plague as its cause; Twigg
argued that a few days is not long enough for an epizootic to develop
and spread among rats.[48] As far as the Justinianic Plague is concerned,
the principal piece of evidence is Procopius' statement that many people dropped dead suddenly after a sudden vomiting of blood.[49] Dols
argued in favor of a high frequency of pneumonic plague during the
Justinianic Plague, also invoking the statement of Rhazes, quoting Ahrun,
that there was often a sudden spitting of blood; others, such as Allen and
Bratton, have denied this.[50] Of course it is impossible to quantify the
Greek word πολλοί in Procopius; as A. H. M. Jones once observed, there

---

[46] Hirst, *Conquest of Plague*, 221, suggested that "the chief effect of cold is to promote the
congregation of human beings together in badly ventilated rooms and so facilitate the
exchange of the microbes of air-borne disease, the climatic conditions being secondary."
A. M. Wakil, cited by Pollitzer, *Plague*, 513, observed that the irrigation system in Upper
Egypt forced farmers to remain inside their houses in March, the peak month for plague
in that region.

[47] Bazin-Tacchella, "Rupture et continuité," discussed Guy de Chauliac. Morris, "Review of
Shrewsbury," 207–8, lists numerous other sources that also provide evidence for pneumonic plague during the early stages of the Black Death.

[48] Twigg, *Black Death: A Biological Reappraisal.*

[49] Procopius, *BP* 2.22.31, pp. 254–55: πολλοὺς δὲ καί τις αὐτόματος αἵματος ἐπιγινόμενος
ἔμετος εὐθὺς διεχρήσατο. Evagrius gives less detail on this point, but his mention of infection going down the throat in some cases is probably also a reference to the pneumonic
form of plague, cf. Leven, "Die 'Justinianische' Pest."

[50] Dols, "Second Plague Pandemic," 169–70; Conrad, "*Ṭāʿūn* and *Wabā*," 294, provided a
translation of Ahrun; Allen, "'Justinianic' Plague"; Bratton, "Identity of the Plague of
Justinian." D. E. Davis, "The Scarcity of Rats" argued for its importance during the Black
Death, although his reason (a supposed scarcity of rats in northern Europe at that time)
is definitely unacceptable (see the main text). Maddicott's essay in this volume offers a
better reason for inferring the presence of pneumonic plague in late seventh-century
England, namely, the sporadic occurrence of plague in winter, e.g., at Lindisfarne in the
680s.

are no ancient statistics. Bratton argued that the statement of Procopius that many doctors visiting patients did not contract the disease themselves militates against the importance of pneumonic plague. However, Evagrius, describing plague epidemics at Antioch, gives a rather different perspective, and Evagrius was a more careful observer. He noted, like Procopius, that some people did not catch the disease at all even though they associated extensively with the sick, but also states that other people became infected through living together or touching each other or sleeping together or meeting in public squares.[51]

It is suggested here that a hypothesis can be formulated by considering the nature of the sources for the Black Death, which is better documented than the Justinianic Plague. The general point should be made first that it is unrealistic to expect any individual source to give us a complete picture of what happened or the full range of contemporary opinions on the observed phenomena. For example, continental sources contemporary with the Black Death stressed astrological interpretations of the disaster. In contrast, English sources for the Black Death, already following the characteristic Anglo-Saxon empiricist fashion, ignored astrology and focused instead on the traditional English obsession with the weather (see the final section).[52] With regard to the Justinianic Plague, we can recall the Arab philologist al-Asm'aī, who gave a list of plagues but did not show any interest in their effects beyond his own hometown of Basra in Iraq.[53] After making this preliminary point, I return to the sources for the Black Death. Guy de Chauliac, doctor to Pope Clement VI, makes it clear that pneumonic plague prevailed during the first two months of the Black Death at Avignon and that thereafter bubonic plague predominated. He estimated that 75% of the population of Avignon died in 1348.[54] John Cantacuzenus similarly testifies to the presence of two

[51] Procopius, *BP* 2.22.23, p. 253; Evagrius, *Ecclesiastical History*, 4.29, pp. 177–78.
[52] Bleukx, "Was the Black Death a Real Plague Epidemic?"
[53] Conrad, "Arabic Plague Chronologies and Treatises," 54–59.
[54] Guy de Chauliac, *Inventarium sive Chirurgia Magna* 2.5, in vol. 1:117–18: "*incepit autem predicta mortalitas nobis in mense Ianuarii, et duravit per septem menses. Et habuit duos modos. Primus fuit per duos menses, cum febre continua et sputo sanguinis, et isti moriebantur infra tres dies. Secundus fuit per residuum temporis, cum febre eciam continua et apostematibus et antracibus in exterioribus, potissime in subasellis et inguinibus, et moriebantur infra quinque dies. Et fuit tante contagiositatis, specialiter que fuit cum sputo sanguinis, quod non solum morando sed eciam inspiciendo unus recipiebat de alio, in tantum quod gentes moriebantur sine servitoribus et sepeliebantur sine sacerdotibus; pater non visitabat filium, neque filius patrem. Caritas erat mortua, spes prostrata . . . et fuit ita magna quod vix quartam partem gencium dimisit.*" Cohn, "Black Death: End of a Paradigm," 717–18, claimed that Guy's account does not fit pneumonic plague because pneumonic plague patients rarely survive for longer than

forms of plague at Constantinople in 1348, one attacking the lungs and the other the head.[55] However, he does not describe the development of the epidemic over time in the way that Guy de Chauliac did. Evidently, the account of a skilful medical observer is superior to that of a plain historian. As far as the Justinianic Plague is concerned, the only extant roughly contemporary sources were written by historians (Procopius, Agathias) or lawyers (Evagrius) or bishops and other men of religion (John of Ephesus, Gregory of Tours, Paul the Deacon, the author of the *Vita* of St. Symeon), in other words, by authors comparable to John Cantacuzenus in respect of their lack of medical expertise. There are no extant descriptions of the Justinianic Plague written by persons with medical expertise comparable to the leading surgeon Guy de Chauliac. Thus, it is arguable that the failure of our non-medical sources for the Justinianic Plague to describe such a progression is simply a reflection of their lack of medical expertise and does not exclude the possibility that the early stages of the Justinianic Plague developed epidemiologically in exactly the same way as the Black Death at Avignon, with a high frequency of pneumonic plague at the beginning, explaining the explosive rapidity of the spread of the disease by direct interpersonal transmission, subsequently giving way to the bubonic form.[56] At least that is the hypothesis

24 hours. However, Pollitzer, *Plague*, 418, noted that the *average* length of life in 1,128 pneumonic plague cases at Harbin in Manchuria in 1921 was 1.8 days. Elsewhere, *Plague*, 442, he stated that untreated pneumonic plague patients rarely survive longer than 2–4 days. The data regarding the duration of pneumonic plague cases presented by Pollitzer are perfectly compatible with Guy's statement that death came *within* 3 days in the first phase of the epidemic at Avignon, *pace* Cohn.

[55] Congourdeau, "La peste noire," discussed the Black Death at Constantinople.

[56] It is sometimes asserted that pneumonic plague cannot spread far because prostrate patients are incapable of spreading the disease, but even pneumonic plague has an incubation period, like all infectious diseases. The latent period from exposure to infection to the development of the first symptoms is most commonly about 4 days, Inglesby et al., "Plague as a Biological Weapon," and sometimes as long as 6 or even 10 days, Pollitzer, *Plague*, 410–11. This is enough time for infected individuals to move around and spread the disease to new localities before developing symptoms themselves. Gill, *Genesis of Epidemics*, 341–42, gives a specific instance of the transfer of pneumonic plague from one town to another in India in 1919 by a traveling person. Moreover, travelers with bubonic plague were particularly likely to develop secondary pneumonic involvement. Petrie and Todd, "Report on Plague Investigations," 131, mention the case of one plague patient who had walked 5 miles to evade quarantine when he was detected, and whose clothing had rat fleas in it. It is also perhaps worth noting at this point that recent work in Madagascar has confirmed the existence of *pestis minor*, cases of plague in which the symptoms are so mild that the patient is able to walk around (Ratsitorahina et al., "Seroepidemiology of Human Plague"). Shrewsbury, *History of Bubonic Plague*, 330–31 and 473, gave historical examples of *pestis minor* in the terminal stages of plague epidemics in London in 1625 and 1645.

that is proposed here. In any event, regardless of the relative importance of the various forms of the disease, the historical documentary evidence overwhelmingly supports the common view that *Y. pestis* did indeed cause the Justinianic Plague.

EVOLUTION AND THE EARLY HISTORY OF PLAGUE

It used to be maintained that plague has been around for millions of years. Fyodorov, following Pavlovsky, suggested that because rodents, the natural hosts of plague, go back millions of years in the fossil record, and because fleas, the vectors of plague, have been found preserved as fossils in amber, it is plausible that plague has also existed for millions of years. This view of plague as a very ancient organism in terms of geological time has encouraged attempts to identify it as the cause of major human epidemics well before the Justinianic Plague.[57] Various historians over the years have tried to find evidence for *Y. pestis* in the Ebers Papyrus from Egypt in the middle of the second millennium BC, in the catastrophes that marked the end of the Late Bronze Age c. 1200 BC, in the so-called "plague of the Philistines" mentioned in the Bible, and in the so-called "plague of Athens" in 430 BC. The hypothesis that plague epidemics caused the collapse of Bronze Age civilization has been proposed more than once, but it is pure supposition.[58] There is no substantial evidence underpinning it that is worth discussing here. Late Bronze Age sources such as the prayer of the Hittite King Mursilis do record epidemics, but there is no detailed description of the symptoms.[59] Similarly, the interpretation of the Biblical text that mentions the "plague of the Philistines" is so difficult that it is impossible to be confident that it was caused by *Y. pestis*, leaving aside the questions of whether there ever was such an event and whether it is wise to try to extract history from every line of the Old Testament.[60] The principal candidates for the role of the pathogen

[57] Fyodorov, "Question of the Existence of Natural Foci," followed by Norris, "East or West?" for example.

[58] Williams, "End of an Epoch"; Walløe, "Disruption of the Mycenaean World."

[59] Archi, "La peste presso gli Ittiti."

[60] Crawfurd, *Plague and Pestilence*, 8–14; MacArthur, "Identification of Some Pestilences"; Blondheim, "The First Recorded Epidemic"; Hirst, *Conquest of Plague*, 6–10; Griffin, "Bubonic Plague in Biblical Times"; Shrewsbury, *Plague of the Philistines*, 13–39, followed Josephus in identifying the plague of the Philistines as dysentery; Biraben, *Les Hommes et la peste*, 23, followed Shrewsbury; Conrad, "Biblical Tradition for the Plague," pointed out all the problems. Mendenhall, *Tenth Generation*, 106–7, attributed the incident at Beth Baal Peor, mentioned in the book of Numbers chapter 25, to bubonic plague.

responsible for the "plague of Athens" are smallpox and typhus; there is nothing in Thucydides' description that points to *Y. pestis*.[61] There are indeed passages in the Hippocratic corpus that mention severe diseases in which fever is associated with the formation of βουβῶνες.[62] However, there is no clear description of an individual case that looks like plague in the Hippocratic texts, still less of a plague epidemic, although it is not inconceivable that the Hippocratic authors had received some vague news from the Greek colonies in Libya about a disease active far away in Africa (see discussion that follows). Arguments that seem plausible are not always correct. It is a mistake to assume that *Y. pestis* had an extremely long history before the time of the Justinianic Plague. This is where molecular biology has recently made a significant contribution to our understanding of plague.

Elisabeth Carniel and her colleagues at the Institut Pasteur in Paris sequenced homologous portions of the DNA sequences of six genes from thirty-six isolates of *Y. pestis* from different geographical regions and from twelve to thirteen strains of *Yersinia pseudotuberculosis* and of *Yersinia enterocolitica*, the two other species in the genus *Yersinia* that are very closely related to *Y. pestis*, to investigate their phylogenetic relationships.[63] In principle, the number of differences between two homologous DNA sequences is a measure of the genetic distance between them; the more distantly related two sequences are, the larger the number of differences between them. Statistical computer programs, such as the DNADIST program in Felsenstein's PHYLIP package, are used to quantify genetic distances. Other programs, using a variety of different algorithms (neighbor-joining, parsimony, maximum likelihood, or Bayesian analysis), can then be used to convert such information into a phylogenetic tree. The results of phylogenetic analysis are initially relative in character. As a further step in the analysis, it is possible to turn a relative chronology into an absolute chronology if independent information is available to estimate mutation rates, in other words, the rate of sequence evolution. In the case of bacteria, many of which reproduce every twenty minutes or so,

---

[61] Williams, "Sickness at Athens" and Hooker, "Buboes in Thucydides?" discussed the hypothesis of bubonic plague at Athens in 430 BC, but the overall account of Thucydides is overwhelmingly hostile to this hypothesis.

[62] Hippocrates, *Aphorisms* 4.55; *Epidemics* 2, sect. 3.5; *Epidemics* 4.61; *Epidemics* 6, sect. 2.2; *On diseases* 4.48; and *On glands* 8, in *Oeuvres complètes*, 4:523, 5:109, 5:197, 5:278, 7:577, 8:563. The text from the *Aphorisms* is given here as an example: οἱ ἐπὶ βουβῶσι πυρετοὶ, πάντες κακοὶ, πλὴν τῶν ἐφημέρων. Hirst, *Conquest of Plague*, 36.

[63] Achtman et al., "*Yersinia pestis*, the Cause of Plague."

mutation rates can be determined experimentally in the laboratory (synonymous mutation rate of about 10^{-9} base^{-1} year^{-1} in the genus *Yersinia*).

The sequencing at the Institut Pasteur revealed that all the various samples of *Y. pestis* from different parts of the world have identical DNA sequences in those parts of the genome that were sequenced. These results suggest that *Y. pestis* evolved very recently because populations that are isolated from each other geographically have not yet diverged from each other at the DNA sequence level. Because of the absence of sequence variation in genes coding for proteins, a different method had to be used to investigate their evolutionary relationships. Many organisms possess stretches of DNA called transposons or insertion elements, sections of DNA that possess, if they are still active, or once possessed, the ability to replicate themselves independently of the whole organism's normal reproductive cycle. These copies can migrate and insert themselves at new locations in the genome. DNA that has originated in this way constitutes a substantial proportion of the entire genomes of many eukaryotic or higher organisms, including humans and maize, for example. This process may be of great evolutionary significance under certain circumstances. For example, if a transposon is inserted inside an important functional gene, it might disrupt the protein coding sequence and so inactivate that particular gene. This process accounts for 51 out of the 149 pseudogenes in the genome of the CO92 strain of the *orientalis* biovar.[64] Insertion elements also function as sites for genetic recombination, leading to rearrangements of the genome of *Y. pestis* that can result in small segments of the genome being deleted in different strains.[65] Over time, different populations of *Y. pestis* will come to possess different insertion patterns. The relationships between these different patterns were investigated using a technique called restriction fragment length polymorphism (RFLP). Analysis of the distribution patterns of the IS100 insertion element in *Y. pestis* strains revealed that one particular group of strains, whose representatives in the Carniel study came mainly from Kenya, is the most divergent and consequently the most ancient group of strains, and therefore presumably the group that was responsible for the first pandemic, the Justinianic Plague.[66] A second group of strains

[64] Parkhill et al., "Genome Sequence of *Yersinia pestis*."
[65] Radnedge et al., "Genome Plasticity."
[66] Analysis of variation at a microsatellite locus also indicated that *antiqua* is the most diverse biovar (Adair et al., "Diversity in a Variable-Number Tandem Repeat") as did ribotyping (RFLP analysis of variation in the 16S and 23S ribosomal genes) – Guiyoule et al., "Plague Pandemics Investigated."

from Kurdistan belong to the *mediaevalis* biovar, the cause of the Black Death, while the third and least divergent cluster of strains come from regions such as Madagascar that are known from documentary sources to have first received plague during the third pandemic. They belong to the *orientalis* biovar.[67]

This analysis yields several important conclusions about the evolution and history of *Y. pestis*. The great similarity among all the isolates suggests that *Y. pestis* originated as a distinct species no more than 20,000 years ago, perhaps even more recently. It has also been demonstrated that *Y. pestis* is most closely related to one particular serotype of *Y. pseudotuberculosis*, serotype O:1b of the O-antigen gene cluster.[68] These two species are so closely related that it is only the historical and medical importance of *Y. pestis* as a human pathogen that enables it to retain its status as a separate species. *Y. pseudotuberculosis* causes a mild enteric disease in humans, with abdominal pain over a period of one or two weeks, but very little diarrhoea. It can survive as a free-living organism for a long time, while *Y. pestis* is generally an obligate parasite. *Y. pseudotuberculosis* is a much more ancient organism than *Y. pestis* because it diverged from the third *Yersinia* species, *Y. enterocolitica*, between 40 and 180 million years ago. Because computer programs for phylogenetic analysis use statistical methods, there is always an error margin in the results, just as there is with radiocarbon dating in archaeology. Absolute dates cannot be obtained by such methods. However, it is clear that *Y. pestis* is a new pathogen not just for humans but also for rodents and the vector fleas. It probably evolved within historical times, and the Justinianic Plague was undoubtedly the first pandemic. These three species of the genus *Yersinia* are so closely related to each other that it is very likely that cross-immunity among them in populations of their natural hosts, wild rodents, played a fundamental role in the rise and decline of historical plague pandemics.

The new data from molecular biology also enable us to reconsider the problem of the place of origin of the Justinianic Plague. According to Procopius, it commenced at Pelusium in Egypt in about July 541 AD and then spread westwards to Alexandria, and then to other areas by sea from Alexandria, and also northwards toward Palestine and Syria, while

---

[67] Motin et al., "Genetic Variability of *Yersinia pestis* Isolates," obtained similar results with IS100. *Orientalis* strains are homogeneous, except for a mutant in Indochina, while *antiqua* strains are diverse.

[68] Skurnik et al., "Characterization of the O-Antigen Gene Clusters."

Evagrius states that it started in Ethiopia.[69] Modern historians have always had the problem of knowing whether the ancient accounts are really accurate. The ancient authors might have simply copied Thucydides' account of the geographical origin of the so-called "plague of Athens," particularly when it is remembered that both the Black Death and the third pandemic started in Asia, not in Africa.[70] Evagrius explicitly says that the Justinianic Plague resembled the "plague of Athens" in some respects, but was very different in others. Nevertheless, the evidence from molecular biology tends to confirm the accounts of Procopius and Evagrius because the most ancient group of strains of *Y. pestis* is well represented in central Africa. The theory of three different biovars was proposed by Devignat.[71] He considered some of the biochemical properties of different groups of strains of *Y. pestis* and noted that one biovar (*antiqua*) possessed the ability to ferment glycerol and to reduce nitrates to nitrites, while a second biovar (*orientalis*) lacked the ability to ferment glycerol, and the third biovar (*mediaevalis*) lacked the ability to reduce nitrates to nitrites. The molecular basis of the glycerol phenotype has now been explained as a ninety-three base-pair deletion in the *glpD* gene, which codes for glycerol-3-phosphate dehydrogenase. This deletion occurs in all strains that lack the ability to ferment glycerol, but does not occur in any strain that can ferment glycerol.[72] Russian scientists once suggested that the ability to ferment glycerol, which is also possessed by *Y. pseudotuberculosis*, was an adaptation to high concentrations of this antifreeze chemical in the body tissues of hibernating rodents.[73] An adaptation to hibernating rodents suggests that *Y. pseudotuberculosis* and subsequently *Y. pestis* (tens of millions of years later) probably evolved in cold regions where rodents hibernate.

[69] Procopius, *BP* 2.22.6, p. 250; Evagrius, *Ecclesiastical History* 4.29, pp. 177–78; John of Ephesus in Pseudo-Dionysios of Tel-Mahrē, *Chronicle*, 77–81, described the plague's progress through Palestine and Asia Minor in more detail on the basis of his own personal experiences during his journey to Constantinople. Morony in this volume considered the evidence of Syriac sources on the question of the place of origin of the Plague of Justinian.
[70] Bornmann, "Motivi Tucididei in Procopio," Meier, "Beobachtungen zu den sogenannten Pestschilderungen," and Samama, "Thucydide et Procope" discussed the relationship between Procopius and Thucydides. There does not seem to be any conclusive evidence for the presence of plague before the Plague of Justinian in India (Sarris this volume). In China, terms referring to plague (*feng zhong du* and *e he zhong*, apparently denoting buboes) first appear in literature during the time of the Sui and Tang dynasties (581–907 AD) according to Dong et al., *Les maux épidémiques*, 55–59.
[71] Devignat, "Variétés de l'espèce *Pasteurella pestis*" and "Comportement biologique."
[72] Motin et al., "Genetic Variability of *Yersinia pestis* Isolates."
[73] Kalabukhov, "Structure and Natural Dynamics of Natural Foci."

Devignat assumed that the second and third biovars have both lost one of these two capacities through mutations inactivating genes responsible for these biochemical functions, and that the biovar that still possesses both functions must be the oldest of the three and consequently responsible for the first pandemic. One significant implication of this analysis is that both *mediaevalis* and *orientalis* are descended independently from *antiqua*, the name given to the most ancient biovar by Devignat. He suggested that *antiqua* spread from a postulated origin in central Asia with the Aryan (or as we might say these days instead, the Indo-European) migrations, as a prehistoric precursor of the movements along the trade routes of Asia along which the Black Death spread in the fourteenth century AD, according to William McNeill. It then spread via "the plague of the Philistines" (accepted by Devignat as caused by *Y. pestis*), ending up in central Africa in antiquity, and then migrating back from Africa to the Mediterranean world as the Justinianic Plague in the sixth century AD.[74] It should be noted that although the *antiqua* strains used in the Carniel study came from Africa, *antiqua* strains are also present in Asia.[75] Indeed, the Asian representatives of this particular biovar seem to be more ancient than the African representatives.[76] Consequently, the molecular evidence does not prove the provenience of the Justinianic Plague from Africa. Nevertheless, the abundance of *antiqua* strains in Africa is congruent with the hypothesis that the Justinianic Plague originated in Africa, supporting the ancient accounts.[77] This remains the case even though the bulk of the molecular evidence indicates that populations of *Y. pestis* as a whole in Asia are more ancient and more diverse than those in Africa.[78] The overall balance of the available evidence still

[74] McNeill, *Plagues and Peoples*, 140–41.

[75] Motin et al., "Genetic Variability of *Yersinia pestis* Isolates," found that *mediaevalis* strains interestingly clustered with *antiqua* strains from southeast Asia. They cited a Russian article by Bobrov and Filippov, "Prevalence of IS285 and IS100," which apparently concluded that some rather unusual strains of *Y. pestis* from Transcaucasia are phylogenetically very ancient. It is not inconceivable that a mountainous region like Transcaucasia could be the ultimate home of plague because it is well placed for both a southward spread toward Egypt and Africa and easterly movements in Asia.

[76] Pourcel et al., "Tandem Repeats Analysis"; Anisimov et al., "Intraspecific Diversity."

[77] Dols, "Plague in Early Islamic History," and Sarris in this volume.

[78] Chinese scientists have recently identified a fourth biovar of *Y. pestis* recovered from some plague foci in China, named *microtus* (D. Zhou et al., "Genetics of Metabolic Variants"). This biovar is characterized by a loss of the ability to ferment arabinose, present in the three other biovars, and by various rearrangements of the genome caused by the activity of insertion elements. However, its most interesting characteristic is that it appears to be avirulent to humans and other large mammals, even though it is still dangerous to rodents. It is possible to speculate that the evolution of a strain of plague that is not dangerous to humans may have played a role in the end of the second pandemic.

supports Devignat's hypothesis proposed about fifty years ago, even though the initial migration of plague from Asia to Africa cannot be traced with the currently available evidence.

The evidence of Rufus of Ephesus, citing previous works by Dionysius the Hunchback in the third century BC and Poseidonius and Dioscorides in the first century BC, is the earliest reasonably secure description of bubonic plague in antiquity.[79] The original works of the three authors cited by Rufus have unfortunately not survived. Dionysius saw bubonic plague (perhaps isolated cases) in Libya, Egypt, and Syria, while Poseidonius and Dioscorides described an epidemic in Libya. Dioscorides is probably to be identified with a doctor who worked at the court of Cleopatra and Mark Anthony in Egypt. It has been suggested that he was sent with Poseidonius to investigate an epidemic that was threatening Egypt in 43 BC.[80] To produce human epidemics of bubonic plague, a triad of organisms is needed: plague itself, the black rat (*Rattus rattus*), and the rat flea *Xenopsylla cheopis*. An Asian origin is still possible for plague itself, while the rat came from southern Asia. However, the flea *X. cheopis* is thought to be native to northeastern Africa.[81] Consequently it is possible, and indeed quite likely, that Egypt or East Africa is where these three organisms came together for the first time. It is not surprising that the Justinianic Plague began in Egypt.

As the entire genomes of two of the three biovars of *Y. pestis* have now been sequenced and published, it has become clear that the inactivation of certain genes, which Devignat observed fifty years ago, is a major component of the recent evolution of *Y. pestis*. Now that these and many other genomes of micro-organisms have been completely sequenced, a general trend in evolution has emerged. When free-living micro-organisms become parasites of specific hosts, or alternatively change their lifestyle as they adapt to a new host, they no longer need some genes that were

---

[79] Rufus of Ephesus, cited in *Oribasii Collectionum* 44.14, pp. 131–32: οἱ δὲ λοιμώδεις καλούμενοι βουβῶνες θανατωδέστατοι καὶ ὀξύτατοι, οἳ μάλιστα περὶ Λιβύην καὶ Αἴγυπτον καὶ Συρίαν ὁρῶνται γινόμενοι. ὧν μεμνημονεύκασιν οἱ περὶ Διονύσιον τὸν κυρτόν. Διοσκουρίδης δὲ καὶ Ποσειδώνιος πλεῖστα διεληλύθασιν ἐν τῷ περὶ τοῦ κατ᾽ αὐτοὺς γενομένου λοιμο῀ ἐν Λιβύῃ. παρακολουθεῖν δ᾽ ἔφασαν αὐτῷ πυρετὸν ὀξὺν καὶ ὀδύνην δεινὴν καὶ σύστασιν ὅλου τοῦ σώματος καὶ παραφροσύνην καὶ βουβώνων ἐπανάστασιν μεγάλων τε καὶ σκληρῶν καὶ ἀνεκπυήτων, οὐ μόνον ἐν ταῖς εἰθισμένοις τόποις, ἀλλὰ καὶ κατ᾽ ἰγνύας καὶ ἀγκῶνας, καίτοι ἐνταῦθα μὴ πάνυ τι γινομένων τῶν τοιούτων φλεγμονῶν. Hirst, *Conquest of Plague*, 10, and Biraben, *Les Hommes et la peste*, 1:24, accepted Rufus' evidence for plague.

[80] Kudlien, "Poseidonios," and Marasco, "Cléopâtre et les sciences," for various views on the identity of Poseidonius; also Thüry, "Zur Infektkette der Pest" on the early history of plague.

[81] Beaucornu, "Diversité des puces vectrices en fonction des foyers pesteux."

essential for their previous lifestyle. Consequently, natural selection no longer operates to eliminate mutations or deletions of bases (or the insertion of transposons) from such genes, which are inactivated and become pseudogenes. *Y. pestis* has about ten times as many insertion elements in its genome as *Y. pseudotuberculosis*. As mutations accumulate over time the sequences of genes that are no longer required may become unrecognizable and eventually even be completely deleted. This process has been observed in several important human pathogens, for example *Mycobacterium leprae* (leprosy), *Rickettsia prowazekii* (typhus), and *Chlamydia trachomatis*, the cause of a variety of human diseases. In the case of *Y. pestis* the complete genome contains 149 pseudogenes. The homologous DNA sequences in *Y. pseudotuberculosis* that correspond to the pseudogenes in *Y. pestis* are nearly all functional genes. *Y. pestis* is losing genes that its close relative *Y. pseudotuberculosis* requires for its lifestyle as an intestinal pathogen, for example, genes coding for proteins required to adhere to the walls of the mammalian digestive system. It is significant that in many cases the mutations in question are still very simple. This indicates that the process commenced very recently. *Y. pestis* probably started to evolve a new way of life not much more than about 2,500 years ago. It is a very good example of evolution in action. In contrast, the degradation process has gone much further in the genomes of *R. prowazekii* and *M. leprae*, which both contain a much larger proportion of redundant and decaying genes than *Y. pestis*. This suggests (assuming a constant rate of evolution) that the agents of typhus and leprosy are more ancient pathogens than plague.[82]

The CO92 strain of the *orientalis* biovar and the KIM strain of the *mediaevalis* biovar of *Y. pestis* have now been completely sequenced.[83] Consequently, it is now possible to compare these two biovars in their entirety. Both possess three small plasmids with important genes for virulence. The single chromosome of KIM is 4,600,755 base-pairs long. CO92 is slightly longer because it contains more insertion elements than KIM. Both genomes are highly conserved at the DNA sequence level,

[82] Parkhill et al., "Genome Sequence of *Yersinia pestis*"; J.O. Andersson and S. G. Andersson, "Pseudogenes"; Cole et al., "Massive Gene Decay"; general review of the theme in Harrison and Gerstein, "Studying Genomes."
[83] Parkhill et al. "Genome Sequence of *Yersinia pestis*," for CO92; Deng et al., "Genome Sequence of *Yersinia pestis* KIM," for KIM. Since the complete sequence of str. 91001, a representative of the *microtus* biovar that was sequenced at the Chinese Academy of Military Medical Sciences, had only just become available at the time of writing this essay, the discussion in the text here focuses on CO92 and KIM.

but there are extensive rearrangements of the order of the genome in CO92 with respect to KIM, owing to recombination principally at the sites of insertion elements. The general process of evolution in *Y. pestis* is that its change of lifestyle led to the redundancy of certain genes needed for its previous lifestyle, permitting their invasion by insertion elements. This in turn creates the possibility of rearrangements of the order of the genome as a result of recombination at the sites of these repetitive insertion elements. KIM has seven operons for ribosomal genes, but CO92 has only six. This difference may partly explain the results of the important experiments mentioned by Devignat fifty years ago, which "appear to indicate a greater power of proliferation of the medieval branches."[84]

Some research performed in the 1980s had pinpointed certain mutations that were then thought to have been important in the evolution of plague virulence, creating separate new strains leading to the various pandemics.[85] This work has subsequently been called into question for various technical reasons.[86] A new view has now emerged according to which there is a wide continuum of strains across a spectrum from *Y. pseudotuberculosis* to *Y. pestis*.[87] Hinnebusch's emphasis on the existence of a broad spectrum of strains is supported by research suggesting that genetic exchanges between different strains of *Y. pestis* are possible in nature. It has been argued that in the case of one particular strain such genetic exchanges have made possible the repair of the inactivated glycerol-3-phosphate dehydrogenase gene.[88] This suggests that the process of genomic degradation described earlier is not necessarily in all respects an utterly irreversible process, an important conclusion for the future prospects of *Y. pestis*. The housekeeping genes in the genome of *Y. pestis* display a certain degree of collinearity with *Escherichia coli*, the favorite workhorse of molecular biologists, despite their very distant evolutionary relationship.[89] The extreme virulence of plague evolved as a means of increasing transmission. Once it had become adapted to transmission by flea, it had to ensure that it would have a high population density to be sucked up by fleas from the rat or human body. A small number of

[84] Devignat et al., "Comportement biologique."
[85] Rosqvist et al., "Increased Virulence of *Yersinia pseudotuberculosis*"; Lenski, "Evolution of Plague Virulence."
[86] Han and Miller, "Reevaluation of the Virulence Phenotype."
[87] Hinnebusch, "Bubonic Plague: A Molecular Genetic Case History."
[88] Motin et al., "Genetic Variability of *Yersinia pestis* Isolates."
[89] Deng et al., "Genome Sequence of *Yersinia pestis* KIM."

genes have been identified as playing crucial roles in this rather unusual lifecycle.[90]

Beyond the investigation of the evolution of plague through comparative analysis of modern DNA sequences, it is also now technically possible to investigate ancient DNA directly. The very important results yielded by such research in relation to plague have been published elsewhere by Drancourt and his colleagues.[91] In relation to the validity of these results, the only comment that needs to be made here is that in the opinion of the current author, based on his personal experience of the ancient DNA field in relation to humans, plants, and pathogens, it is inherently extremely likely that positive results for polymerase chain reaction amplification of DNA sequences with a very low copy number (number of copies per genome), like most bacterial DNA sequences, from ancient human skeletal remains will be sporadic because the quantity of exogenous pathogen DNA in the infected person is usually orders of magnitude smaller than the quantity of endogenous human DNA. This is compounded by DNA degradation after death and poor subsequent preservation of residual pathogen DNA.[92] The sporadic nature of results from research on ancient DNA is inevitable but should not be allowed to detract from the validity and significance of the positive results that have been obtained. These results confirm that the plague of Marseilles in 1720 and the Black Death were indeed caused by *Y. pestis* and confirm the widely accepted interpretation of the historical documentary sources for these epidemics.[93]

EPIDEMIOLOGY OF PLAGUE

First, some general observations need to be made. It may be very difficult to identify a disease in specific individual patients, but under those

[90] Cornelis, "Molecular and Cell Biology"; Darby et al., "Plague Bacteria." Drancourt and Raoult, "Molecular Insights"; Hinnebusch, "Bubonic Plague: A Molecular Genetic Case History"; Hinnebusch et al., "Role of Yersinia Murine Toxin"; Prentice et al., "*Yersinia pestis* pFra"; Brubaker, "Recent Emergence of Plague."

[91] Drancourt et al., "Detection of 400-year-old *Yersinia pestis*"; Raoult et al., "Molecular Identification"; Drancourt and Raoult, "Molecular Insights"; and McCormick in this volume for speculation about future possibilities.

[92] Sallares and Gomzi, "Biomolecular Archaeology."

[93] There is also now another independent, unpublished report of a positive identification of ancient DNA from *Y. pestis* in a skeleton from London attributed to the Black Death; see McKeough and Loy, "Ring-A-Ring-A-Rosy: DNA Analysis," 145. Pusch et al., "Yersinial F1 Antigen," have also reported success in finding *Y. pestis* biomolecules in skeletons from Stuttgart in Germany.

circumstances it may still be possible to detect a distinctive epidemiological pattern at a regional or population level. That is why the epidemiological approach to disease identification is interesting. For example, the periodic intermittent fevers that are the hallmark of malaria only occur in a minority of cases; in many cases, there is a quotidian fever instead that is easily confused with several other diseases. However, the footprints of malaria can still be recognized even if it is difficult to identify it in individual cases because it was the only major disease transmitted by mosquitoes in Europe in the past and, consequently, the only major disease that had an epidemiological association with mosquito breeding sites in wetland environments.[94] With regard to plague, Scott and Duncan have claimed in a recent book that the epidemiology of historical plague epidemics in Europe is incompatible with the epidemiology of the third pandemic in India in modern times. They have invented a new disease, which they call "haemorrhagic plague," and also invented a new pathogen (a new virus) as its cause. *Y. pestis* is relegated to a minor role.[95] The intention here is to reconsider the relationship between the epidemiology of ancient and modern plague epidemics.

This leads to the second general observation, the breadth of the exercise. It has been argued that later epidemics are irrelevant to the Justinianic Plague. For example, Harrison wrote: "A main problem in studying plague is the impossibility of using modern epidemics as equivalents of historical ones."[96] The relevance of later epidemics depends to some extent on the purpose of the exercise. If one's main preoccupation is to write a history of the sixth to the eighth centuries AD, or to solve the problem of the alleged "early medieval crisis," as Harrison characterized the preoccupations of many historians, then it is arguable that data from other periods of history are irrelevant. However, if the Justinianic Plague is regarded as a topic in medical history, and the aim of the exercise is to write a history of plague, as such, then it is perfectly legitimate to compare the Justinianic Plague with more recent plague epidemics. It is only by doing so that it is possible to discover what might be unique about the Justinianic Plague and find out which features it shares with subsequent pandemics. Comparative history can focus on patterns of significant differences, not just on similarities. Indeed, it is only by comparative analysis

---

[94] Sallares, *Malaria and Rome*, 10–11.
[95] Scott and Duncan, *Biology of Plagues.*
[96] Harrison, "Plague, Settlement and Structural Change," 19; contrast Biraben, "Rapport," 122, expressing the view that the epidemiology of later pandemics should be relevant to the Plague of Justinian.

of all the pandemics that it is possible to consider the significance of the Justinianic Plague for the history of plague.

In the third general observation, the leading skeptics, Twigg and Scott and Duncan, claim that the biology and mode of transmission of *Y. pestis* impose *severe constraints* on plague. It is necessary to consider whether this is the most appropriate perspective on the problem. I suggest instead that acquisition of fleas as an intermediate host and vector has actually *multiplied the possibilities* open to the plague pathogen (compare malaria and typhus), leading the pathogen not just to new individual hosts but also to new host species, while eliminating the need for direct contact between individual hosts, and creating chances of survival for a time (for example in rodent burrows) even if there is no immediate access to a host.[97] The spread of *Y. pestis* around the world during the third pandemic indicates that it is a highly successful organism. Indeed it should be regarded as one of the success stories of the twentieth century. Scott and Duncan say that historical epidemics can legitimately be compared with modern plague epidemics because *Y. pestis* is antigenically stable.[98] This is indeed true, as we have just seen, because all known populations of *Y. pestis* are extremely similar at the DNA sequence level (this is also another rejoinder to Harrison's claim that it is inappropriate to compare different epidemics). However, the fact that different plague epidemics were caused by essentially the same organism at the DNA sequence level does not necessarily mean that the epidemiology of plague must always be the same, under all circumstances, because the rodents, fleas, humans, and other factors such as the climate introduce additional variables into the equation. I argue next that the epidemiology of plague can and does vary, despite the shortage of genetic variation in *Y. pestis*.

It hardly needs saying that the Justinianic Plague spread over a very wide geographical area. That is why it is classified as a pandemic. Procopius stated that it affected the whole world. In a later passage, he specified that it invaded the Persian as well as the Byzantine Empire and attacked all the other barbarians as well. John of Ephesus wrote that all the regions of the Near East through which he traveled on his journey to Constantinople (Palestine, Syria, Cilicia, Cappadocia, Galatia, Mysia, Iconium, Asia, and Bithynia) suffered from the divine chastisement

---

[97] Experiments in four houses at Kôm Ombo in Upper Egypt showed that the period of infectivity from fleas lasted for nearly a month after the houses had been abandoned by their human inhabitants; see Petrie and Todd, "Report on Plague Investigations."

[98] Scott and Duncan, *Biology of Plagues*, 53.

of plague.[99] The Justinianic Plague decimated the populations of the largest cities such as Constantinople, Antioch, and Alexandria, but it is also arguable that rural populations were severely affected (see discussion that follows). Zachariah the Rhetor of Mytilene adds Italy, Africa, Sicily, and Gaul. Corippus recorded its impact on North Africa. The minor chroniclers also comment on the passage of the plague to the western Mediterranean. The Auctariam Marcellini records that a great epidemic struck Italy, the Orient, and Illyricum, and other sources such as Gregory of Tours and Paul the Deacon yield further information of great interest.[100] The question of whether the Justinianic Plague had severe effects in northern Europe as well as the Mediterranean is very controversial. Unfortunately, there are no detailed descriptions of the symptoms of the various epidemics in Britain mentioned by Celtic and Anglo-Saxon sources, such as the *Pestis Flava* or "Yellow Plague," but obviously this does not prove that none of them could have been plague caused by *Y. pestis*; it simply means that the question cannot be answered one way or the other. It is chronologically quite possible and intrinsically very likely that the epidemic called *blefed*, which struck Ireland in 544 AD according to the Irish Annals, was the last ripple of the first wave of the Justinianic Plague moving across Europe.[101]

Despite the scarcity of evidence for plague in northern Europe, which may simply be a reflection of the lack of sources (the epithet *Dark Ages* is surely still an appropriate description of this period), there is no doubt

[99] Procopius, *BP* 2.22.1, 3, 6, 21, pp. 249–50, 253; John of Ephesus in Pseudo-Dionysios of Tel-Mahrē, *Chronicle*, 80.
[100] Zachariah, *Syriac Chronicle*, pp. 312–13; Corippus *Iohannidos* 3.347–393, pp. 60–62; *Auctarium Marcellini*, p. 107; Kulikowski on Spain in this volume; Grmek, "Les conséquences de la peste" on Illyricum.
[101] Bede, *Life of St. Cuthbert* 8 in *Two Lives of St. Cuthbert*, 180–81 (*tumor qui in femore parebat*), with reference to the epidemic of 664, is the best piece of evidence for plague in Anglo-Saxon England, cf. Bede, *EH* 3.27 and 4.1, pp. 310–15, 328 and Maddicott's essay in this volume for a lengthy discussion, as well as Dooley in this volume on plague in Ireland, also Russell, "Earlier Medieval Plague"; see also MacArthur, "Identification of Some Pestilences" and "Medical Identification of Some Pestilences" and Shrewsbury, "Yellow Plague" suggesting relapsing fever and smallpox, respectively, as the identity of the "Yellow Plague." It is uncertain if the archaeological evidence adduced by Russell, *Control of Late Ancient and Medieval Population* – discussed by Harrison, "Plague, Settlement and Structural Change" – is of any relevance to the Plague of Justinian. Literary sources indicate that many of the plague's victims did not receive formal burial at all (see Sarris in this volume.) For example Gregory of Tours, *Historia Francorum* 4.31, p. 168 says that 10 or more corpses would be buried in a single grave: cf. the much more massive problem of disposal of the dead at Constantinople as described by Procopius and John of Ephesus.

that plague achieved a very broad geographical spread in Mediterranean latitudes. However, the much more significant point to note here for understanding the epidemiology of the Justinianic Plague is that the very same sources that record its extensive geographical spread also make it clear that plague did not occur everywhere but had a patchy distribution, both on a regional level and from district to district and even from house to house inside cities. This is inconsistent with the patterns of major viral infectious diseases that are transmitted directly from person to person by the respiratory route (e.g., influenza, measles, and smallpox). Such diseases basically occur everywhere (once certain population density requirements are reached if the virus induces immunity in survivors), and the virus hypothesised by Scott and Duncan should have behaved in this way if it spread by direct interpersonal transmission, as they suppose. However, the patchy distribution of the Justinianic Plague is precisely the general pattern observed in arthropod-borne diseases such as bubonic plague, typhus, and malaria because the vectors (and also other host species, if there are any) are not equally distributed everywhere. Several illustrations of the patchy nature of the Justinianic Plague can be found in the sources.

The most general illustration is Procopius' statement that plague later returned to areas that it had bypassed or scarcely touched during the initial onslaught.[102] This clearly implies that some areas did escape the initial onslaught. Milan, which escaped the Black Death but was severely affected by later plague epidemics, for instance in 1524 and 1630, is one later parallel; Bohemia is another example.[103] Gregory of Tours provides a specific illustration of this general principle at the regional level during the Justinianic Plague. He describes how the province of Arles in southern Gaul was ravaged by bubonic plague in 543 AD, while Clermont and the Auvergne were spared.[104] Gregory ascribed the saving of Clermont to divine intervention following the prayers of Bishop Gallus, but this

---

[102] Procopius, *BP* 2.22.8, pp. 250–51: ἦν δέ πού τινα καὶ παρήλασε χώραν, ἢ μὴ ψαύσασα τῶν ταύτῃ ἀνθρώπων ἢ ἀμωσγέπως αὐτῶν ἀψαμένη...

[103] Carmichael, "Contagion Theory and Contagion Practice," 232–50; Lastufka, "Bohemia during the Medieval Black Death" on Bohemia.

[104] Gregory of Tours, *Liber vitae patrum* 6.6, p. 684: *"Cum autem lues illa quam inguinariam vocant per diversas regiones desaeviret et maxime tunc Arelatensim provinciam depopularet . . . cum autem regiones alias, ut diximus, lues illa consumeret, ad civitatem Arvernam, sancti Galli intercedente oratione, non attigit."* Cf. Gregory's *Liber in gloria martyrum* 50, pp. 522–24 and *Liber de virtutibus S. Iuliani* 46a, p. 582, also *Historia Francorum* 4.31, p. 168, recording the impact of plague on the Auvergne during the 571 AD epidemic.

episode is a clear illustration of the patchy nature of an arthropod-borne disease.[105] If malaria in Europe in the past, for example, is considered as a parallel, it was quite possible to have intense malaria in one locality and no malaria at all in another locality just a few miles away, because even though the mosquito vectors of malaria can fly, they are weak fliers and rarely fly far, and mosquito breeding sites do not occur everywhere, yielding a patchy distribution.[106] The distribution of plague was patchy because the black or house rat (*Rattus rattus*) does not migrate far from its home, like mosquitoes, and consequently the rapid long-distance movement of plague depended most probably on the chance transport of infected fleas in grain, cloth, or other merchandise by humans, an erratic process.[107]

The life of St. Symeon the Younger gives a good description of the patchy nature of plague at the local level, within the city of Antioch. The progress of the epidemic is described as it moved from one district of the city to another; starting in the quarter of the Syrian gate it moved to the vicinity of the gate of Daphne, then to the locality called Cheroubim, then on to Rhodion, Kerateon, and finally the area around the southern gate leading to Seleucia. However, part of the city escaped the epidemic altogether.[108] Not surprisingly, this was ascribed once again to divine intervention in response to the saint's prayers. Similarly Evagrius described in general terms the patchy nature of the Justinianic Plague at the local level:

Whereas some cities were stricken to such an extent that they were completely emptied of inhabitants, there were parts where the misfortune touched more lightly and moved on ... there were places where it affected one part of the city but kept clear of the other parts, and often one could see in a city that was not diseased certain households that were comprehensively destroyed. And there are

[105] For one more recent parallel consider once again the observations of Jahangir on plague: *Tūzūk-I-Jahāngīrī*, 2:65. The emperor observed that in 3 successive years plague was active in Agra and the surrounding villages, but it failed to reach the town of Fathpur, located within a day's march of the area where plague was prevalent.
[106] Sallares, *Malaria and Rome*, 265.
[107] McCormick, "Bateaux de vie, bateaux de mort," 52–65 and "Rats, Communications, and Plague" rightly emphasized the relationship of the spread of plague to trade routes in the Mediterranean.
[108] The *Vita* of St. Symeon Stylites the Younger, ch. 126–29, in *La vie ancienne*, 1:112–22, does not describe the symptoms of this later epidemic (perhaps to be dated to the second wave of the Justinianic Plague), although the earlier text in ch. 69 clearly refers to bubonic plague in 543. The progress of the epidemic from district to district of Antioch recalls the gradual spread of the plague of London in 1665: see Appleby, "Disappearance of Plague," 164.

places where, although one or two households were destroyed, the rest of the city has remained unaffected.[109]

Where other sources, such as Procopius and John of Ephesus, simply paint a picture of utter devastation everywhere, Evagrius, a better observer, provides a more subtle account of the varied effects of plague. The pattern that he described is not the epidemiological pattern of a viral disease transmitted directly from person to person by the respiratory route (influenza, to give an obvious example, does not restrict itself to one or two households in a city). It is the epidemiological pattern of arthropod-borne diseases, and naturally matches the epidemiological pattern of sylvatic plague.[110] Scott and Duncan analysed in great detail plague epidemics in early modern England and traced chains of infection linking person to person and household to household. They claimed that their data indicate direct interpersonal transmission of the pathogen, and excluded *Y. pestis* as the cause of historical plague epidemics. However, in such observations from historical records, it is difficult to discriminate at the individual or household level between direct interpersonal transmission and transmission mediated by an arthropod vector, and Scott and Duncan have failed to do this convincingly. Although a person infected with a virus transmitted by the respiratory route is more likely to infect other members of his own household than to infect people in the house across the road or ten houses down the street, it is equally true that once an arthropod-borne disease is established in a particular house, it is more likely to infect people in the same household than to infect people in the house across the road or ten houses down the street. Although it is not possible to discuss this problem in detail here, the patterns of infection described by Scott and Duncan for historical plague epidemics in Britain seem to the current author to be extremely similar to the observed historical patterns of infection in Britain of typhus, a disease that is curiously almost entirely absent from their book but offers a very interesting parallel to bubonic plague because it is another arthropod-borne disease.

---

[109] Evagrius, *Ecclesiastical History* 4.29, pp. 177–78: καὶ πολλάκις ἦν ἰδεῖν ἐν οὐ νοσούσῃ πόλει ἐνίας οἰκίας ἐς ὑπερβολὴν φθειρομένας. ἔστι δὲ οὖμιᾶς ἢ δύο φθαρεισῶν οἰκῶν τὸ λοιπὸν τῆς πόλεως ἀπαθὲς μεμενήκει. Hirst, *Conquest of Plague*, 126 noted the significance of Evagrius' remarks.

[110] Baltazard et al., "Le foyer de peste du Kurdistan," 449, quoted Meyer: "focal occurrence and discontinuous distribution is apparently one of the characteristics of sylvatic plague." Panzac, *La peste dans l'Empire ottoman*, 366, reckoned that many rural areas of the Ottoman Empire in fact escaped various plague epidemics and so were able to repopulate the cities.

For example, MacLagan analyzed the epidemic of typhus at Dundee in Scotland in 1872–1873.[111] He was able to recognize a chain of transmission of the disease from person to person that seems very similar to the interpersonal transmission networks described by Scott and Duncan for plague epidemics in England, yet typhus is now known to be transmitted by human lice, not directly from person to person. The point of this argument is not to claim that the major plague epidemics were actually caused by typhus because descriptions of the symptoms and the ancient DNA evidence point to *Y. pestis*. Rather, the point is that the epidemiological patterns described by Scott and Duncan are after all compatible with the class of arthropod-borne diseases in general, to which both plague and typhus belong. Consequently, there is no need to invent a new virus with bizarre properties to explain historical plague epidemics. Fleas and lice are sufficiently similar as vectors to make it likely on a priori grounds that there should be, not a complete identity of patterns, but nevertheless some parallels between bubonic plague and epidemic typhus, and such parallels are obvious. In London, it was observed that typhus often remained localized in one or two houses in a street, a situation that recalls Evagrius' comments on the Justinianic Plague.[112] Even in the case of malaria in Europe in the past, it was quite possible for one part of a small town to be more severely affected than other parts because mosquitoes do not fly far.[113] The conclusion reached here is that the patchy distribution of the Justinianic Plague and later plague epidemics is precisely what is to be expected from an arthropod-borne disease and so is perfectly compatible with *Y. pestis*.

Of course, the most important difference between typhus and plague is that typhus was usually a purely human pathogen in Europe in the past (even though it may have reservoirs in other animals in other parts of the world, such as flying squirrels in the United States), while another animal, the rat, was essential for plague pandemics. Endemic sylvatic plague is primarily a disease of certain species of wild rodents such as tarbagans,

---

[111] MacLagan, "Early Cases." It should be noted that this account postdates the definitive identification of typhus as a specific disease and its clinical differentiation from typhoid fever and other diseases in 1847–1851 by Jenner and others. Consequently, there is no doubt that MacLagan was actually observing a typhus epidemic. The solitary reference to typhus by Scott and Duncan, *Biology of Plagues*, 355 is unsatisfactory. The tracing of chains of infection has a very long history as a line of inquiry. It was practised by the health magistrates of Italian cities in the early Renaissance period, for example at Milan in 1468 (Carmichael, *Plague and the Poor*.)

[112] Hardy, "Urban Famine or Urban Crisis?" 411.

[113] Sallares, *Malaria and Rome*, 55–6.

marmots, ground squirrels, and gerbils, which may be fairly resistant to it, with as many as eighty different species of fleas acting as the vectors. Plague epidemics either occur at or follow cyclical population peaks of its usual hosts. In Kazakhstan, plague epidemics follow population peaks of the great gerbil (*Rhombomys opimus*) with a two-year time lag.[114] The periodicity of human plague epidemics, for example, the fact that they often roughly followed the Byzantine fifteen-year indictional cycle in the sixth century AD according to Evagrius, may ultimately be a distant reflection of population cycles among these animals.[115] Plague sometimes overflows into rats, which are more susceptible than its normal hosts, and then it occasionally spreads from rats into human populations. However, there are genetic bottlenecks at these inter-species transitions, as shown by the observation that only part of the genetic diversity of *Y. pestis* in rats successfully made its way into humans during the epidemics in India in 1994.[116] Humans are largely incidental to *Y. pestis*, indeed an undesirable dead-end in the case of bubonic plague, which is normally not transmitted directly from person to person.

There are foci of endemic sylvatic plague in every continent now (except Australia and Antarctica), and human plague cases still occur practically every year in Madagascar, the Congo, Brazil, Peru, the United States, Myanmar, and Vietnam, with less frequent human cases in more than thirty other countries.[117] However, there are no foci of sylvatic plague in Europe today. It has been suggested that there may have been some endemic foci among wild rodents such as *Apodemus sylvaticus* and *Citellus citellus* in eastern Europe in the past. Panzac identified a temporary focus of rural plague in mountainous terrain in Albania and Epirus in the eighteenth century.[118] Crete was perhaps the most interesting case for the

[114] Elton, "Plague and the Regulation of Numbers," cf. Gill, *Genesis of Epidemics*, 348; Panzac, *La peste dans l'Empire ottoman*, 123, mentioned a record of a population explosion of these wild rodents accompanying a human plague epidemic in Ilghun, a village in eastern Anatolia, in 1836. See Davis et al., "Predictive Thresholds for Plague," on Kazakhstan; Girard et al., "Differential Plague-Transmission Dynamics."

[115] Evagrius, *Ecclesiastical History* 4.29, pp. 177–78. See Stathakopoulos in this volume on the periodicity of the approximately 17 different waves of the Justinianic Plague.

[116] Shivaji et al., "Identification of *Yersinia pestis*," showed that plague isolates from humans were less diverse than those from rats, an important conclusion. Only a fraction (possibly no more than 1 or 2 clones) of the genetic diversity of plague among rodents reached humans during these recent plague outbreaks in India.

[117] Dennis et al., *Plague Manual*.

[118] Fyodorov, "Question of the Existence of Natural Foci"; Panzac, *La peste dans l'Empire ottoman*, 109–16 on the Balkans. Keeling and Gilligan, "Bubonic Plague" and "Metapopulation Dynamics" presented computer simulations suggesting that *Y. pestis* can persist

possible survival of semiendemic plague in Europe since, as an island, it must have received the pathogen by sea, but there is a multiplicity of rodent populations there that could conceivably support endemic plague. Not only do both *Rattus rattus* and *Rattus norvegicus* occur on Crete today, but also other rodents such as *Acomys minus* (a member of an African rodent genus occurring nowhere else in Europe) and *Apodemus sylvaticus*, which might have the potential to support plague. Nevertheless, plague epidemics on Crete during the second pandemic never lasted longer than three or four years.[119] It even seems to be possible for *Y. pestis* to survive in the ground for periods of years.[120] However, the historical evidence strongly suggests that plague epidemics in Mediterranean and northwestern Europe were generally the result of introductions by sea from outside Europe.[121]

Procopius states that the epidemic always commenced at the coast and then moved into the hinterland.[122] Similarly, John of Ephesus records that plague "crossed the sea [i.e., from Alexandria] to Palestine and the region of Jerusalem."[123] Pope Gregory the Great made several references to the great plague epidemic at Rome in January–April 590 AD,

in rat populations for a long time. This finding could help to explain some of Panzac's temporary plague foci, e.g., the focus in Istanbul from 1919 to 1929, as well as the plague focus in East Anglia in England from 1906 to 1918 (Black, "Plague in East Suffolk"). Nevertheless, the historical evidence indicates that plague was generally imported to Europe, rather than being endemic.

[119] Sfikas, *Birds and Mammals of Crete*, 18–19; Panzac, *La peste dans l'Empire ottoman*, 207. Hirst, *Conquest of Plague*, 210, concluded that "rat plague is liable to spontaneous decline within a period of decades at most." The various reports of the Plague Commission in India yielded conflicting evidence concerning the possibility of chronic plague infection in rats (*Reports*, II, XIX, XXXIV: "Existence of Chronic Plague," "Natural Occurrence of Chronic Plague" and "Resolving (Chronic) Plague in Rats.") See Stathakopoulos in this volume on the *Vita* of Andrew of Crete as possible evidence for the Justinianic Plague on Crete.

[120] Panzac, *La peste dans l'Empire ottoman*, 87–88 and Rose et al., "Survival of *Yersinia pestis*," concluded that *Y. pestis* can survive for several days on exposed surfaces.

[121] Maddicott in this volume argues cogently that the rate of overland spread that would have been required suggests that there were multiple introductions of plague by sea to England in 664 AD. In comparison, it is interesting that Bleukx, "Was the Black Death a Real Plague Epidemic?" p. 67, observed that the contemporary sources for the arrival of the Black Death in England give several different names for the port where the disease landed. Perhaps the Black Death too had multiple introductions by sea to England, cf. Shrewsbury, *History of Bubonic Plague*, 488, for the possibility of multiple introductions of the great plague in 1665.

[122] Procopius *BP* 2.22.9, p. 251: ἀρξαμένη δὲ ἀεὶ ἐκ τῆς παραλίας ἡ νόσος ἥδε, οὕτω δὴ ἐς τὴν μεσόγειον ἀνέβαινε χώραν.

[123] John of Ephesus, in Pseudo-Dionysios of Tel-Mahrē, *Chronicle*, 77.

which killed his predecessor, Pelagius II.[124] The timing of this particular epidemic, starting in winter, suggests that pneumonic plague played an important part in it. The disease had evidently arrived at Rome's port of Porto by sea and been carried inland. It was then transported still further up the Tiber Valley, as is suggested by a letter from the pope to the bishop of Narni referring to great loss of life at Narni in Umbria.[125] It is interesting that even during a major plague epidemic, Gregory's principal preoccupation was ensuring the triumph of the catholic faith over heresy and paganism. This area around Narni in southwestern Umbria has recently yielded archaeological and biomolecular evidence for a malaria epidemic in the fifth century AD. The combination of plague and malaria was active during the reign of Gregory, whose rule, marking the transition between the ancient and the mediaeval worlds in the city of Rome, was marked by a heavy disease burden.[126] It was not unusual for plague to be transported along trade routes up river valleys from the sea, as McCormick demonstrated in the case of the Rhône Valley in France.[127] In this respect also, plague paralleled malaria, which spread along river valleys when floods created mosquito breeding sites. The very last wave of the Justinianic Plague was first noticed on the northern side of the Mediterranean sea in Sicily, Calabria, probably Naples, Rome, Monemvasia in Greece, and the Aegean islands before it ended up in Constantinople in 746 AD, evidently traveling by sea.[128] The Black Death traveled in exactly the same way. Both John Cantacuzenus and Nicephoros Gregoras noted that it spread along the coasts from the Crimea. During the Ottoman period

---

[124] Gregory the Great, *Dialogues* 4.19.2, 27.6, 37.7, 40.3, in vol. 3:72–73, 90–91, 128–31, 140–41; Paul the Deacon, *Historia Longobardorum* 3.24, pp. 104–5 and Gregory of Tours, *Historia Francorum* 10.1, pp. 406–9 on the epidemic of 590–91 (the fourth wave), cf. Gregory the Great *Dialogues* 4.27.10, in vol. 3:92–93, and Paul the Deacon, *Historia Longobardorum* 2.4 & 26, pp. 74, 86–87 on the epidemic of 571 (the third wave.)

[125] Gregory the Great, *Epistolae* 2.2, PL 77:540–41: *"Gregorius Praejecto episcopo Narniensi. Pervenit ad nos, peccatis imminentibus, in civitate vestra Narniensi mortalitatem omnino grassari, quae res nos nimis adduxit. Quamobrem salutantes fraternitatem tuam modis omnibus, suademus ut a Langobardorum sive Romanorum, qui in eodem loco degunt, admonitione sive exhortatione nulla ratione cessetis, et maxime a gentilium et haereticorum, ut ad veram rectamque fidem catholicam convertantur. Sic enim aut divina misericordia pro sua eis forsitan conversione, et in hac vita subveniet; aut si eos migrare contigerit, a suis, quod et magis optandum est, transient facinoribus absoluti."* This letter is dated to September 591.

[126] Sallares, *Malaria and Rome*, 230–31.

[127] Biraben, *Les Hommes et la peste*; McCormick, "Bateaux de vie, bateaux de mort," 59; Eckert, *Structure of Plagues*, demonstrated that plague also had the capacity to spread along overland trade routes in early modern central Europe.

[128] Theophanes, *Chronographia*, pp. 422–23, discussed by Turner, "Politics of Despair"; McCormick in this volume on John of Naples.

plague epidemics regularly spread by sea from the harbor area at Istanbul to the Balkans, Black Sea region, and Alexandria in Egypt.[129] It is well known that the third pandemic spread by sea around the world from 1894 onward.

Skeptics have doubted the role of *Y. Pestis* in the long-distance dispersal of plague by sea. For instance, it has been found strange that the disease did not develop on board the ships that brought the Black Death to Italy.[130] However, in the case of the Justinianic Plague, John of Ephesus does record that entire crews of ships at sea died.[131] Moreover, the researchers who studied the plague epidemics in Bombay in India did express the view that plague is sometimes transmitted in the company of people who do not develop it themselves, and Evagrius expressed a similar view with regard to plague in his time: "and some who have fled from diseased cities have remained unaffected, while passing on the disease to those who were not sick."[132] Scott and Duncan argued that the rapid spread over long distances suggests that bubonic plague was not a major component of the Justinianic Plague. Yet again, however, it should be observed that the researchers who studied the early

---

[129] Panzac, *La peste dans l'Empire ottoman*, 117–19. A major weakness of Scott and Duncan, *Biology of Plagues*, is their failure to pay attention to the abundant evidence for plague epidemics in the Ottoman Near East, for which see Panzac, *La peste dans l'Empire ottoman*, (see also Scheidel, *Death on the Nile*, esp. 187–94). Of course, in the Near East the second pandemic did not end in the eighteenth century, as it did in western Europe (there were sporadic abortive introductions later, e.g., the last recorded cases in Italy were in the lazaretto in Venice in 1818: del Panta, *Le epidemie*, 180). In the Near East it continued unabated until toward the middle of the nineteenth century. Consequently, detailed historical accounts of the second pandemic (e.g., the epidemic in Egypt in 1834–1835) are available that are much more recent than those that Scott and Duncan considered. These accounts make it absolutely certain that the disease active at the end of the second pandemic was the very same disease active at the beginning of the third pandemic only 50 years later and that this disease was indeed capable of causing very high mortality rates, a point unreasonably doubted by Scott and Duncan.

[130] Twigg, "Bubonic Plague," 383; Scott and Duncan, *Biology of Plagues*, 86.

[131] John of Ephesus in Pseudo-Dionysios of Tel-Mahrē, *Chronicle*, 75. Similarly Lerner, "The Black Death and Western European Eschatological Mentalities," 77, cited the German chronicler Mathias von Neuenburg, *Chronica*, pp. 263–264 for entire ship crews dying during the Black Death. Shrewsbury, *History of Bubonic Plague*, 158, expressed skepticism about such accounts, but see McCormick, "Bateaux de vie, bateaux de mort," 62–65.

[132] Evagrius, *Ecclesiastical History* 4.29, pp. 177–78: ἔνιοι δὲ ἐκ νοσουσῶν πόλεων πεφευγότες ἀπαθεῖς μεμενήκασι, τοῖς οὐ νοσοῦσι τῆς νόσου μεταδόντες. Cf. Hankin, "Epidemiology of Plague," 53: "there is no doubt that plague is, not infrequently, carried from place to place by persons who themselves escape the disease or who are not the first attacked in the places to which they have carried the infection. This curious fact is however not simply a feature of the Bombay plague. It was noticed both in the Justinianic Plague and during the Black Death."

development of the third pandemic did not share this opinion of the way that plague spreads. For example, Thompson, discussing plague at Sydney, Australia in 1900, wrote "distance is an incidental accompaniment, without real significance, and of very little practical importance."[133] The rapid spread of the Justinianic Plague over long distances is not a reason for doubting the identity of the pathogen, but is quite simply testimony that there was a significant enough volume of maritime trade in the Mediterranean during the sixth to eighth centuries to disseminate the pathogen.[134]

A large quantity of historical evidence from the second pandemic, supported by the conclusions of the researchers who studied the third pandemic, indicates that plague was frequently transported long distances (by infected rat fleas *Xenopsylla cheopis*) in grain, clothing, or other merchandise. The grain trade was probably particularly important for plague because rats love grain and so does *X. cheopis*.[135] In India, buildings used by grain dealers were frequently the starting points of epidemics.[136] During the Second World War, the notorious Unit 731 of the Japanese army spread plague in China by dropping from aircraft containers of wheat and rice with infected fleas among the grains. These activities provided experimental proof that the transport of infected fleas in grain is indeed an effective way of spreading plague.[137] Petrie and Todd, studying the plague epidemics in Upper Egypt in the early twentieth century, reached the following conclusion: "We believe that the people themselves are largely responsible for the spread of the infection by their movements to and fro and by the removal to distant parts of the town of relatives who are ill or of bundles of clothing or other articles."[138] This was also the main conclusion of the Plague Research Commission in India.[139] Under such circumstances, the epidemiology of plague may well come

[133] Scott and Duncan, *Biology of Plagues*, 5–6; contra Thompson, "Epidemiology of Plague," 544; Hirst, *Conquest of Plague*, 145–50; cf. Curson and McCracken, *Plague in Sydney*, for a more recent account of plague in Australia.
[134] McCormick in his *Origins of the European Economy* has assembled the evidence for this trade in a monumental fashion.
[135] Hirst, *Conquest of Plague*, 242 and 308.
[136] Hankin, "Epidemiology of Plague," 72; Pollitzer, *Plague*, 497. Over most of India, plague tended to disappear at the end of each season. It was probably not truly endemic in most parts of the country. Gill also made the interesting ecological observation that wheat-growing regions in India suffered from plague, but areas where rice was cultivated did not (Gill, *Genesis of Epidemics*, 318 and 324).
[137] J. Watts, "Victims of Japan's Notorious Unit."
[138] Petrie and Todd, "Report on Plague Investigations," 140.
[139] Gill, *Genesis of Epidemics*, 330.

to approximate the epidemiology of diseases spread by direct person-to-person transmission. Although there is very little direct evidence available for the Justinianic Plague, there is every chance that Gregory of Tours was right to ascribe the origin of the epidemic at Marseilles in 588 AD to contaminated merchandise that was imported from Spain on board a ship and sold to many of the citizens, just as the plague of 1720 in Marseilles originated from infected fleas in cotton, muslin, and silk on board the ship *Grand Saint Antoine,* which had arrived from the Levant. At the beginning of the twentieth century, rat fleas were frequently found on board ships at Marseilles.[140]

Plague spreads in two ways: first, rapidly by human transport over long distances, and second, slowly over short distances, as rat epizootics develop.[141] The first process is essential for pandemics, but the second process is essential for human epidemics at the local level because bubonic plague is normally not transmitted directly from person to person (although the epidemiology may tend to give this appearance, as explained earlier). *R. rattus* does not move far, as noted earlier.[142] Experimental research in Upper Egypt on rat psychology demonstrated that rats show no awareness of illness among other rats and so do not even attempt to flee an epizootic (unlike humans!).[143] Consequently, rat epizootics tend to advance extremely slowly.[144] John of Ephesus described

[140] Gregory of Tours *Historia Francorum* 9.22, p. 380; Hirst, *Conquest of Plague,* 307–20; Rothschild, "Note on the Species of Fleas Found upon Rats."

[141] Eckert, *Structure of Plagues* and "Retreat of Plague" distinguished between *maritime phases* and *internal* (or *continental*) phases of plague epidemics.

[142] Petrie and Todd, "Report on Plague Investigations," 124, concluded that in Upper Egypt most of the movements of *R. rattus* were "oscillations between contiguous houses, and doubtless represent sorties in quest of food from nests and burrows situated in the foundation of walls that were common to adjoining houses." Similarly, the Plague Research Commission in Bombay "failed to find the slightest evidence" for the migration of rats during epizootics (*Reports,* XXII: "Epidemiological Observations Made by the Commission," 755–56). This is why the point made by Scott and Duncan, *Biology of Plagues,* 280–81, that quarantine measures would not have stopped rats moving around, is not a serious objection to *Y. pestis* as a cause of the early modern plague epidemics.

[143] Petrie and Todd, "Report on Plague Investigations," 126. Although a rat is not motivated to migrate by illness among other rats, it may be impelled to move by natural phenomena that it can feel itself, such as floods or earthquakes, cf. the great Tiber flood in Rome in December 589, which preceded an epidemic of bubonic plague.

[144] The Plague Research Commission in India concluded that plague was spread among rats in Bombay not by the movements of *R. rattus,* but principally by *R. norvegicus,* which is more mobile (*Reports,* XXII, "Epidemiological Observations Made by the Commission").

the slow progress of bubonic plague depending on rat epizootics in the Near East during the Justinianic Plague:

God's providence informed [us] about it in such a way that [news] was sent to every place in advance, and then the scourge arrived there, coming to a city or village and falling upon it as a reaper, eagerly and swiftly, as well as upon other [settlements] in its vicinity, up to one, two or three miles [from it]. And until what had been ordered against [one city] had been accomplished, [the scourge] did not pass on to enter the next. In this way it laid hold on [cities and villages] moving slowly.[145]

The slow movement of rats is why plague was often highly localized in the past. Nevertheless, the presence of rats was essential for bubonic plague epidemics among humans.[146] One major objection made by the skeptics who doubt that *Y. pestis* caused the historical pandemics has been a supposed lack of rats, firstly in terms of archaeological discoveries of rat bones, and secondly a shortage of references in written sources to rat mortality in association with plague epidemics. Writers belonging to previous generations tended to argue that the Justinianic Plague must have been restricted to Mediterranean countries because there was no archaeological evidence for rats in northern Europe.[147] This argument from silence has turned out to be completely misleading. The techniques in use on archaeological sites until the 1970s were generally unsatisfactory for the recovery of small mammal bones. However, rat bones are now routinely being recovered from archaeological sites dating to the time of the Black Death in the fourteenth century.[148] Evidence for earlier periods is still thinner, but nevertheless is accumulating year by year. There have been a series of scattered finds of rat bones stretching from Isin and Uruk in Mesopotamia and the Hyksos capital Tell el-Dabaa in Egypt in the second millennium BC, Corsica in the Hellenistic period, Quseir el-Qadim on the Red Sea coast of Egypt, Stobi in Macedonia, to as far north as Lincoln, London, Wroxeter, and York in England during the time of the Roman Empire, and Zanzibar and Naples in the sixth century AD.[149]

---

[145] John of Ephesus in Pseudo-Dionysios of Tel-Mahrē, *Chronicle*, 85–86.

[146] As Ell, "Interhuman Transmission," 501, observed, "the mechanism of the great plague pandemic of sixth-century Europe is hard to explain without *R. rattus.*"

[147] E.g., Bonser, "Epidemics During the Anglo-Saxon period"; Shrewsbury, *History of Bubonic Plague,* 7–16; Davis, "The Scarcity of Rats"; Scott and Duncan, *Biology of Plagues,* 47–49, 55–57 and 80.

[148] Audoin-Rouzeau, "Le rat noir."

[149] Hirst, *Conquest of Plague,* 122–26, thought it "probable that true rats were well known in Anglo-Saxon England"; Girard, "A quelle époque?"; Rackham, "*Rattus rattus*"; Davis, "Palaeoecological Studies at Stobi"; Driesch and Boessneck, "A Roman Cat Skeleton";

However, the recovery of evidence is still impeded by attitudes among archaeologists, particularly classical archaeologists operating in Mediterranean lands. There is no doubt that the distribution map of rat finds in Europe given by Coram-Mekkey in 1997 tells us more about archaeologists than it does about rats.[150] Classical archaeologists are trained to appreciate Greek and Roman sculpture, pottery, architecture, and vase painting, not rat bones. I believe that the scattered finds of rat bones that have been made in Europe dating to the classical and early medieval periods are sufficient to demonstrate that there were enough rats around at the time of the Justinianic Plague, probably even in northern Europe as well as in southern Europe.

The second part of the rat problem is the scarcity of references to rats in association with plague epidemics. There are in fact at least five plague epidemics where rats are explicitly associated with the disease in historical sources: the epidemic at Beijing in China in 1792 described by Hung Liang-chi; an epidemic at Leeds in England in 1645; the diary of the Emperor Jahangir (the *Tuzuk-i-Jahangiri*) recording the death of a rat or mouse preceding human plague in a household at Agra in the Punjab in 1616; the Black Death at Constantinople as described by Nicephoros Gregoras, who mentioned rats dying in houses; and the Justinianic Plague according to John of Ephesus.[151] John specifically mentions rats dying with swollen tumors. This seems as good evidence as we can hope to get from sources of this period.[152] Even if, just for the sake of argument, we did not have such explicit evidence for both the Justinianic Plague and the Black Death, would it be significant that there is a lack of references to rats (and fleas) in connection with plague epidemics? Coming to plague after spending years working on the history of malaria, I cannot see any

---

Armitage et al., "New Evidence of Black Rat in Roman London"; Armitage, "Unwelcome Companions"; Audoin-Rouzeau, "La peste et les rats" and "Le rat noir"; Audoin-Rouzeau and Vigne, "La colonisation de l'Europe par le rat noir"; O'Connor, "On the Lack of Bones"; McCormick, "Bateaux de vie, bateaux de mort," 56–57 for Naples; Ervynck, "Sedentism or Urbanism."

[150] Coram-Mekkey, "Peste et rat."

[151] Dong et al., *Les maux épidémiques*, 57, and Benedict, "Bubonic Plague in Nineteenth-Century China," 119; Shrewsbury, *History of Bubonic Plague*, 406–7; Jahangir, *Tūzūk-I-Jahāngīrī*, 2:65–67; Ansari, "Account of Bubonic Plague"; Nicephorus Gregoras, *Historiae Byzantinae* 16.1, PG 74:517–18: καὶ εἴ τινες ἐν τοῖς τῶν οἴκων τοίχοις οἰκοῦντες ἔτυχον μύες; John of Ephesus in Pseudo-Dionysios of Tel-Mahrē, *Chronicle*, 87; Scott and Duncan, *Biology of Plagues*, 78.

[152] For the second pandemic there is also iconographic evidence, e.g., Poussin's painting *Philistins frappés de la peste* (dating to c. 1630), now in the Louvre, which shows dead rats among the human corpses (Blanchard, "Notes historiques sur la peste," 633).

problem whatsoever with the shortage of references to rats in descriptions of plague epidemics. A huge mass of historical references and scientific research in recent times demonstrates that malaria flourished in many parts of Europe for more than 2000 years, but throughout that time hardly anyone mentioned mosquitoes in connection with it.[153] People in the past were not aware that malaria was transmitted by mosquitoes and consequently had no reason whatsoever to mention mosquitoes when they were writing about malaria. Similarly with typhus; no one suspected that the ubiquitous lice carried a deadly disease. The situation with plague was exactly the same. People were simply not aware of the role of the rat as a host for *Y. pestis* (or the role of fleas as its vector), and therefore there was no reason why they should mention rats (or fleas) when they were writing about human plague epidemics.[154] It is only a "problem" if modern historians impute to people in the past modern knowledge that they did not possess.[155] This point is a good illustration of how certain "problems" that appear to some writers considering the history of plague in isolation to be rather mysterious become quite easily comprehensible features of the history of arthropod-borne diseases in general, if a broader perspective is adopted.[156]

Plague epidemics did undoubtedly sometimes have utterly devastating effects on very large urban human populations, even if numbers

---

[153] Sallares, *Malaria and Rome*, 45, 49.

[154] Hirst, *Conquest of Plague*, 121, wrote as follows: "the conception of the rat origin of outbreaks of bubonic plague has now become familiar to students of modern medicine and even to the educated laity; so much so that it is difficult to realize how strange and improbable this thesis seemed to the majority of epidemiologists at the end of the nineteenth century and with what hesitation it was eventually accepted."

[155] Even when rat mortality was noticed prior to a human epidemic, archaic systems of thought were capable of accounting for this phenomenon without needing any notion of a transfer of infectious material from rat to man. For example in China, Wu Xuanchong argued that miasma arising from the ground affected rats in their burrows underground before affecting humans above ground (Benedict, "Bubonic Plague in Nineteenth-Century China," 138). According to the miasmatic theory it was quite logical to observe rats dying before humans! Such conclusions illustrate why it took such a long time for the miasmatic theory to be overthrown.

[156] Even during a modern epidemic in which people are aware of the nature of plague as a disease and are deliberately searching for dead rats, it is not always easy to find them. In the epidemics at Mahajanga in Madagascar in the 1990s. 43.1% of the laboratory-confirmed plague patients did *not* notice dead rats in or around their homes (Boisier et al., "Epidemiologic Features"). This difficulty arises because sick rats tend to retreat to their burrows or other hideouts and die in inconspicuous places. Excavations of areas that were not readily accessible had to be undertaken to locate many of the dead rats in Upper Egypt (Petrie and Todd, "Report on Plague Investigations in Egypt," 128, 131) and in Ceylon (Hirst, *Conquest of Plague*, 148).

found in historical sources are often exaggerations. John of Ephesus claimed that more than 300,000 bodies were removed from the streets of Constantinople.[157] Such figures have sometimes encouraged the view that human plague is primarily an urban phenomenon.[158] Shrewsbury doubted that plague epidemics were possible in the north of England after the Black Death because the human population density was too low. However, because plague is primarily a disease of rodents, not of humans, density-dependence should operate principally at the level of rat and flea populations rather than human populations. This implies that plague epidemics among humans are possible in areas of low human population density, if there are enough rats and rat fleas around.[159] There is now abundant evidence for intense plague in rural areas during the second pandemic in various parts of Europe and the Near East as well as in India during the third pandemic. Benedictow found that in the diocese of Cilento near Salerno in Italy, plague completely penetrated a rural environment during the epidemic of 1656–1657 (the last major plague epidemic in Italy), producing very high morbidity and mortality rates in small villages. He reached the conclusion that "plague stands out as a disease with unique powers of diffusion."[160] Panzac found that many of the temporary plague foci in the Ottoman Empire (e.g., the western Balkan and Anatolian foci) occurred in thinly populated regions and estimated that many of these areas had low human population densities (about 5–15 inhabitants per km^2).[161] Hankin wrote about India: "all the known plagues of western India resemble the Black Death and the epidemics to which it gave rise in showing a high degree of intensity at one time over a

---

[157] John of Ephesus in Pseudo-Dionysios of Tel-Mahrē, *Conquest*, 87.

[158] Hirst, *Conquest of Plague*, 12, wrote as follows: "human plague is essentially an affair of urban communities. Without gross aggregations of population there can be no major epidemics" – a view followed by the current author in previous writing on this question (Sallares, *Ecology of the Ancient Greek World*, 270) and by Benedict, "Bubonic Plague in Nineteenth-Century China," 111, in her research on plague in China. According to Ibn Khaldūn, plague was more frequent in overpopulated cities such as Cairo in the fourteenth century (cited by Congourdeau & Melhaoui, "La perception de la peste," 119).

[159] Shrewsbury, *History of Bubonic Plague*, 53, suggested that bubonic plague epidemics in England required a human population density of 60 persons per square mile, but it is hard to see why this should have been so because humans are largely incidental to plague.

[160] Benedictow, "Morbidity in Historical Plague Epidemics," 413–16, on Italy, and *Plague in the Late Medieval Nordic Countries* reaching similar conclusions for Norway (discussed by Brothen, "Population Decline and Plague").

[161] Panzac, *La peste dans l'Empire ottoman*, 247–8.

large area, and in the relatively high rate of mortality that they produced in villages as compared to towns. The two groups of outbreaks also resemble one another in their power of spreading with facility from village to village." He made the comparison with Simon de Couvin's observation that the Black Death was particularly severe in the small towns (*suburbia*) of Europe.[162] Similarly in Madagascar recently 68.9% of human plague cases occurred in remote villages.[163] Benedictow explained the empirical data by arguing that the ratio of rats and rat fleas to humans was higher in the countryside than in cities.[164] Malaria in Europe in the past yet again offers an interesting parallel to plague. It required extremely large mosquito populations to flourish, and mosquito-breeding sites were more likely to be abundant in the countryside than in the middle of large cities. Consequently malaria too had a rural character in many parts of Europe where it occurred, with the ratio of mosquitoes to humans being higher in the countryside than inside large cities. Once again we are looking at a

---

[162] Hankin, "Epidemiology of Plague," 57–58; Renardy, "Un témoin de la grande peste" on Simon de Couvin; the Plague Research Commission in India found that there was no relation between human overcrowding and the frequency of plague in Bombay (*Reports*, XXII: "Epidemiological Observations Made by the Commission," 780–81). Cohn, "Black Death: End of a Paradigm," 714, accepted that the Black Death caused very high mortality rates in at least some rural areas.

[163] Chanteau et al., "Current Epidemiology of Human Plague."

[164] Benedictow suggested that the higher incidence of plague in rural than urban areas is incompatible with Biraben's theory (following Baltazard, "Déclin et destin d'une maladie infectieuse" and Karimi et al., "Sur l'écologie des puces") that plague was primarily transmitted not by rat fleas (*Xenopsylla cheopis*), but by human fleas (*Pulex irritans.*) Even where interhuman transmission by the human flea has been claimed, for example, in Morocco in recent times, plague had a sporadic character. The human flea seems to be an inefficient vector of plague because it lacks a proventriculus in which a mass of plague bacilli can accumulate awaiting regurgitation. Consequently, it probably did not play an important role in plague epidemics in most areas in the past (Girard, "Les ectoparasites de l'homme"). Very high population concentrations of human fleas could conceivably lead to plague transmission even if the individual human flea is an inefficient vector (Hirst, *Conquest of Plague*, 186–87). This is one possible explanation (pneumonic plague being the main alternative) for the apparent phenomenon of plague without rats on Iceland (Karlsson, "Plague without Rats"). Large numbers of human fleas have been discovered in recent archaeological excavations on Greenland (Buckland and Sadler, "A Biogeography of the Human Flea"; Buckland et al., "Insect Remains from GUS"), which is said to have been affected by the Black Death. However, Chanteau et al., "Current Epidemiology of Human Plague" noted that human fleas are common on Madagascar and concluded that there would have been far more plague on Madagascar than there has been recently if the human flea really played an important role in plague transmission. Baltazard apparently used a type of trap that catches human fleas efficiently but not rat fleas, leading him to underestimate the frequency of rat fleas (Hirst, *Conquest of Plague*, 242–43).

common feature of arthropod-borne diseases, not at something unique or specific to plague.

In the light of these considerations, it is plausible that the Justinianic Plague could have penetrated thinly populated regions, certainly in southern Europe, North Africa, and the Near East, perhaps even in northern Europe too.[165] Consequently, the various sources that record devastation in the countryside should be taken seriously. Procopius claimed, with some exaggeration, that it did not leave any inhabited island, cave, or mountain ridge untouched.[166] Paul the Deacon described the desolation of the Italian countryside; grain and grapes were not harvested, flocks lost their shepherds, the countryside was silent, there were no travelers, not even brigands, only human corpses everywhere. John of Ephesus drew a very similar picture for the Near East.[167] Theophanes recorded that the last wave of the Justinianic Plague in 747 annihilated the population not only of Constantinople but also of the surrounding region.[168] Kulikowski (in this volume) has suggested that the four plague sermons in a seventh-century AD homiliary from Toledo provide evidence that plague penetrated very deeply into the interior of the Iberian peninsula, besides affecting the Mediterranean coastal towns, which have yielded some archaeological evidence that can plausibly be linked with the Justinianic Plague.[169] Similarly, Conrad has argued that the Justinianic Plague had profound effects in the countryside as well as the cities in the Near East, although it affected only sedentary, not nomadic, populations. He exploited the poetry of Hassan ibn Thābit to uncover evidence for extensive activity of an epidemic disease, probably plague, in the countryside south of Damascus in Syria in the late-sixth century AD.[170] Even as far north as Britain, the sources suggest extensive penetration of rural environments, as Maddicott argues in this volume, because Bede and Adomnán use words such as *villa*, *vicus*, and *viculus* for

---

[165] Seger, "Plague of Justinian and Other Scourges" argued that the Justinianic Plague has left a detectable mark on the archaeological record in Finland.

[166] Procopius, *BP* 2.22.8, pp. 250–51.

[167] Paul the Deacon, *Historia Longobardorum* 2.4, p, 74; John of Ephesus in Pseudo-Dionysios of Tel-Mahrē, *Chronicle*, 81.

[168] Theophanes, *Chronographia*, p. 423.

[169] Grégoire, *Les homéliaires du Moyen Âge*, 214–22, for the *sermones de clade*, discussed by Orlandis, *Hispania y Zaragoza*, 115–22, and translated in the appendix to the essay by Kulikowski in this volume.

[170] Conrad, "Epidemic Disease in Central Syria" and "Die Pest und ihr soziales Umfeld im Nahen Osten," 93–102; Kennedy in this volume for the archaeological evidence.

some of the settlements affected by plague.[171] Sarris (in this volume) has shown that the numismatic, legal, and papyrological evidence strongly support the idea of large-scale agrarian depopulation.

Procopius and John of Ephesus indicate that the first wave of the Justinianic Plague affected all age groups and both sexes equally.[172] Nicephoros Gregoras expressed the same opinion with reference to the Black Death at Constantinople. In some of the later waves of the Justinianic Plague, the sources hint at differing effects of plague on different segments of the population. For example, Agathias wrote that young men were particularly badly affected, while women suffered much less, in the epidemic of 558 AD at Constantinople.[173] It is difficult to know the correct interpretation of such a statement, when so little evidence is available, because several different interpretations are possible. Even for more recent epidemics there are many contradictory views regarding possible age- and sex-specific effects of plague.[174] The impression that young men were worse affected could be an artifact created by a lack of interest in or a tendency to conceal women. Thus, the data collected by the Plague Research Commission in India recorded a higher number of cases among men in Bombay, but the authors of the report felt that plague cases in women were concealed from the authorities more frequently than cases in men.[175] The impression that young men were worse affected than women could alternatively be a true reflection of the situation, but even so, different explanations for such a statistical trend

---

[171] See the essay by Maddicott in this volume.

[172] Procopius, *BP* 2.22.3, pp. 249–50; John of Ephesus in Pseudo-Dionysios of Tel-Mahrē, *Chronicle*, 74 and 95.

[173] Agathias, *Historiae* 5.10.4, p. 176. Theophanes, *Chronographia*, p. 232 also observed its effects on the young.

[174] Carmichael, *Plague and the Poor*, 12, suggested that reports of high mortality specifically among children might have been the product of smallpox epidemics. She cautioned against using such reports as evidence for long-lasting immunity among the survivors of previous plague epidemics. In general, human immunity acquired after bacterial infections is weaker than the immunity acquired after many viral infections. Immunity among the survivors of previous plague epidemics was probably not an important factor in the historical epidemiology of plague. Ell, "Immunity as a Factor of Medieval Plague," discussed this problem. Cohn, "Black Death: End of a Paradigm," 727–28 and 734–35, argued that European populations adapted rapidly to the "pathogen of the Black Death" in the following hundred years and used the apparent spread of acquired immunity as an argument against attributing the Black Death to *Y. pestis*, but this argument relies on the unlikely assumption that *all* the epidemics that followed the Black Death had the same causative agent as the Black Death. Moreover, Cohn's argument rests on highly selective citations of the available documentary evidence (McVaugh, Review of Cohn).

[175] *Reports*, XXII: "Epidemiological Observations Made by the Commission," 764.

are possible. Ell is the main advocate of the hypothesis that iron deficiency hinders the growth of *Y. pestis*.[176] Consequently women, losing
iron in menstruation, should be less vulnerable to plague than men. This
is a real possibility, but it must be remembered, as Procopius observed,
that pregnant women are exceptionally vulnerable to plague (just as they
are to other acute infectious diseases such as malaria).[177] On the whole,
another view is preferable; namely, that both sexes and all age-groups are
equally susceptible to plague, but that age-specific or sex-specific effects
are sometimes observed in practice because of differing degrees of access
to sources of infection.[178] It is possible that men may be infected more
often than women, for example, simply because men visit certain types of
environment that are sources of infection more frequently than women.
Differential access to the sources of infection is a very important theme
to which we return shortly.

Although Scott and Duncan try to give the impression that the epidemiology of historical plague epidemics in Europe was utterly incompatible
with the epidemiology of the third pandemic in India, it is important to
note that this opinion was not entirely shared by the members of the
Plague Research Commission in India, as the earlier quotation from
Hankin demonstrates. However, there was one significant difference
between plague in India and Europe that requires consideration. This
was a pattern of one case per household on average in India compared
to a very high infection rate per household in Europe. For example,
the *Eulogium historiarum*, a chronicle dating to 1360–1370, estimates that
only a fifth of the total population of England perished during the Black
Death, the lowest estimate given by any English source, but states that most
of the individuals in affected households died.[179] Clearly, this implies a

[176] Ell, "Iron in Plague Epidemics." (1985).
[177] Procopius, *BP* 2.22.35–36, p. 255; Pollitzer, *Plague*, 418.
[178] Attempting to search for age- or sex-specific effects of plague in the archaeological record by studying human skeletal remains from cemeteries introduces another set of complex problems that cannot be discussed here in detail, beyond observing that it is unlikely that any historical population repeatedly affected by major plague epidemics would have demographic patterns similar to those of any modern or model popula- tion (Sallares, *Malaria and Rome*, 284). For various views on the feasibility of such an enterprise see Paine, "If a Population Crashes in Prehistory," Waldron, "Plague Pits," Roberts and Grauer, "Commentary," and Margerison and Knusel, "Paleodemographic Comparison," cf. Hollingsworth and Hollingsworth, "Plague Mortality Rates."
[179] Bleukx, "Was the Black Death a Real Plague Epidemic?" 80–82, discusses this passage in the *Eulogium Historiarum* 184, vol. 3:213: "*nec civitatem nec villam nec capham nec etiam nisi raro domum relinquens quin majorem partem vel totum interfecit, ita quod quinta pars hominum et mulierum ac infantum in tota Anglia sepulturae traditur.*"

very patchy distribution of the Black Death across England as a whole, a phenomenon that has already been discussed, but the disease was lethal where it did occur, with a very high death rate within the household. Similarly, John Cantacuzenus states that entire households were destroyed at Constantinople during the Black Death. The fragments of evidence available for the Justinianic Plague yield a similar picture. The testimony of Evagrius about certain households being completely destroyed even in towns where the overall effect of the plague was slight has already been mentioned. Similarly, John of Ephesus mentioned: "houses large and small, beautiful and desirable, that suddenly became tombs for their inhabitants and in which servants and masters at the same time suddenly fell [dead], mingling their rottenness together in their bedrooms, and not one of them escaped who might remove their corpses out from within the house."[180]

Gregory of Tours gave a fascinating description of the development of the epidemic at Marseilles in 588 AD.[181] He wrote that many of the citizens bought merchandise from a ship that had arrived from Spain. The epidemic started in one particular household, all eight of whose members died. However, it did not spread immediately to the rest of the town, but only after the lapse of a certain period of time.[182] It is now easy to recognize that this was the time required for an epizootic to develop among rats. Similar observations were made in India by Simond, one of the great pioneers of modern plague research. It is worth quoting Hankin's description of Simond's observations in India in full to show

[180] John of Ephesus in Pseudo-Dionysios of Tel-Mahrē, *Chronicle*, 74, cf. Theophanes, *Chronographia*, p. 423 saying that entire households were destroyed during the last wave of the Justinianic Plague at Constantinople in the summer of 747.
[181] Gregory of Tours, *Historia Francorum* 9.22, p. 380: "*navis ab Hispania una cum negotio solito ad portum eius adpulsa est, qui huius morbi fomitem secum nequiter deferebat. De qua cum multi civium diversa mercarentur, una confestim domus, in qua octo animae erant, hoc contagio interfectis habitatoribus, relicta est vacua. Nec statim hoc incendium lues per domus spargitur totas; sed, interrupto certi temporis spacio, ac velut in segetem flamma accensa, urbem totam morbi incendio conflagravit.*" Compare Bertrand, *A Historical Relation of the Plague* and Drancourt et al., "Detection of 400-year-old *Yersinia pestis*," for the Marseilles epidemic in 1720; Hirst, *Conquest of Plague*, 125; Shrewsbury, *History of Bubonic Plague*, 19, 22; Biraben, *Les Hommes et la peste*, 1:42–43; Stoclet, "Entre Esculape et Marie" and in this volume on plague in early medieval France.
[182] A good later parallel is the progress of plague in Milan in 1468 as described by Carmichael, "Contagion Theory and Contagion Practice," 232–33; it started with several cases in one large household in March, then 22 days passed until the next officially confirmed plague case (a girl who lived next door to the large household), then more cases in May, but all concentrated in two districts of the city.

how closely it matches Gregory's account of the epidemiology of the Marseilles plague in 588:

The typical mode of development of an outbreak of known history is as follows. The person bringing the infection is, usually, himself attacked, and also a varying number of those in contact with him, within a few days of his arrival, and within the probable incubation period of the disease. The virus then remains quiescent for a long period, generally for about twenty days, but sometimes as little as ten days, and sometimes for a longer period extending to three or more months. The first sign of its renewed activity may be the death of rats, human beings only falling victims after these rodents have been killed off. In other cases rats and men are attacked simultaneously, or lastly only men may be attacked.[183]

The length of the initial latent period is not surprising because not only must the rat itself have the infection and die to force its fleas to desert it and search for a new host, but also two weeks or more may have to pass, after a rat flea (*X. cheopis*) has become infected, before the plague bacilli have multiplied sufficiently within it to form a mass capable of blocking its proventriculus and so making it possible for the flea to transmit plague.[184] Consequently, it is inevitable that bubonic plague epidemics will have a long serial generation time, even though the period of acute clinical symptoms is very short, only about five days. It is very important to note that the combined latent and infectious period before symptoms of thirty to thirty-five days, followed by a period of symptoms of five days, which was determined by Scott and Duncan for their hypothetical "haemorrhagic plague," is in fact perfectly compatible with the known behavior of plague caused by *Y. pestis*. Thompson observed in 1906 that intervals of about thirty-five days between human cases were regularly observed in the early stages of plague epidemics at the beginning of the twentieth century.[185]

---

[183] Hankin, "Epidemiology of Plague," 63.

[184] Hirst, *Conquest of Plague*, 160. Regurgitation of infectious organisms after blocking of the vector's digestive system is an unusual transmission method only observed elsewhere in the sandflies that transmit leishmaniasis.

[185] Scott and Duncan, *Biology of Plagues*, 128; Thompson, "Epidemiology of Plague," 561. Scott and Duncan, "Biology of Plagues," 385, suggested a filovirus, like Ebola or Marburg viruses, as the cause of historical plague epidemics in northwestern Europe. However, the properties of these viruses do not fit the requirements because, for example, Marburg virus has a short incubation period of only 3–9 days (Bell et al., *Zoonoses*, 133). Equally there is no evidence that such viruses have ever been active in Europe (outside laboratories). They appear to be incapable of causing human epidemics covering large geographical areas and have no vector for transmission from person to person. Scott and Duncan, "Biology of Plagues," 352–53, claimed that the CCR5 gene 32-base pair deletion may have given resistance to their hypothetical "haemorrhagic plague" and so

There is no doubt that in the past, living conditions were frequently extremely unhygienic.[186] Houses, particularly those belonging to the poor, were often crowded with fleas, lice, mosquitoes, and other undesirables in addition to their human occupants, not to mention dirt, rubbish, and rats.[187] The investigations of the plague epidemics at Kôm Ombo in Upper Egypt revealed that fourteen out of twenty-seven houses studied had more than 120 rat fleas (*X. cheopis*) in them, while the most infested house yielded no fewer than 1,005 rat fleas.[188] Why then have some modern plague epidemics in other parts of the world yielded a pattern of only one case per household? This is a fundamental question to which the literature on plague does yield some potential answers. Answering it would eliminate the main obstacle to reconciling the epidemiology of the Justinianic Plague and the Black Death with bubonic plague's modern epidemiology in India.

been selected by the Black Death. However, it has since been demonstrated experimentally that CCR5Δ32 is unlikely to give any resistance to plague (Mecsas et al., "CCR5,"). Moreover, plague epidemics probably persisted for too short a time to explain the current frequencies of CCR5Δ32 (Schliekelman et al., "Natural Selection"). There are alternative hypotheses to explain the spread of this mutation. Galvani and Slatkin, "Evaluating Plague and Smallpox" suggested an association with another disease, smallpox. Lucotte, "Distribution of the CCR5 Gene" suggested that because CCR5Δ32 reaches its highest frequencies in Scandinavian populations, it was probably dispersed to the rest of Europe during the Viking migrations, i.e., in between the first and the second pandemics, in which case it would have nothing whatsoever to do with plague. Other hypotheses linking human genetic mutations to plague have also been proposed. Cassano, "Cystic Fribosis" suggested that cystic fibrosis is the result of an adaptive response to plague.

[186] Zupko and Laures, *Straws in the Wind*, described the attempts of legislators to grapple with hygiene problems in the city states of late medieval northern Italy; Conrad, "Die Pest und ihr soziales Umfeld im Nahen Osten" on hygiene in the Near East.

[187] John of Ephesus in Pseudo-Dionysios of Tel-Mahrē, *Chronicle*, 86 emphasized that the poor were the first people to be attacked in Constantinople during the Justinianic Plague, although Nicephorus Gregoras *Historiae Byzantinae* 16.1, *PG* 74:517–18, said that the Black Death affected rich and poor equally. *The Brut* (an English chronicle of the late fourteenth century) states that the Black Death affected the poor more than the elite (Bleukx, "Was the Black Death a Real Plague Epidemic?", 82–83). The Plague Research Commission also reached the conclusion that plague was commoner among the poor than the rich in Bombay in India (*Reports*, XXII: "Epidemiological Observations Made by the Commission," 784), cf. Shrewsbury, *History of Bubonic Plague*, 4 and 405, for England. Benedictow, "Morbidity in Historical Plague Epidemics," 416–17, discussing the epidemic at Basel in Switzerland in 1609–1611, quoted Greslou's conclusion that "plague was a disease of the poor," cf. Dyer, "Influence of Bubonic Plague." Only the rich could afford to flee and had somewhere else to go. Of course it was the same in the case of malaria in Europe in the past (Sallares, *Malaria and Rome*, 174, 180–81, 197 and 228).

[188] Petrie and Todd, "Report on Plague Investigations," 130.

An interesting article on plague in Australia in 1900 by Thompson points the way forward.[189] There was a series of sporadic cases of bubonic plague across the city of Sydney among unrelated people. There was almost always only one case per household. The explanation of the apparently sporadic distribution pattern emerged when the researchers considered not where the infected individuals *lived*, but where they *worked*. It became clear that multiple infections were in fact occurring in certain workplaces. The infected individuals went home after work and became ill at home. There were no infected rats in the household precisely because the source of infection lay outside the household, and there was no further spread of the disease within each household from the original case because bubonic plague is not normally transmitted directly from person to person. That is how the pattern of one case per household was generated in Sydney. The significance of the Sydney epidemic is that it suggests that the location of the source of infection can play a critical role in the epidemiology of plague. If the point of infection lies outside the household, only one case per household would be expected. However, if there is a rat epizootic within the household, then we might well expect to see multiple cases of plague infection among the human occupants of that household. These considerations suggest that human plague epidemics can in fact display quite different epidemiological patterns under different circumstances, and Scott and Duncan failed to consider these possibilities in their book. Consequently, the fact that the epidemiology of European epidemics of plague in the past did not match its epidemiology in India during the third pandemic in respect of the household effective contact rate is not a fatal objection to identifying *Y. pestis* as the cause of both the Justinianic Plague and the Black Death.

The Plague Research Commission noted that the general response to the recognition of a single case of plague in a household in India was to abandon that house immediately.[190] It might be expected that this habit would have restricted further infections among the members of that particular household. In contrast, in Europe in the past, the authorities often tried to force people to remain where they were by quarantine and similar procedures (cf. the famous plague epidemic at Eyam in England). Flight certainly did occur and contributed to depopulation of settlements, for example in the Near East during the Justinianic Plague as Conrad has argued.[191] Paul the Deacon noted that so many

[189] Thompson, "Epidemiology of Plague."
[190] Discussed by Benedictow, "Morbidity in Historical Plague Epidemics," 427–28.
[191] Conrad, "Arabic Plague Chronologies and Treatises," 89.

people abandoned the city of Ticinum (modern Pavia) in Italy during
the plague epidemic in 680 AD that the forum and squares of the city
became overgrown with grass and other plants.[192] Similarly, during the
last great plague epidemic in Italy in 1656–1657 many people who fled
from Rome never subsequently returned, leaving the city depopulated
for a generation afterward.[193] The waves of the Justinianic Plague might
sometimes have moved people around rather than kill them. However,
Paul's description of the epidemic in 680 also makes it clear that many
whole families did perish at Rome. Unfortunately, there is no quanti-
tative evidence available that would enable us to evaluate the relative
importance of death and flight as components of depopulation during
the Justinianic Plague. Nevertheless, explaining the high infection rates
per household during the first and second pandemics in Europe requires
the presupposition that people sometimes did not flee to quite the same
extent as they have done in India recently. In the only bubonic plague
epidemic in England in the twentieth century, in a single household in
Suffolk in December 1909–January 1910 in which all seven members of
the household were infected, at intervals of three to six days, the infection
rate would presumably have been lower if the house had been abandoned
after the first case appeared.[194] Of course, the inhabitants of Europe and
the Near East in 541–544 AD and the years of the Black Death had no
previous personal experience of plague; subsequent generations were
able to benefit from experience. The European practice of quarantine
may well have restricted the geographical spread of epidemics during the
later course of the second pandemic, as many historians have argued, but
it may well have also increased infection and mortality rates in affected
areas.[195] Quarantine worked by restricting the movement of infected fleas
in merchandise.

[192] Paul the Deacon, *Historia Longobardorum*, 6.5, p. 166. It was during this epidemic that
the cult of St. Sebastian as the patron saint of plague became established. See Gelpi,
"Saint Sebastian and the Black Death" and the essay by Little in this volume.

[193] Sallares, *Malaria and Rome*, 273–75.

[194] Black, "Plague in East Suffolk." Three survived and four died. Cf. Shrewsbury, *History
of Bubonic Plague*, 181 and 343, for single households being ravaged by plague in the
villages of Glapthorne in Northamptonshire in 1545 and Malpas in Cheshire in England
in 1625.

[195] For example Del Panta, *Le epidemie*, emphasized the importance of quarantine in the
elimination of plague from Italy. See McCormick in this volume for Desiderius of Cahors,
Epistolae 2.20, pp. 74–75, c. 640 AD in Gaul, for the only evidence for the concept of
quarantine during the Justinianic Plague. The letter shows that it had already been
surmised only a century after the initial wave of that pandemic that plague spread in
contaminated merchandise.

There is one other major possible explanation for the apparent lower infectivity of plague during the third pandemic relative to the first two pandemics that requires consideration. This explanation involves taking the apparent discrepancy in the behavior of plague at face value and postulating that biovar *orientalis* is in fact less efficient at airborne transmission today than biovars *antiqua* and *mediaevalis* were in the past. It has already been seen that the frequency of cervical buboes produced by tonsillar plague indicates a high frequency of infection by the respiratory route in late medieval plague epidemics, while on the contrary it was often observed in India at the beginning of the twentieth century that plague's infectivity was so low that a plague hospital was a safe place to stay during a plague epidemic, as Cohn noted.[196] However, it is not necessary to follow Cohn's inference that the pathogens responsible for the second and the third pandemics must be different organisms, because he did not consider the possibility of differences among the three biovars. At this point, it should be recalled that Devignat carried out experiments fifty years ago that suggested that the *mediaevalis* biovar has a faster rate of reproduction and so is more virulent than biovar *orientalis*. Although the genomes of these two biovars are very similar, as was discussed earlier, it still remains possible that a small number of genetic differences between them could have conferred higher infectivity upon *mediaevalis* (and *antiqua*), since it is now known for sure that changes in just a handful of genes, or the acquisition of a small number of genes from other bacteria by horizontal transfer, can transform the lifestyle of *Y. pestis* (for example, the genetic changes that made transmission by fleas possible). It is suggested here that *antiqua* and *mediaevalis* were indeed more infectious than *orientalis*, and consequently infection by the respiratory route was more important during the Justinianic Plague and the Black Death than it has been during the most recent pandemic. By chance, it is even possible to offer a precise parallel to such a course of evolution from another very important species of pathogenic airborne bacteria, namely, *Mycobacterium tuberculosis*. Like plague, the numerous strains of human tuberculosis have been divided into three evolutionary groups, and it has been argued that the group of tuberculosis strains that evolved most recently exhibits reduced powers of infectivity compared with the other two groups that evolved earlier.[197]

The seasonality of the disease is another major objection made by the skeptics to *Y. pestis* as the cause of the pandemics. Procopius states

---

[196] Cohn, "Black Death: End of a Paradigm," 712.
[197] Sreevatsan et al., "Restricted Structural Gene Polymorphism."

that the first wave of the Justinianic Plague occurred in all seasons of the year, as did the Black Death.[198] However, later waves of both the first and second pandemics tended to follow a seasonal pattern. A summer peak is recorded for some of the later waves of the Justinianic Plague. For example, Paul the Deacon noted that the epidemic in 680 in Italy occurred in July, August, and September.[199] Likewise Theophanes indicates that the final wave of the Justinianic Plague arrived at Constantinople in September 746, was quiescent during the winter, reactivated itself in the spring, but raged during the summer of 747.[200] This summer peak was the regular pattern observed in late medieval epidemics. In Florence, for example, plague epidemics generally lasted from May to September. The Bills of Mortality show that in London deaths from plague peaked in late summer and then decreased sharply. Even during the Black Death in 1348, plague peaked in summer in most areas (except in Avignon and Marseilles among major western Mediterranean cities), as Cohn has shown.[201] Similarly, plague epidemics in modern times have tended to be confined to certain seasons.[202] This periodicity is explained above all by the requirements of the vector fleas, which require certain humidity levels for a long lifespan as well as certain temperature levels (neither too cold nor too hot) for reproduction. The plague season occurs earlier and earlier in the year with decreasing latitude.[203] Thus in England plague peaked in late summer and did not coincide with the season of typhus, a winter disease, enabling Shrewsbury to propose his theory that typhus epidemics in winter regularly succeeded summer plague epidemics in England. However, in Upper Egypt the plague season coincided with the typhus season from January to March.[204] Nevertheless, regardless of its seasonality, the peak period for plague in each region was always the time of year when rat flea populations reached maximum levels. In Upper Egypt, this happened in March each year.

[198] Procopius, *BP* 2.22.5, p. 250; Evagrius, *Ecclersiastical History* 4.29, pp. 177–78; Patlagean, *Pauvreté économique*, 92–94, on seasonal mortality in the Byzantine world.
[199] Paul the Deacon, *Historia Longobardorum* 6.5, p. 166.
[200] Theophanes, *Chronographia*, p. 423, describing an example of what Kunhardt (cited by Pollitzer, *Plague*, 495) termed an "incomplete" plague outbreak because it reached Constantinople too late in 746 to run through the entire rat population before the onset of winter.
[201] Cohn, "Black Death: End of a Paradigm," 718–25.
[202] Van Loghem, "Plague of the 17th Century."
[203] Gill, *Genesis of Epidemics*, 326.
[204] Shrewsbury, *History of Bubonic Plague*; Petrie and Todd, "Report on Plague Investigations"; Pollitzer, *Plague*, 487–90, listed data on the plague seasons in various countries.

Twigg claimed that it is "biologically impossible" for plague to have caused epidemics as far north as England because it is too cold for flea reproduction so far north. There are indeed conflicting reports in scientific literature regarding the possibility of rat flea (*X. cheopis*) reproduction in northern Europe. However, the bulk of the evidence indicates that rat fleas can reproduce easily inside a house in summer as far north as England, as suggested by experiments in London in 1935, because the optimal temperature range they require is 20–25°C.[205] An indoor rat flea simply requires a rat that loves life indoors, like *R. rattus*, to flourish in England, as Hirst pointed out. Conversely *R. norvegicus* is unsuitable because it prefers to live outdoors, away from man. At the time of writing, the temperature inside an unheated house in Manchester in the north of England on a cool, overcast day in early July was 21.1°C. Rat flea reproduction so far north seems quite plausible with the temperature requirements generally given in the literature.[206] Moreover, it is important to remember that plague epidemics did not occur every year. As far as the Justinianic Plague is concerned, favorable environmental conditions once every dozen or so years would have sufficed. Consequently, the *average* levels of temperature (and other climatic variables) are irrelevant.[207] According to the Annals of Clonmacnoise, the summer of 664 AD, the first reasonably well-documented plague epidemic in England, was exceptionally hot.[208] Again, a parallel with malaria is instructive. Gill had already noted that the effects of humidity on fleas are so similar to its effects on mosquitoes that some of what he had previously written about malaria could be applied verbatim to plague.[209] *Plasmodium malariae*, the pathogen that causes quartan fever, has, according to the textbooks, temperature requirements for completion of its development inside mosquitoes, which should permit it to occur only in the hottest

[205] Hirst, *Conquest of Plague*, 272–75 and 341; Shrewsbury, *History of Bubonic Plague*, 3. For a different view see Beaucournu, "Diversité des puces vectrices en fonction des foyers pesteux."

[206] Duncan, "Possible Influence of Climate" discussed the relationship of climate to plague in Scotland.

[207] This is the fundamental weakness of the argument of Cohn, "Black Death: End of a Paradigm," 725, namely, that the hot dry summers of Mediterranean cities are hardly ideal for rat fleas. Humid conditions do sometimes occur in Mediterranean cities in summer (to give a specific instance, the current author experienced very unpleasant high humidity levels while attending a conference in August 1999 in Barcelona, one of the cities mentioned by Cohn), and that is all that is needed for plague epidemics to occur occasionally.

[208] See the essay by Maddicott in this volume.

[209] Gill, *Genesis of Epidemics*, 371.

parts of Europe. However, a mass of evidence demonstrates that it had a much wider distribution in the past.[210] The balance of probability is that the situation was much the same with plague as it was with mosquitoes and malaria parasites in northern Europe in the past; it *was* warm enough inside houses for *R. rattus* and *X. cheopis* to reproduce, certainly in summer, perhaps occasionally even in winter.[211] Of course in southern Europe and the Near East there was no problem.

These considerations adequately account for the normal seasonal periodicity of plague. It is still necessary to try to explain the lack of seasonality of the initial wave of the Justinianic Plague. The conclusion that weather parameters are important to the epidemiology of plague naturally creates the possibility that unusual weather conditions could lead to unusual occurrences of plague. This seems to be the best path toward an explanation (in conjunction with the presence of virgin-soil populations of rats with no immunity to plague) because there is evidence for unusual weather conditions at the time of both the Justinianic Plague and the Black Death. In the case of the Black Death in England, sources such as Ranulph Higden's *Polychronicon*, Thomas Walsingham, and the chronicle called *The Brut* all record very heavy rainfall continuously from June 24 until the end of the year 1348.[212] Presumably this indicates the prevalence of humid westerly winds. Modern research has confirmed that increased precipitation is correlated with an increased frequency of plague.[213]

Keys linked the origin of the Justinianic Plague to the dust-veil event of 536, an extraordinary climatic event of uncertain cause marked by the second narrowest tree ring in the past fifteen hundred years, indicating an exceptionally cold and dry summer. The tree rings for 540–541 and several of the succeeding years are also very narrow.[214] Keys postulated that

---

[210] Sallares, *Malaria and Rome*, 102, 131–36 and 218.

[211] Of course, as Hirst, *Conquest of Plague*, 276, pointed out, "the micro-climate of the rat hole or rat burrow may be much more important to the epidemiologist than the macroclimate of human dwellings."

[212] All quoted by Bleukx, "Was the Black Death a Real Plague Epidemic?", 78–79 and 82–85.

[213] Parmenter et al., "Incidence of Plague"; Enscore et al., "Modeling Relationships Between Climate"; Hirst, *Conquest of Plague*, 26, had already observed that unusual dampness and warmth promotes the spread of plague in temperate regions.

[214] Keys, *Catastrophe*, 35–45, building on Stothers, "Mystery Cloud," and Baillie, "Dendrochronology Raises Questions"; see also Stothers, "Volcanic Dry Fogs," Gunn, *Years Without Summer*, and D'Arrigo et al., "Spatial Response to Major Volcanic Events" for evidence for the impact of this event outside Europe. According to L. B. Larsen, the Greenland ice-cores yield evidence for a major event in 527 ± 1, but no sign of anything unusual in the 530s and 540s (abstract of conference paper in *Environmental Catastrophes and Recovery in the Holocene*, ed. S. Leroy and I. S. Stewart, London: Brunel

severe drought followed by increased rainfall in eastern Africa caused a population explosion of plague's usual rodent hosts, such as gerbils. This was followed by an explosion of plague itself, which was then transported by ships carrying ivory from Zanzibar, where bones from *R. rattus* as well as Mediterranean pottery have been excavated at the port of Unguja Ukuu in archaeological strata dated to the sixth century AD, to the Red Sea, and Egypt. This theory is certainly plausible, although in view of the evidence of Rufus of Ephesus that plague was already present in the vicinity of Egypt centuries before the Justinianic Plague, it still remains possible that the origins of the Justinianic Plague lay closer to the Mediterranean world than Zanzibar.

If the information of Dionysius the Hunchback about plague cases in Libya, Egypt, and Syria in the third century BC is taken at face value, it is possible that there were already scattered foci of sylvatic plague in these areas well before the Justinianic Plague, in which case its commencement at Pelusium, a rather unexpected location for the beginning of a pandemic, may be easier to explain. The important evidence of Aretaeus should also be considered. Aretaeus, who came from Cappadocia in Anatolia and sometimes refers to the medical situation in Syria and Egypt in his writings, mentioned "pestilential and very malignant buboes."[215] Although this reference is very brief, it should be remembered that Aretaeus was the most accurate observer of diseases in Roman times; he has given us, for example, the best extant ancient description of lepromatous leprosy, as well as pioneering descriptions of coeliac disease and diabetes. It is hard to imagine anything to which he could be referring when he mentioned "pestilential and very malignant buboes" except bubonic plague. Consequently Aretaeus' evidence strengthens the case for believing that there were already foci of sylvatic plague somewhere in Libya,

University, 2002). If the ice-cores are accurately dated, this information may indicate that the 536 event was the product of a relatively minor volcanic eruption that generated an acid dry fog in the troposphere rather than the higher stratosphere (Grattan and Pyatt, "Volcanic Eruptions"). Koder, "Climatic Change" also discussed the climate of the sixth century. Cassiodorus, *Variae* 12.25, pp. 381–82, described the climate of these years.

[215] Aretaeus, *Acute Diseases* 2.3.2, in *Extant Works*, p. 270: Βουβῶνες μὲν οἱ λοιμώδεες ἥπατος καὶ σφόδρα κακοήθεες, ἐξ ἄλλου δὲ γίγνονται οὐδενός. Hude in his more recent edition for the *CMG*, p. 22, preserved the manuscript reading ἥπατος, but the textual emendation ἥβης considered by Adams, following Wigan, is highly plausible. Unfortunately the date of Aretaeus is rather uncertain. Oberhelman, "On the Chronology and Pneumatism of Aretaios," suggested the mid-first century AD, the acme of the Pneumatist school of medicine.

Egypt, perhaps Syria too, well before the Justinianic Plague, giving rise
to occasional small-scale epidemics among humans. As was noted earlier,
pneumonic plague, a form of the disease that generally prefers cold conditions, has manifested itself with surprising frequency in modern times
in Upper Egypt, normally a hot region.[216] It is not inconceivable that
the exceptionally cold conditions in 540–541 AD turned one of these
frequent small-scale and highly localized epidemics of the airborne form
of the disease in a region of sylvatic plague, somewhere in the vicinity of
Libya, Egypt, or the Levant, into a massive epidemic of pneumonic plague
affecting humans on a large scale for the first time. That would help to
explain the extraordinary mortality near the epicenter of the epidemic;
for instance the statement of John of Ephesus that the entire populations
of two cities on the borders between Egypt and Palestine were annihilated to the extent that there was not a single survivor (bubonic plague
is usually not quite so deadly).[217] The hypothesis proposed here is that
sylvatic *Y. pestis* had already been around for several centuries by the time
of the Justinianic Plague but had interacted with humans only occasionally on a small scale. It took an extraordinary climatic event to transform
occasional localized contact into massive contact. The precise details of
the origin of the Justinianic Plague will probably always remain a mystery. However, it is now indisputable that it commenced at a time of very
unusual climatic conditions, which would have created the possibility of
an unusual epidemiology of plague. Consequently, the lack of seasonality
of the first wave of the Justinianic Plague is not an insuperable obstacle
to identifying *Y. pestis* as its cause.

The immediate effects of the Justinianic Plague on early medieval
history have been surveyed in other essays in this volume.[218] Suffice it to
say here that it undoubtedly played a major role in undermining the old
order of the sub-Roman world and paved the way for the immigration of
less Romanized newcomers. As long ago as 1948 Mirko Grmek suggested
that the effects of the Justinianic Plague in Illyricum permitted the Slav

[216] A. W. Wakil, cited by Pollitzer, *Plague*, 509, "believed that an increased susceptibility of
the dark-skinned inhabitants of Upper Egypt to lung affections in general was partly
responsible for the high incidence of pneumonic plague in that region," although
Pollitzer observed that the same correlation was not observed in other areas.
[217] John of Ephesus in Pseudo-Dionysios of Tel-Mahrē, *Chronicle*, 77–80.
[218] Riché, "Problèmes de démographie historique," 47–48, suggested that the Plague of
Justinian was as bad as the Black Death. For the effects of the Black Death on Europe,
out of a vast literature, see Carpentier, *Une ville devant la peste* and Bowsky, "The Impact
of the Black Death."

invasion from 545 onward.[219] The Byzantine emperor Constantine VII Porphyrogenitus explicitly stated that it cleared the way for the Slavs to penetrate into Greece.[220] Plague weakened the Visigothic kingdom in Spain and so assisted the Arab invasion, it facilitated the movement of the Lombards into Italy as Paul the Deacon realized, and it may well have weakened the indigenous Romano–British states and so helped the progress of the Anglo-Saxons in England.[221]

The Justinianic Plague certainly had considerable short-term effects on the economy. For example, the widespread reversion to handmade pottery in many regions in the second half of the sixth century AD, after centuries in which wheelmade wares had been regularly used, indicates a certain contraction in long-distance trade.[222] There have also been interesting speculations by economic historians regarding more long-term effects of the Justinianic Plague. For example, it has been suggested that great epidemics such as the Justinianic Plague and Black Death might have introduced a stochastic element into the timing of the Industrial Revolution in Europe. Another suggestion is that because it is difficult to use economic theory to explain transitions from one epoch to another, exogenous factors such as great epidemics are required as a stimulus. A third idea is that some observed fluctuations in the atmospheric concentrations of carbon dioxide over the last 1,500 years can be attributed to forest regrowth after land abandonment following plague epidemics; in other words, human interactions with the natural environment may have led to fluctuations in the levels of greenhouse gases long before the

---

[219] Grmek, "Les conséquences de la peste."

[220] Constantine VII Porphyrogenitus, *De thematibus* 2.6, pp. 90–91: ἐσθλαβώθη δὲ πᾶσα ἡ χώρα καὶ γέγονε βάρβαρος, ὅτε ὁ λοιμικὸς θάνατος πᾶσαν ἐβόσκετο τὴν οἰκουμένην.

[221] Although the idea that the Justinianic Plague severely weakened the indigenous populations and thereby facilitated the spread of the Anglo-Saxons across England is certainly not a new idea (see e.g., Sawyer, *From Roman Britain to Norman England*, 18; Burgess, "Population, Climate and Upland Settlement"), its significance is greatly enhanced if it is linked to recent research on the historical genetics of the population of England. Weale et al., "Y Chromosome Evidence" showed that Y chromosome haplotypes from central England are indistinguishable from those of Frisia, while the populations of both north Wales and Norway have different genetic patterns. This suggests that the bulk of the modern male population of England is indeed descended from people who migrated across the North Sea, not from the indigenous Romano-British population. The predominance of the genes of the migrants is easy to explain if the indigenous population had just been decimated by the Justinianic Plague. This also correlates very strongly with the lack of evidence for any significant indigenous cultural influence upon the Anglo-Saxons, for example, the scarcity of Celtic loan words in English.

[222] E.g., Gutiérrez Lloret, "Eastern Spain in the Sixth Century."

modern industrial period. One ancient historian has suggested a disease-based model for the substantial population reduction in Late Antiquity, in which the so-called Antonine "plague" (smallpox) in the second century AD initiated a decline, which was aggravated by other non-disease factors, culminating in the Justinianic Plague in the sixth century.[223]

For the purposes of this essay, it is more important to consider the significance of the Justinianic Plague for the history of plague itself. Medical historians have put great effort into devising theories to explain the end of the second pandemic: the spread of the practice of quarantine, increasing immunity to *Y. pestis* among rats, methods of house construction that excluded rats, improvements in human nutrition, the replacement of *R. rattus* by *R. norvegicus*, the introduction of arsenic as a rat poison, the spread of cross-immunity to *Y. pestis* owing to interactions with other micro-organisms (*Y. pseudotuberculosis*, *Y. enterocolitica*, tularaemia, salmonella) – these are some of the theories that have been proposed (this list is not intended to be comprehensive).[224] However, there is an almost complete absence of theories to explain the end of the first pandemic, the Justinianic Plague, in about 750.[225] It is clear that most of the theories proposed to explain the end of the second pandemic cannot possibly be applicable to the end of the first pandemic as well. For example, Hirst argued that the key to the disappearance of plague from Britain was the replacement of the combination of an indoor rat (*R. rattus*) with an indoor flea (*X. cheopis*) by the combination of an outdoor rat (*R. norvegicus*) with an outdoor flea (*Nosopsyllus fasciatus*), breaking the close contact between humans and rats.[226] The logic of his argument seems impeccable; nevertheless, the explanation cannot possibly work for the eighth century AD because there is no evidence that *R. norvegicus* was present in Europe or the Mediterranean world then, and if (just for the sake of argument) it had already arrived in the eighth century AD, the

[223] Lagerlöf, "Diseases and Growth"; Findlay and Lundahl, "Demographic Shocks"; Ruddiman, "Anthropogenic Greenhouse Era"; Liebeschuetz, *Decline and Fall,* 52–54, 390–92.

[224] For some discussion of these various theories see Appleby, "Disappearance of Plague"; Biraben, *Les Hommes et la peste;* Del Panta, *Le epidemie;* Eckert, "Retreat of Plague"; Hirst, *Conquest of Plague;* Loosjes, "Brown Rat"; Slack, "Disappearance of Plague."

[225] Morony in this volume suggests that plague epidemics continued in the Near East after c. 750 AD. This is not impossible. Evidently *Y. pestis* did not vanish off the face of the earth c. 750 AD; foci of sylvatic plague undoubtedly continued to exist and might have given rise to localized epidemics. However, there is no evidence for plague epidemics in Europe between the middle of the eighth century AD and the Black Death, and to that extent it is certain that plague did retreat in the middle of the eighth century.

[226] Hirst, *Conquest of Plague,* 333.

explanation would not work for the end of the second pandemic. Similarly, there is no evidence at all for the widespread application of quarantine procedures, changes in house construction methods, improvements in human nutrition, or the use of rat poisons in response to plague (or great changes in the human flea [*Pulex irritans*] population for those who believe in its importance as a vector of plague) in the middle of the eighth century AD. The Justinianic Plague invalidates nearly all the theories about the decline of the second pandemic as general explanations for the decline of pandemics.

Because all the other hypotheses are evidently unsatisfactory as general explanations of pandemics, by default, we are left with the question of immunity. Gill suggested that the essential cause of the long-term periodicity of plague is the rise and fall of herd immunity among rodents.[227] Although he did not consider the complications now known to be caused by cross-immunity between *Y. pestis* and the other *Yersinia* species and other micro-organisms, it seems that only an explanation along these lines can provide a unified explanation for the rise and fall of all the pandemics.[228] The alternative is to assume that there is a different reason for the rise and the fall of each pandemic; in other words, there are multiple pathways along which plague pandemics can develop. This is also quite possible. Plague has still to divulge many of its secrets. There is still room for further research on the Justinianic Plague, and still the possibility of a fourth pandemic in the future.

[227] Gill, *Genesis of Epidemics*, 378; Pollitzer, *Plague*, also emphasized this idea.
[228] Fukushima et al., "*Yersinia enterocolitica* O9," showed that in one natural focus of sylvatic plague in Yanchi in China, *Y. pestis* is endemic among wild rodents, but in another part of the country (Haiyuan) where plague is absent, *Y. enterocolitica* is the species found among wild rodents. They speculated that the third pandemic failed to become established in Europe because infection with *Y. pseudotuberculosis*, generating cross-immunity to *Y. pestis*, had become endemic in rodents in Europe by the time that the third pandemic started in the Far East.

12

Toward a Molecular History of the Justinianic Pandemic

Michael McCormick

Disease has a deep history. Modern "plagues" have made historians sensitive to the problem of human illness and suffering in the past, and even the broader public is drawn to questions of catastrophic change, disease, and the decline of the ancient world.[1] Historians have long used the medical science of their day to illuminate historical records of plague.[2] Medical research of the first half of the twentieth century underpinned Biraben's pioneering work on both the Justinianic and the medieval plagues. In no small part, Benedictow challenged some of that analysis because of medical progress forced by the outbreaks of bubonic plague (*Yersinia pestis*) during the American war in Vietnam.[3] A decade later, the advances of molecular biology are assuming revolutionary proportions and oblige us to consider the issues anew.

Every passing week deepens biologists' understanding of DNA, how it works, and its implications for all life forms. The development of the PCR (polymerase chain reaction) procedure allows swift and accurate

---

[1] See the path-breaking synthesis of McNeill, *Plagues and Peoples*. Although aspects of their methodology and conclusions may fail to satisfy some specialists, Keys, *Catastrophe*, and Baillie, *Exodus to Arthur*, deserve credit for bringing to light new data and questions of great importance for understanding the sixth century. This essay was written in the winter of 2001–2002; I tried to take into account the fast-breaking work in molecular biology and ancient biomolecules published while the book awaited publication, as well as Sallares' valuable essay in this volume. Unfortunately, I did not have the time to overhaul the essay's fundamental conception, which reflects the date of its original composition.

[2] And vice versa, as for instance the early Italian medievalist Lodovico Antonio Muratori (1672–1750) reminds us with his *Del governo della peste*.

[3] See Biraben, *Les Hommes et la peste*; Biraben and Le Goff, "Plague in the Early Middle Ages," and Benedictow, *Plague in the Late Medieval Nordic Countries*.

amplification and sequencing of DNA from very small quantities. This makes possible the identification of the genomes of various organisms, and that illuminates the molecular processes of disease and life itself. New outbreaks of plague add to the clinical and epidemiological data. Even leaving aside the problem of bioterrorism, the World Health Organization has classified bubonic plague as a newly reemergent disease. Over the fifteen years from 1989 to 2003, 38,310 cases (2,845 deaths) were reported worldwide, and plague has made unexpected reappearances in India (1994 and 2002), Indonesia (1997), and now for the first time in fifty years, Algeria (2003).[4]

Today, for example, sylvatic or wild (as opposed to urban) *Y. pestis* is endemic in the southwestern United States. It is time to reassess what we know about the disease and its potential implications for understanding the historical phenomenon of the Justinianic Pandemic, a phenomenon whose impact seems to loom larger as investigation deepens.[5] The implications of the disease allow us to formulate a series of observations and questions, inspired by and addressed to researchers working in biology, medicine, and the brand new field of molecular archaeology.

The problems posed by the Justinianic Pandemic are daunting.[6] But microbiology contributes mightily to articulating the issues. To fully address so complex a phenomenon will require archaeologists and historians to look beyond microbes to larger life forms, and to investigate rats and fleas against a broader backdrop. Answers will come but slowly, and the issues will interrelate in ways intricate and unforeseen. Some questions raised here may seem to outstrip our current scientific or archaeological tools, but if we fail to ask them today, we risk missing the opportunity of discovery tomorrow. Who, just a few years ago, dreamed of recovering traces of the great plagues from the bodies of the victims themselves, centuries after the infection so unexpectedly ended their

---

[4] *Weekly Epidemiological Record*, no. 33 (August 13, 2004): 302, available at http://www.who.int/wer/2004/wer7933/en/.

[5] Among recent discussions, see, e.g., Grmek, "Les conséquences de la peste," and Sarris, "Justinianic Plague."

[6] Even the historian who has been privileged to enjoy the counsel of generous scientists runs risks in such new and highly technical territory. That I have not erred more often is largely due to the patient advice of my friends Professor Thomas L. Benjamin, of the Harvard Medical School, and Dr. Charles U. Lowe, formerly of the National Institutes of Health, who kindly read and critiqued this essay; Dr. Lowe also offered bibliographical advice in the final stage of revision. I am equally grateful to Professor Markus Meister and my other colleagues for the stimulating discussion that followed a version of this essay at Harvard University's Center for Genomic Research.

historical existence? Still, it bears emphasizing that this essay is mostly about potential, not actual data, about questions, rather than answers. We have only begun looking for molecular evidence of the pathogen of the Justinianic Pandemic. Even if answers lie far in the future, three big questions seem to me critical in appraising the Justinianic Pandemic's impact on world history.

First, what pathogen, exactly, caused the Justinianic Pandemic? Second, what light can biology cast on the origins and course of the Justinianic Pandemic? Third, where did it go? Why did the pandemic end? We have, I think, no real idea why it stopped after c. 750 (or perhaps as late as 766).[7] For each of these three broad questions, we need to identify the main options for exploration and explanation.

Was the Justinianic Pandemic in fact due to *Y. pestis*? The question has to be posed, front and center. For the initial outbreak, the features we can piece together from the written texts suggest that the pathogen was indeed *Y. pestis*: the symptoms, especially the buboes, the timing, the rodent mortality,[8] the apparent correlation with classic modes of sea-borne transmission, and the mortality levels all seem to point in the same

---

[7] As Biraben and Le Goff, "Plague in the Early Middle Ages," 60, 63, and 77, note, the latest attestation comes from John of Naples, *Gesta episcoporum neapolitanorum* 42, *MGH, SRL*, 425.15–19: "*In eo siquidem anno, quo Paulus episcopus defunctus est, irato Deo, tanta desaevit clades in Neapoli, quae a medicis inguinaria vocatur, ut patris interitum mors subsequeretur filiorum, et ad sepeliendum rarus superstes inveniretur; unde etiam prope omnes clerici eiusdem episcopii vitam finirent.*" John was writing c. 900, using good local sources: see e.g., McCormick, *ODB* 2: 1065–6. This outbreak appears to be completely isolated. Caution may be called for, given the author's distance from the event (although he is generally reliable) and his manifest desire to justify the election of the secular duke of Naples as its bishop. It is not impossible that an error could have arisen in copying the date from a paschal table (normally arranged in cycles of nineteen years), leading John erroneously to link plague devastation and the duke's uncanonical episcopal election. If indeed Bishop Paul died in March 766, a nineteen-year displacement of the date of the plague would place it in 747, i.e., at the height of the last great wave documented outside Naples: see McCormick, *Origins of the European Economy*, 870, no. 153. On the other hand, recent mathematical modeling of rodent epidemics conceivably might explain such an isolated outbreak, if the eighth-C. rat and human population of Naples were large enough to sustain that hypothetical pattern of recurrent plague: see Keeling and Gilligan, "Bubonic Plague." There the model is shown for a rat population of 60,000, which may have been larger than what Naples could have sustained at this date.

[8] Notwithstanding the occasional scholarly observation to the contrary, an eyewitness does record bubonic rodent mortality during the first wave of the Justinianic epidemic: John of Ephesus, *Historiae ecclesiasticae fragmenta*, fragmentum G, 234.20–4, rendered here as *mures*, i.e., "rodents"; cf. the English translation of this passage as preserved in Syriac in *CZ*,105, rendered as "mice." Judging from Greek and Latin, the ancients did not distinguish clearly between mice and rats: see McCormick, "Rats, Communications and Plague," 4.

direction. For most of the subsequent episodes, the textual evidence is much thinner. In any case, some medical and historical researchers challenge this identification for the Justinianic Pandemic, and more throw into question the diagnosis for the incomparably better documented second pandemic, the medieval Black Death.[9] For the Black Death, however, early molecular evidence appeared to confirm the identification of the pathogen as *Y. pestis*, while a more recent study challenges these results. This brings us to the promise and problems of ancient DNA, or aDNA.

Deoxyribonucleic acid, or DNA, is the genetic material of all living things. It is, to quote *Britannica Online*, an "organic chemical of complex molecular structure that is found in all . . . cells and in many viruses." DNA codes genetic information for the transmission of inherited traits. It exists in cells as a double helix, a kind of twisted ladder, whose rungs are formed by the bonds linking two out of four different molecules (chemical complexes), conventionally termed "bases," and designated by the letters A, G, C, and T. These four bases pair with each other in predictable fashion – A always pairs with T, and G with C to form a sequence comprising, sometimes, millions of pairs of bases, or "rungs" on that twisted ladder. Although there are some zones on these ladders that are highly conserved (i.e., shared) across the evolution of organisms, the total sequence of the pairs of bases that make up DNA is unique to a particular organism. What we call a "gene" corresponds to some sequence of base pairs (abbreviated "bp") in the double helix of DNA that transmits instructions for the production of a particular protein. In the last twenty years, it has been shown that unlike protein molecules, DNA molecules, although subject to various degrees of decay, are remarkably tough and can survive for centuries, even millennia.[10]

---

9 Three recent examples: Scott and Duncan, *Biology of Plagues*, 6, on the Justinianic Plague: "It is not possible to be certain from the evidence available, but the rapid spread over great distances, the heavy mortality and other features of the pandemic suggest that bubonic plague was not the major component, but that some other infectious disease, spread person-to-person, was responsible." Their monograph uses epidemiological methods to argue that the medieval pandemic was chiefly some form of unknown viral hemorrhagic fever, although they allow that the new molecular evidence indicates that some bubonic plague was present: e.g., 49 and 340. Herlihy, *Black Death and the Transformation of the West*, 25–31, challenged the identification of the pathogen, but left the question open. Cohn, *Black Death Transformed*, denies that the disease was caused by *Y. pestis*, but refuses to offer an alternative. For a detailed critique of these positions, see Sallares, in this volume.

10 Audic and Béraud-Colomb, "Ancient DNA is Thirteen Years Old;" for a sober survey of results and problems, see Hofreiter et al., "Ancient DNA."

Because DNA lies at the very basis of all living cells, including the bacterium that is *Y. pestis*, it is capable of conveying a tremendous amount of information that we are just beginning to understand; molecular archaeologists are applying these advances to studying DNA from ancient humans. This is no easy task. For various reasons, contamination by extraneous DNA is potentially a great problem for all DNA analysis. Moreover, aDNA is usually degraded, that is, it is partially broken down, or fragmentary. It often survives in segments of only about 100 bp, complicating the design of uniquely identifiable sequences. Modern DNA, on the other hand, is, literally, everywhere and abundant. This makes contamination problems, in the ground as in the lab, loom all the larger.[11] Lastly, various factors that appear of little relevance to modern DNA seem to inhibit the enzymatic reactions that are essential to PCR, and so stall laboratory work at an early stage.[12]

In 1998, a team at the University of Marseilles announced the recovery of the early modern aDNA of *Yersinia pestis* from the relatively well-isolated human remains that are teeth. They subsequently took their analysis a step further back in time, analyzing dental pulp of twenty-three teeth taken from three individuals in a collective "catastrophic" burial in Montpellier, dated archaeologically to the fourteenth century.[13]

For all three individuals, they reported that the PCR procedure and subsequent sequencing yielded distinctive fragments of DNA uniquely identifiable as that of *Y. pestis*. Recent studies arguing that the Black Death was due to some pathogen other than *Y. pestis* appeared seriously challenged, at least for the fourteenth-century infection at Montpellier.[14]

[11] Kolman and Tuross, "Ancient DNA Analysis," esp. 16, with respect to possible contamination of the aDNA of *Y. pestis*; cf. Cooper and Poinar, "Ancient DNA."
[12] For a concise account of aDNA and its challenges, see Delefosse and Yoder, "Ancient DNA"; more details on inhibition in Hummel, *Ancient DNA Typing*, 104–5.
[13] They use the burial's stratigraphic position (on top of a thirteenth-C. wall, and "behind" a fourteenth-C. one), and observe that different parts of the whole cemetery (which comprises 800 excavated graves dating from the ninth to the seventeenth C.) were dated by means of "historical records, stratigraphy, the study of 7,059 ceramic remnants and fourteenth-C. data." Raoult et al., "Molecular Identification," here 12800; cf. Drancourt and Raoult, "Molecular Detection"; see also Drancourt et al., "Detection of 400-year-old *Yersinia pestis*."
[14] Scott and Duncan, *Biology of Plagues*, 49, note that the chronology of the cemetery where the victims were located might extend into the thirteenth C., and suggest that they therefore did not necessarily come from people who died during the Black Death. It is true that the description of the stratigraphy of the graves is not completely clear, but the suggestion that this lack of clarity might in fact mean that the bubonic plague appeared in unrecorded fashion a few generations before 1348, and that the recorded epidemic was not bubonic plague, is hard to follow.

A more recent study questions these results. Tests by a well-known laboratory specializing in ancient biomolecules at Oxford has failed to replicate the earlier outcome on a larger but different set of sixty-one late medieval and early modern victims, excavated in five different suspected plague burials in northern Europe (Angers, Copenhagen, two in London, and Verdun).[15] Of course the absence of evidence is not evidence of absence. Nevertheless, the Oxford results are extremely valuable, for they underscore the fragility of early results in a new type of investigation for which consensus is still developing on proper procedures, methods, and expectations.[16] At the same time, they make imperative the multiplication of testing of and explanations for the validity of different techniques and procedural details as applied to various ancient evidence and its biomolecules, including those thought to be connected with the medieval plague. A recent report out of Germany only underscores this point.[17] The power of molecular research to recover the evidence,

---

[15] Gilbert et al., "Absence of *Yersinia pestis*," Drancourt and Raoult, "Molecular Detection"; Gilbert et al., "Response to Drancourt." There is some lack of clarity in Gilbert et al., "Absence of *Yersinia pestis*," concerning the nature of several of the burials that provided the tested teeth. The 34 individuals tested from the Copenhagen site come from a "Plague pit" (343, Table 1), but the discussion in the text (342) refers to a total of fifty-seven individuals in fifty-four graves at this eighteenth-C. site. This seems to indicate that individual burials prevail at this site, which would not be the expected pattern at the height of a plague epidemic (see notes 23–24). No dating evidence is given for the mass grave discovered at Angers in 2001, whereas the 14Carbon dating of the part of the Spitalfields, London cemetery that supplied remains of five individuals "assigns them to the late thirteenth century." No parameters are given for the radiocarbon results. If the late thirteenth-C. date holds, that obviously would exclude the Black Death, which reached London in 1348: Biraben, *Les Hommes et la peste*, 1: 82. Although circumstantial evidence seems to make the thirteen individuals from mass burials at Verdun good candidates for early modern plague victims, Drancourt and Raoult, "Molecular Detection," also report negative results from different teeth from the same Verdun burial place. This leaves the eight individuals and their twenty-seven teeth from the Royal Mint (London) as the most compelling source for the negative results. For a contradictory report of other tests on evidence from the Royal Mint, see note 17.

[16] The absence of clear consensus on the details of procedures that most reliably produce authentic results seemed manifest from the public discussions among practitioners of the new field at the stimulating conference "Archaeozoology and Genetics. First scientific meeting," organized by Jean-Denis Vigne at the Muséum national d'histoire naturelle, Paris, June 14–15, 2004.

[17] At least five more reports concerning the identification of *Y. pestis* from aDNA merit mention. At Munich, Garrelt and Wiechmann, "Detect of *Yersinia pestis* in early and late medieval burials," and Wiechmann and Grupe, "Detection of *Yersinia pestis* DNA," present positive results from individuals from a fourteenth-C. mass grave and a sixth-C. multiple grave in Bavaria. At Tübingen, Pusch et al., "Yersinial F1 Antigen," have reported using two different methods to successfully identify *Y. pestis* in the remains

including aDNA, of ancient pathogens is not in question.[18] Rather than discouraging more testing, the *non liquet* resulting from the contradictory results of the first two series of experiments argues for systematic analysis of multiple specimens from multiple sites, following the nascent standards of authentication, in as many independent laboratories as is possible.

There is no theoretical obstacle to applying the same procedure to aDNA from the first pandemic because 1,500 years is well within the range of DNA survival.[19] Concretely, we need to find plague victims from the Justinianic Pandemic. An undisturbed tomb with an inscription stating that its occupant died of the plague in the reign of Justinian would be ideal. This is, however, unrealistic, given that the rapid and devastating onset of the epidemic quickly preempted normal funerary practices.[20] There are nonetheless plenty of graves that can be assigned to the sixth, seventh, or eighth centuries. Among them we find the sort of mass burials that evoke a great epidemic. The next step must be careful and systematic analysis of multiple specimens from multiple sites, given that the preservation of aDNA is unpredictable, and that there will be no certainty that a given mass burial, even of the appropriate date, reflects a plague epidemic. Multiple testing is all the more important in this case because the specimens will be a millennium or more older than those analyzed for the

---

of twelve putative 17th-C. victims of the plague from Stuttgart. While a PCR approach yielded only a 17% success rate, an innovative antigen test gave positive results from 83% of specimens. McKeough, "Ring-A-Ring-A-Rosy," reported that a slightly modified version of Drancourt's method successfully identified the aDNA of *Y. pestis* from one of six bones analyzed from the London Royal Mint site; incomplete publication precludes assessment of the validity of these results, insofar as they can be deduced from the summaries published in *Australian Archaeology*, 52 (2002): 48; and online at http://www.australianarchaeologicalassociation.com.au/conference/2001/HTML/PostersAbstractsMZ.html#mckeough and http://www.australianarchaeologicalassociation.com.au/postergallery/images/mckeough_poster.pdf. Finally, in an early study not often cited by later specialists, Hummel et al., "aDNA-Ein neuer Zugang," 60–61, gave a preliminary report of possible amplification of a *Yersinia* sequence from the femur of an individual buried in a medieval plague cemetery in Lübeck. In a conversation in June 2004, Dr. Hummel kindly confirmed to me that she is skeptical of that result today.

[18] E.g., Gilbert et al., "Absence of *Yersinia pestis*," 342; see the survey of Zink et al., "Ancient Microbial Infections."

[19] E.g., Hofreiter et al., "Ancient DNA," 353.

[20] So far the only explicit epigraphic record of a plague death is a building inscription for a church in the Hauran, at Azra'a, which records the decease from inguinal and axillary buboes of the bishop involved in the church: ed. Koder, "Ein inschriftlicher Beleg."

second pandemic, and because a warmer Mediterranean environment in general appears to be less favorable to aDNA preservation than a cooler northern European one.[21]

If the identity of the pathogen can be definitively resolved, we will need to tackle its extent: How far did it spread? The written sources' potential for tracking even the relatively well-documented first outbreak in 541–542 is woefully limited; thereafter, the lights dim nearly to darkness. Modern claims have been made that the infection reached Scandinavia, Finland, Poland, and the British Isles, far beyond the Mediterranean shores on which it is most securely attested.[22] To settle these questions and reconstruct the first pandemic, the first thing we need is a critical inventory of late antique, early medieval, and early Islamic mass graves that are potential plague burials. What we should expect can be deduced from sixth-century descriptions of burial conditions, reinforced by early modern accounts and excavation of charnel pits from the Black Death and later. Individuals were placed in collective graves without the customary burial customs of their time and place; in some cases, efforts were made to cram the maximum number of cadavers into the available space.[23] It remains to be seen whether systematic scrutiny of such collective tombs yields a reliable typology that would discriminate plague graves from those due to other catastrophic illnesses. It is not impossible that plague burials display a distinctive demography, compared with other, contemporary cemeteries. Early evidence from a medieval plague pit is inconclusive, despite some archival and modern evidence for a distinctive age and sex distribution of plague mortality.[24] Thus, one analysis of

---

[21] Höss et al., "DNA Damage."

[22] Scandinavia and Finland: Seger, "Plague of Justinian and Other Scourges," with further references; he hypothesizes (192) a plague connection with mass graves at Käldamäki (Vörå) and Levänluhta (Isokyrö), Finland, hitherto identified as sacrificial or slave burials. Poland: careless, multiple burials (two, three, or five individuals) in a "Germanic" cemetery assigned to the fifth century near Wrocaw: Franz, "Zur Bevölkerungsgeschichte," a reference that I owe to the kindness of Joachim Henning. British Isles: Dooley and Maddicott in this volume.

[23] See Procopius, *BP* 2.23.1–12, pp. 256.9–258.4; John of Ephesus, *Historiae ecclesiasticae fragmenta*, fragmentum G, 236.30–237.5, on Justinian's arrangements for mass graves for, supposedly, 70,000 victims, across the Golden Horn in Galata; cf. *CZ*, 108. Similarly the extract from the *Megas chronographos, Chronik 1* 9, 1:42, 5–16.

[24] Waldron, "Plague Pits"; and Roberts and Grauer, "Commentary," 109–10. Waldron's aim was to test the hypothesis that plague pits offer more accurate portrayals of the demographic structure of a population than normal cemeteries. Comparing this London Black Death pit (602 burials) to a normal medieval cemetery directly overlaying it,

detailed data from a poor London parish in the plague of 1603 shows the mortality was sharply skewed toward males, and hit youths aged five to twenty-four especially hard.[25] John of Ephesus' claim that Justinian commanded the excavation of gigantic pits capable of receiving 70,000 cadavers each may suggest that in some cases, sheer size could be a valuable indicator.[26] More scrutiny of collective graves from the second pandemic that archival evidence identifies as plague burials should refine the typology of this kind of entombment.[27] But certainty will come only from using modern molecular methods to find irrefutable evidence of the pathogen.

I am preparing a provisional inventory of potential Mediterranean plague pits from the first pandemic. By way of example, I might cite four sites featuring twelve collective graves. All appear in places that certainly or probably were afflicted by plague; at least two or three of those sites are indubitably from the right time.[28] Two such, so far unpublished, occur on the southeastern coast of Asia Minor, at Anemurium, and seem to date around 600 AD. The Necropolis Church contained a collective grave of at least thirteen children, ranging in age from infants to ten- to twelve-year-olds; the Central Church contained a grave with the remains of at least thirty-one individuals, which appear to have been set afire.[29] At Naples, excavators have explicitly raised the possibility of a small plague

Waldron concludes that the patterns are so similar that the hypothesis fails, and that his expected patterns of plague mortality are not evident in the pit. Regardless of the merits of this hypothesis, I note two potentially significant divergences from the "control" cemetery. Infant and juvenile burials (which typically are less well preserved, and under represented in medieval cemeteries) are somewhat better represented in the plague pit (29.46%, N = 177) than in the cemetery (23.2%, N = 55), and so closer to the expected normal infant and juvenile mortality. Dental pathologies were also significantly lower (28%) in the pit than in the control group (43.5%).

[25] Hollingsworth and Hollingsworth, "Plague Mortality Rates." They plausibly link the pattern to cultural factors – playing in streets, exposure to places with rats – rather than biological ones. It may not therefore translate directly to Late Antiquity. Note however the similar pattern in Madagascar in 1998: Migliani et al., "Résurgence de la peste," 117.

[26] John of Ephesus, *Historiae ecclesiasticae fragmenta*, fragmentum G, 236.30–237.5.

[27] See, for example, Signoli and Dutour, "Etude anthropologique."

[28] A coastal town across from Cyprus, Anemurium is in the province of Isauria, which was created out of and neighbors Cilicia. John of Ephesus explicitly mentions that the first epidemic ravaged Cilicia, and reports delusions that accompanied the infestation at Ascalon: *Historiae ecclesiasticae fragmenta*, fragmentum F, 231.20–22 and fragmentum E, 229.26 respectively; cf. *CZ*, 99 and 96, respectively. Naples, 8th C. John of Naples, *Gesta episcoporum neapolitanorum* 42, p. 425.15–19.

[29] Personal communication of Prof. James Russell, University of British Columbia, for which I am deeply grateful.

pit. This eighth-century collective grave contained at least seven children. They ranged in age from around four months to four-and-one-half years, displayed no signs of trauma, and seem to have been covered with quicklime at burial.[30] Four more tombs in the vicinity of Ascalon have been reported as filled with remains and "transformed into an emergency charnel pit."[31] Another set of five mass graves that has come to light in southern Italy, at Venosa, may date from the eighth century. It presents an age and possibly a sex profile that resembles seventeenth-century plague mortality in London.[32]

A second, potentially rewarding avenue of investigation is now opening up. Although underwater archaeology has already made fundamental contributions to our knowledge of ancient and medieval seafaring, the natural conditions yield human or animal remains only very exceptionally. That is about to change, judging from the discovery in 2000 of a late Roman ship, perfectly preserved by the anoxic conditions that prevail in the Black Sea below approximately 200 m. The entire wooden vessel, the mast, even some of the rigging, still lie intact at a depth of 320 m. AMS radiocarbon analysis yielded a calibrated date of 410–520 for the ship.[33] The vigor of ancient and medieval Black Sea shipping combines with the prevailing anoxic conditions to imply that countless shipwrecks and their organic contents survive where the bottom conditions are undisturbed. The new discovery, and others like it surely to come, herald a new source of ancient human or, perhaps more likely, rodent remains that will have been trapped below deck at sinking. They should be better preserved than even the best land burials; whether the particular submerged conditions also allow the preservation of useful molecules, remains to be discovered.

An expanding inventory of mass graves and other mammal remains potentially linked to the Justinianic Pandemic will allow more extensive

[30] Arthur, ed., *Il complesso archeologico*, 58 and 74–5.

[31] Abu Juwei'îd (c. 15 km east of Ascalon), three tombs, apparently all filled with remains: Dauphin, *La Palestine byzantine*, 3:872, site 10/187; cf. 2:512; 2: Fig. 13; and Khirba al Sharaf (anc. "Saraphia"), episcopal see c. 6 km south of Ascalon, c. 4 km from the present coast; 1 km west of the ancient town, a chamber tomb, apparently originally intended as a family burial place, was "transformed into an emergency communal charnel pit," filled with a "large number" of burials: ibid., and 3:876, site 10/236; of "Byzantine," i.e., late Roman date, according to Holy Land archaeological convention.

[32] Macchiarelli and Salvadei, "Early Medieval Human Skeletons." The sex distribution is twenty-three males, twelve females, but thirteen individuals are of undetermined sex. I am grateful to Luca Bondioli for alerting me to these graves, and to Maurizio Tosi also.

[33] See Ballard et al., "Deepwater Archaeology," here 619–21.

laboratory testing for molecular traces of the suspected pathogen. The fundamental scientific principle of replicable results will require analyses to be duplicated in multiple laboratories. Establishing that (or whether) the victims discovered at such and such a site did indeed die of such a pathogen will be a real breakthrough. But it will be only the first step. The next will be to build up, case by case, a map of the certain geographic diffusion of the first pandemic that is independent of, more reliable, and almost certainly, more extensive than what the sparse written records reveal. If confirmed, the Marseilles molecular investigations indicate that we should expect to find DNA of *Y. pestis* in the teeth of some victims who died of the plague. Some, but not all. Medical reasons, as well as diagenetic changes, that is the changes undergone over time by buried materials, suggest that we should expect a moderate success rate at best.

Victims who succumbed to the toxins of *Y. pestis* before septicemia set in, that is, before plague bacteria overwhelmed their bloodstream, may not present its DNA in the blood-rich pulp preserved in the dental core.[34] And not every tooth will test positive, even for those who did die of plague: three of four teeth of one fourteenth-century victim tested negative in one Marseilles investigation.[35] The Oxford results were negative for as many as 108 teeth from 61 possible plague victims.[36] And those tests were directed, in part, to relatively well-documented plague pits, whereas our investigation will have much less to go on. Furthermore, opinion varies widely among practitioners as to the likely success rate for ancient DNA analyses, even given apparently promising looking materials, and it seems prudent to anticipate a high proportion of negative results.[37] The investigation will have to proceed by trial and error and accept that some, perhaps many, of the multiple graves we are in the process of identifying may not preserve useful ancient nucleic acids, while other victims will have succumbed to other infections and sickness encouraged by the generally catastrophic health and dietary conditions prevalent during an epidemic. Others still may have expired from different forms of mass death, arising from other infections, or other events. Clearly, we will have to be patient

---

[34] As Dr. Lowe points out to me.

[35] Raoult et al., "Molecular Identification," 12801.

[36] Gilbert et al., "Absence of *Yersinia pestis*."

[37] Kolman and Tuross, "Ancient DNA Analysis," 19, for a sobering assessment, with respect to human aDNA. It is essential to record success rates for probes. For example, discussion at the Archaeozoology and Genetics conference (above, note 16), reported success rates ranging from a truly exceptional 96% to, more commonly, between 10% and 40%.

and focus at least our early tests on areas where the infection is securely attested and the archaeology advanced. But in the long term, we will have to take into account that the first pandemic of plague attained truly global proportions, to judge from an account of it in China in 610.[38]

What about the remains of survivors who overcame the infection? In the hypothesis of *Y. pestis*, previous infection leaves clear serological traces in living human and animal survivors of the disease.[39] Sera – essentially, body fluids – will not normally survive in ancient human remains. Is there any conceivable evidence other than serological that could identify individuals who survived the disease? First, if there were, comprehensive demographic and palaeopathological analysis of cemeteries would allow us to reach beyond plague pits in mapping the geographic extent of the epidemics. Second, we might be able to get a handle on infection and, possibly mortality rates in a particular population by comparing plague pits and survivors and studying the results in the light of historical and modern rates. Indeed, one might look for some genetic factor that links survivors but is lacking in victims. That sort of finding would resonate far beyond historical investigation, as suggested for instance by the ongoing debate about a genetic link between surviving the Black Death and resistance to HIV in modern Europeans.[40]

In sum, a database of the ancient biomolecules derived from the inventoried plague pits should make conceivable new questions of great significance to historians and not without interest for microbiologists and specialists of infectious diseases. If the ancient pathogen's identity with *Y. pestis* should be confirmed, the issues of microbiology with greatest historical implications seem to me to be those of evolutionary and geographic origins, as well as the pathogen's molecular characteristics.

Molecular investigation of the evolutionary origin of *Y. pestis* addresses chronology. It is now clear that *Y. pestis* evolved from a relatively innocuous gastrointestinal pathogen, *Y. pseudotuberculosis*. This bacterium has an animal reservoir, causes gastroenteritis, including severe diarrhea, and is transmitted among humans through food and water.[41] Calculations

[38] McNeill, *Plagues and Peoples*, 147.
[39] Migliani et al., "Résurgence de la peste"; Chanteau, "Current Epidemiology of Human Plague"; Ratsitorahina, "Seroepidemiology of Human Plague."
[40] Stephens et al., "Dating the Origin"; cf. also Altschuler, "Plague as HIV Vaccine Adjuvant." The evidence is presently running against this particular link: Mecsas et al., "CCR5 Mutation," with Elvin et al., "Ambiguous Role of CCR5."
[41] U.S. Food and Drug Administration, *Foodborne Pathogenic Microorganisms*, s.v. "*Yersinia enterocolitica.*"

based on "molecular clock" have provided the first independent dates
for the evolutionary origin of *Y. pestis*. Essentially, molecular clock refers
to the rate of fixation of mutations in DNA, which allows estimates of the
approximate age of a particular organism. This rate indicates that *Y. pestis*
evolved out of *Y. pseudotuberculosis* somewhere between 20,000 and 1,500
years ago.[42] It is more distant, genetically, from a third *Yersinia*, *Y. enterocolitica*.[43] In other words, molecular clock allows – but of course does not
prove – the identification of the Justinianic pathogen with *Y. pestis*. Will
future microbiological research make it possible to refine the molecular
clock and get a more precise date for the emergence of *Y. pestis*? If, for
example, *Y. pestis* had already been around for several centuries, historians will have to scrutinize with renewed vigor what exactly was new in the
540s that made the epidemic outbreak possible.[44]

The geographic origin of the Justinianic Plague remains unknown.
Molecular investigation should clarify that. Based on their fermentation
characteristics, three variant types or biovars, three lineages of *Y. pestis*,
were identified in 1951. Biomedical literature has repeatedly connected
these three biovars with the three great pandemics: biovar *Antiqua* is
thought to be the strain of the Justinianic Plague and, so far, has been
found especially in Africa and Asia. Biovar *Medievalis*, assumed to be
the 1347 strain of the pathogen, is linked with Central Asia (perhaps
Kurdistan). Biovar *Orientalis* is well documented. It corresponds to the
pandemic that reached international attention in 1894, and stems from
East Asia. *Orientalis* presently occurs in Vietnam, Africa, the United States,
and South America. Recently, molecular evidence has been adduced
in support of the identification of the three biovars, which seems also
to indicate ages for them that conform to this schema.[45] Nevertheless,
the limited genetic markers deployed to differentiate the biovars to date
may yet prove insufficient. A substantial amount of research conducted
in the former Soviet Union and China indicates a more complex picture of strains than those on which western researchers have hitherto

[42] Achtman et al., "*Yersinia pestis*, the Cause of Plague."
[43] E.g., Alonso, "Interactions écologiques," summarizes the distance at 60% DNA relatedness, whereas *Y. pseudotuberculosis* shows 90% DNA relatedness, which implies that it
really is not a different species from *Y. pestis*.
[44] See Sallares, in this volume, on the earlier evidence from Greek medical literature of
apparent isolated plague outbreaks.
[45] Achtman et al., "*Yersinia pestis*, the Cause of Plague"; also Guiyoule et al., "Plague Pandemics Investigated"; cf. Lucier and Brubaker, "Determination of Genome Size," and
esp. Prentice et al., "*Yersinia pestis* pFra."

concentrated, and a fourth biovar has been proposed.[46] For historians, the geographic origins and spread of the Justinianic Pandemic are of great interest, for they tell us much about the communications networks and economic organization of the later Roman Empire and its neighbors.

Our main witnesses concur that the plague first reached the Roman Empire in Egypt. The well-connected contemporary, Procopius, states that it began in the Nile's eastern mouth, at Pelusium. From there it spread to Alexandria, the greatest shipping center of the empire, and hence around the Mediterranean, reaching Constantinople in the mid-spring of 542.[47] Now for the historian, this seems strange: Why should the infection have reached the Mediterranean at Egypt's second port, Pelusium, rather than at Alexandria, her greatest and most active sea city? This should be connected with communication patterns between the Egyptian delta and the source of the infection. One is tempted to think of some sort of link with the Red Sea, the royal road to the Roman Empire's well-documented trade with southeast Asia, as well as with eastern Africa. That route to the Orient will have been particularly favored when the overland caravan corridor via Mesopotamia became insecure. In fact, the Persians invaded Roman Syria in the spring of 540, and must have disrupted traffic across the Mesopotamian frontier precisely at the crucial moment.[48]

The implication may be a south Asian origin or transmission of the Justinianic contagion. If the ancient canal linking the Red Sea and the Nile were operational in late 541, ship-borne rats could have transported the pathogen directly. Otherwise, it would have come with an overland caravan. Infected fleas are surprisingly long-lived, even in bundles of textiles, and could well have created the fatal link.[49] Whichever way the pathogen traveled, in the preceding decades, Justin

---

[46] Radnedge et al., "Genome Plasticity"; Anisimov et al., "Intraspecific Diversity," summarize some key conclusions from the research done in the former Soviet Union, and make clear how complex the situation may be; cf. for a new biovar from Chinese data: D. Zhou, et al., "Genetics of Metabolic Variations."

[47] Procopius, *BP* 2.22,6, p. 250.13–18; John of Ephesus, *Historiae ecclesiasticae fragmenta*, fragmentum E-H, 227–38. For the chronology of the outbreak, Stein, *Histoire du Bas-Empire*, 2: 758–9 and 841; Conrad, "Plague in the Early Medieval Near East," 99–119; Kislinger and Stathakopoulos, "Pest und Perserkrieg bei Prokop."

[48] Procopius, *BP* 2.5,1, p. 167.1–7.

[49] The canal may also have been the route by which the black rat first reached the Mediterranean: McCormick, "Rats, Communications and Plague," 8–9; live fleas and dead rats were commonly found in sacks of grain and packets of textiles during the third pandemic: Audoin-Rouzeau, *Les chemins*, 223–27; cf. 51–52 for the longevity of fleas and the bacillus.

I and Justinian had been evangelizing and building political relations with eastern Africa and southern Arabia, the pivot for trade with India. Justin I even supplied ships to the ruler of Axum (Ethiopia) for his campaign to subjugate the Himyarites of the Arabian peninsula. When the plague appeared, this area (modern-day Yemen) was under the control of an ally of Justinian, Abraha (535–558), the Christian former slave of a Roman trader.[50] This political, religious – the Axumites were Monophysites, under the patriarchate of Alexandria – and commercial nexus supplies a context for another statement, from a fragment attributed to John of Ephesus, that the Justinianic infection started "first in the inland peoples of the regions southeast (!) of India, that is, of Kush, the Himyarites, and others." Kush designates the African territory beyond the boundaries of Egypt, presumably along the Sudanese Nile, and the Himyarites of course refer to Yemen.[51] If the *Antiqua* biovar has been correctly identified with the first plague pandemic, then the phylogenetic features of the *Y. pestis* of Kenya might argue in favor of African antiquity, and therefore the African origin of *Y. pestis* from *Y. pseudotuberculosis.*[52] On the other hand, the close contacts between Africa, Yemen, and the southeast Asian trade as well as mounting genomic research militate for an Asian origin.[53] In any case, if *Y. pestis* is indeed the pathogen, ancient biomolecules should one day confirm whether the *Antiqua* biovar was in fact the cause of the Justinianic Pandemic. Should this prove to be the case, we could look forward to conclusive determination of its geographic origin.[54] The historical implications for early Byzantine relations and communications systems with eastern and central Africa, compared to those with the Orient and East Africa, will become clearer from this microbiological research.

After evolutionary and geographic origin, the second question for our future data bank of aDNA of the Justinianic pathogen relates to its molecular identity and characteristics. The genomes of the *Medievalis* and the *Orientalis* biovars of *Y. pestis* have been fully sequenced, and

---

[50] See, in general, Munro-Hay, *Aksum,* and, for more recent finds and bibliography, Phillips, "Punt and Aksum," here 449–56; Jones et al., *Prosopography* 3: 4–5, "Abraha."

[51] *Chronique de Michel le Syrien* 9.28, 2:235–36; for Kush, Munro-Hay, *Aksum,* 16.

[52] Achtman et al., "*Yersinia pestis,* the Cause of Plague," fig. 2, and pp. 14047–48.

[53] See the wider assortment of strains (and geography) discussed by Radnedge et al., "Genome Plasticity," and Anisimov et al., "Intraspecific Diversity." For the importance of the antiqua biovar in China: D. Zhou et al., "DNA Microarray Analysis," and particularly Pourcel et al., "Tandem Repeats."

[54] See Achtman et al., "*Yersinia pestis,* the Cause of Plague."

studies of them are proceeding rapidly.[55] Some parts of the genome show a high mutation rate. This may have implications for changing virulence among and within varying strains.[56] One critical question is whether the devastating ancient and medieval infections were more potent than the already imposing *Orientalis* biovar with which physicians and public health officials have been dealing since 1894. So far, the evidence from aDNA is mixed. The segments of the aDNA from the sixteenth- and eighteenth-century phases of the medieval pandemic that the Marseilles researchers believe they have sequenced were identical to those of modern *Y. pestis*. But of course, they analyzed only two sequences of 133 and 300 bp out of what we now know is a genome comprising 4.65 m bp, as well as three plasmids of c. 100, 70 and 9.5 kilobases.[57] On the other hand, for the fourteenth-century adults and child, the picture seems more mixed. The 147 bp sequence of the characteristic and important segment (from the Pla gene) of the *Y. pestis* DNA that infected the child was 100% identical to the corresponding segment identified by the genome project. However, the 148 bp sequenced for the two adults uncovered a mutation. This could be significant if confirmed because this potential fourteenth-century mutation concerns a gene associated with the virulence factor.[58]

The high rate of mutation observed in other segments of the *Y. pestis* genome *might* hold particular promise for a phylogenetic approach. Because mutations accumulate and are transmitted to each succeeding generation of the bacteria as, over time, the DNA works its way through a population, the accumulating mutations constitute a kind of trail; by examining those mutations, one can reconstruct the genealogy of an individual strain of infection, using the biostatistical techniques that make up phylogenetic analysis. Precisely such a phylogenetic analysis led to the molecular classification of forty-nine strains of the family tree into the three biovars of *Y. pestis*.[59] Certainly genetic analysis of the DNA of *Y. pestis* in associated victims of a recent outbreak seems to show high but not perfect genetic identity, even as it throws light on the roles of subpopulations of rodent vectors. In this case, only a small subset of the infected

---

[55] Deng et al., "Genome Sequence of *Yersinia pestis* KIM"; Parkhill et al., "Genome Sequence of *Yersinia pestis*."

[56] Perry and Fetherston, "*Yersinia pestis*," here 37.

[57] Parkhill et al., "Genome Sequence of *Yersinia pestis*," 523.

[58] Raoult et al., "Molecular Identification," 12801–2.

[59] Achtman et al., "*Yersinia pestis*, the Cause of Plague" fig. 2. See also note 46.

rodents actually transmitted the pathogen to humans.[60] One wonders
whether the recently observed phylogenetic power of a sequence phenomenon known as VNTRs (variable number tandem repeats) in the *Y.
pestis* genome might extend to aDNA?[61] Although the task would be complex and difficult, given the denatured character of the aDNA and the
fairly short segments that result, it is theoretically possible that a phylogenetic analysis could be applied to the aDNA of *Y. pestis* recovered from
individual victims of the Justinianic infection.

   Y. pestis DNA mutates easily and often. The perspective opened by a
phylogenetic approach that capitalizes on this fact is as dizzying as it is
arduous. If the data proved rich enough, it would not be surprising to
discover that the DNA of *differing waves* of the pandemic displays *differing
constellations of mutations*. Recent data on the *Orientalis* biovar is encouraging on this score because it has now been shown that even within the
last 100 years, significant changes have occurred in the genome.[62] In
other words, the *Y. pestis* DNA of an individual victim might, in and of
itself, assign that victim, and others in the same grave, to a particular
wave of the pandemic. The data from the particular strain of DNA could
be compared to the independent chronological evidence of stratigraphy,
burial goods, and Carbon-14.[63] It thus may prove possible to improve
the resolution of our aDNA map of the plague between 541 and the
eighth century, and to map with precision individual waves of the pandemic. It is conceivable that, pursued on a large scale, such phylogenetic
analyses could produce still more insight. If we can get enough samples of sufficient quality, they might show, for instance, that the DNA of
Y. pestis of a particular set of victims in Carthage displays not only the
mutations identified for the third wave of infection at Alexandria, but
additional mutations that are known only for the third wave of infection
at Constantinople. Such a pattern would imply that the pathogen of that
wave reached Carthage from Alexandria only through the intermediary
of Constantinople. Behind such a pattern, we could sense the ghostly

[60] Shivaji et al., "Identification of *Yersinia pestis.*"
[61] Adair et al., "Diversity in a Variable-Number Tandem Repeat." Analysis of VNTRs has in
   fact allowed a detailed reconstruction of the spread of plague among Arizona prairie
   dog colonies in 2000–1: Girard et al., "Differential Plague-Transmission"; cf. also Pourcel
   et al., "Tandem Repeats."
[62] Radnedge et al., "Genome Plasticity," 1697.
[63] For our period, AMS 14C dating should give a ± 35–40-year date from a single bone
   sample; the situation implicit in a mass plague grave should create ideal circumstances
   for refining that date from a statistical analysis of multiple samples of identical date of
   death: see e.g., Evin et al., eds., *Les méthodes*, here 112 and 115.

shapes of ships that once sailed from Egypt to the imperial capital, and of other ships sailing from the capital to the African metropolis, as the death-dealing rodents scurried in their holds. It is just imaginable that beyond the broad routes and patterns of long-distance transmission of the plague pathogen, we might be able to discern the changing constellations of long-distance ship movements in the late Roman and early Islamic empires with a precision and detail that would render obsolete my own recent efforts to do so from the written and archeological sources.[64]

These observations and questions barely scratch the surface of the rapidly accumulating knowledge that illuminates the biology and history of *Y. pestis*, as of so many other infectious diseases. There is much more that calls out for deeper discussion at the frontiers of biology and history. For instance, recent work reinforces the trend to downgrade the demographic impact of the pneumonic expression of infection with *Y. pestis*.[65] We are learning more about the hosts and vectors that foster the pathogen, and every advance opens new questions. The ancient history of the black rat is crucial to any study of plague in antiquity. After all, *Y. pestis* is at base a rodent disease that affects humans only coincidentally, hence the significance of research into the routes, extent, and means of the black rat's colonization of the Roman world. How exactly, and how far did they penetrate inland, where boats could not take them, and how does that story relate to the competition between Roman carts and medieval pack animals, that is, the debate about the camel versus the wheel? Here too, molecular techniques have their part to play in clarifying the history of the rat.[66] The changing built environment, ecology, and waste management affected late Roman rat demography and predators, and therefore shaped the preconditions for an explosion of *Y. pestis.*

---

[64] McCormick, *Origins of the European Economy.*

[65] The champion of the demographically devastating impact of the pneumonic plague is Le Roy Ladurie, "Un concept," but see also the Scandinavian historians criticized by Benedictow, *Plague in the Late Medieval Nordic Countries*, 214–27. Although its 100% mortality is indeed terrifying, clinical data for the modern strains of *Y. pestis* that confirm the high contagiousness and lethality of the primary pneumonic form of the disease qualify the impression of it as a uniquely devastating epidemic form of the disease. This is essentially because it does not spread as easily as has been imagined. Benedictow, *Plague in the Late Medieval Nordic Countries*, 25–37, with citations of earlier scientific literature; Dennis et al., *Plague Manual*, 45–46 or http://www.who.int/emc-documents/plague/whocdscsredc992c.html, with further references. A new outbreak in 1997 confirms this view: Ratsitorahina et al., "Epidemiological and Diagnostic Aspects," which estimates the infection rate in the contact population at 8.4%.

[66] McCormick, "Rats, Communications and Plague," 9, and in general, Audoin-Rouzeau and Vigne, "La colonisation de l'Europe par le rat noir."

Earlier Roman cityscapes were far from trash-free. But the accumulation
of trash in urban sites may have accelerated in the declining cities of
Late Antiquity. Thus around 450, some rooms of a large, early-imperial
apartment block (*insula*), as well as the contiguous segment of the city
street, began to serve as a garbage dump in downtown Naples. Black rats
appear in the next stratigraphical sequence, c. 500.[67] Wars and earthquakes are known to expand rat populations, and need another look
from this angle.[68] The newly demonstrated epidemiological link between
abnormally wet weather and bubonic plague turns our attention to climate history.[69] Periods of above-normal precipitation produce increases
in plague outbreaks; conversely, periods of exceptional dryness have the
opposite effect. That link operates by means of a trophic cascade – a surge
in sustenance all along the plant, insect, and rodent food chain.

Blood-sucking insects are the other, crucial part of the host-vector
equation. The early results of archaeoentomology invite specialists to
address this essential aspect of ancient health conditions and epidemics.
Biologists dismiss any possible role on the northern rim of the Mediterranean of the historians' favorite plague vector between rodent and
man, the oriental rat flea, *Xenopsylla cheopis*, despite its prominence in
the third pandemic.[70] The archaeological evidence for other potential
arthropod vectors is beginning to emerge in northwestern Europe. Thus,

[67] P. Arthur, in Arthur, ed., *Il complesso archeologico*, 73. Absence of waste removal was incrim-
inated as an important factor in the rise of plague in Vietnam in the 1960s and 1970s:
Butler, *Plague and other Yersinia Infections*, 37–38. See, in addition to McCormick, "Rats,
Communications and Plague," Thüry, *Müll und Marmorsäulen*.

[68] Warfare: Becker, *"Rattus rattus,"* here 388. The earthquake that hit a region in India
in 1993, thanks largely to "unlimited energy inputs," i.e., food, allowed a gradual but
steady growth in rodent populations over the next eight to ten months, implying a
rupture of equilibrium among the various populations, and explaining an outbreak of
plague there the following year: Saxena and Verghese, "Ecology of Flea-Transmitted
Zoonotic Infection," (cited from the abstract in *Biosis*); see also Shivaji et al., "Identification of *Yersinia pestis*," for definitive confirmation of the *Y. pestis* diagnosis from
rDNA.

[69] A major study from the American southwest has conclusively proven the link at multiple highly local levels (the regional level analysis also yielded positive correlations, but
they fell below the statistical threshold of significance): Parmenter et al., "Incidence of
Plague."

[70] E.g., Beaucournu, "Diversité des puces vectrices," here 420, dismisses for ecological
reasons the possibility that *X. cheopis* factored in the second pandemic in France. Today
this flea is distributed, approximately, between 35° N. and 35° S.: Gordh and Headrick,
Dictionary of Entomology, 646. Cf. the distribution implied by the collection data in Hopkins
and Rothschild, *Illustrated Catalogue*, 1:238–61. It is a pleasure to thank my colleague
Naomi E. Pierce for her generous advice on fleas.

human fleas (*Pulex irritans*), once a leading suspect, have now been definitively established to have reached France by the fourth millennium BC.
Another sort of rat flea, a *Nosopsyllus* (probably but not certainly identified as *fasciatus*), *P. irritans*, and the dog flea are looking increasingly well
documented in Roman and medieval (ninth-century and later) sites in
England and France, as well as in the Viking world, even as the archaeological absence of *Xenopsylla cheopis* grows more glaring.[71]

The interaction between historical and medical research offers a sobering example of how the imperfect knowledge both of the Justinianic
Pandemic and of the older scientific literature combined to sidetrack
modern medical understanding on an unprofitable byway. One could
scarcely wish for a better example of the relevance of historical investigation to the modern life sciences. Empirical and experimental evidence
had already shown in the early twentieth century that *Nosopsyllus fasciatus*,
the type of rat flea common in Europe, was an efficient vector of *Y. pestis*.
Even so, the erroneous belief that there were no Roman rats converged
with the conviction that the Justinianic Plague was indeed bubonic to stimulate French researchers to seek another arthropod vector. The result was
a theory championing the role of human-to-human infection transmitted
by the human flea (*P. irritans*), based initially on research in North Africa
in the 1940s. The empirical and experimental basis for that theory has
now been definitively ruined. In its place stands the recognition that *N.
fasciatus* could well have played the key role in transmitting *Y. pestis* from
infected rodents in Europe.[72] But even allowing for the part played by *N.
fasciatus*, careful attention will have to be paid to the delicate interactions
of climate and ecology that are indispensable to understanding insect
vectors.[73]

---

[71] Archaeoentomology: e.g., Panagiotakopulu, *Archaeology and Entomology*, 111, for uniden-
tified Siphonaptera (fleas) from the Roman site of Mons Claudianus in Egypt. For the
splendid work on Roman and medieval York, see e.g., Hall and Kenward, *Environmental
Evidence*, which documents the human, dog, and rat flea. For the history of *P. irritans*, see
Buckland and Sadler, "A Biogeography of the Human Flea," as updated by Yvinec et al.,
"Premiers apports," who also emphasize the absence of archaeological evidence for *X.
cheopis* in northwestern Europe, and argue for the role of *P. irritans* in transmitting ancient
and medieval plague. Opinions continue to divide about *P. irritans*. Although some clas-
sify it as a "possible or probable" vector (Gratz, "Rodent Reservoirs," here 66–67), others
reckon it to have only "very poor" capacity to transmit the pathogen to humans: Perry
and Fetherston, "*Yersinia pestis*," 53, and still others champion it: Beaucournu, "Diversité
des puces vectrices." The debate nevertheless appears to be over: see next note.

[72] Audoin-Rouzeau, *Les chemins*; cf. the experimental data of Burroughs, "Sylvatic Plague."

[73] For a helpful summary of the ecological aspects of insect vectors, see Cavanaugh and
Williams, "Plague: Some Ecological Interrelationships," esp. 247–50.

Rats and fleas lead, sooner or later, to the last big question. Where did the Justinianic Plague go? Do archaeology, changing ecological conditions, and molecular biology point to local or broader extinctions of rat populations? Some have thought that rat colonies disappeared. After Late Antiquity, securely dated archaeological evidence for rats in Europe emerges, so far, only in the ninth century.[74] Whether such a hypothetical extinction would have been due to the plague itself or occurred in concert with other factors, it could explain the disappearance of the contagion in the second half of the eighth century.[75] There has also been some indication that rats develop immunity to *Y. pestis*; if that occurred on a scale sufficient to foster herd immunity in the affected regions, it might explain why the pathogen ceased attacking the human populations of the Mediterranean.[76]

We need also to think about the possibility that plague may have helped drive into the countryside the human survivors of Late Antiquity's dwindling cities, just as similar epidemic experiences emptied ancient Iroquois towns in seventeenth-century North America.[77] Paul the Deacon describes how the inhabitants at least temporarily abandoned Pavia during a seventh-century attack of plague.[78] Rural flight would have deprived rodent colonies of the human mass the rodents need to thrive in the large numbers that foster plague reservoirs. The evidence for *de facto* or real quarantines and isolation policies around the early medieval Mediterranean would benefit from renewed scrutiny, because some specialists of the second pandemic ascribe to such policies a major role in ending the medieval and early modern plagues.[79] Contemporaries were aware of

---

[74] McCormick, "Rats, Communications and Plague," 23, note 36.

[75] Armitage, "Unwelcome Companions," here 233–34; Audoin-Rouzeau and Vigne, "La colonisation de l'Europe par le rat noir," 139.

[76] See e.g., Audoin-Rouzeau, *Les chemins*, 164, and 220, note 51.

[77] See A. Taylor, *William Cooper's Town*, 34–35. From AD 1000 to 1500, Iroquois Indians constructed "extensive fortified villages scattered on hilltops." "They abandoned the fortified villages during the seventeenth century, when they proved to be deathtraps; their inhabitants were vulnerable to attacking Europeans and, especially, to disease pathogens that afflicted crowded populations. As their number shrank from war and disease, the survivors moved into smaller, more decentralized villages strung along the riverbanks. The new villages were easier to flee from when danger approached or epidemics spread. Assuming the Iroquois had always lived in small, dispersed, riverside villages, Americans were mystified by the abandoned earthworks."

[78] *Historia Longobardorum* 6.5, p. 166, 25–77.

[79] For quarantines and the end of the second pandemic, Slack, "Disappearance of Plague," and Eckert, "Retreat of Plague."

the connection between arriving ships, moving merchandise, and the outbreak of plague. The Gazans' belief that magic ships spread the infection on the beaches implies such a link, and Gregory of Tours' description of the arrival of the plague with a merchant ship from Spain makes it explicit.[80] The establishment of a quarantine on Gaul's roads leading to the sea is directly attested by a letter alerting the bishop of Cahors to an outbreak of plague at Marseilles, c. 640, and urging him to block travel, especially of merchants.[81] If the slack administrative structures of Merovingian Gaul deployed a cordon sanitaire against plague, the more bureaucratized Byzantine and Arab empires could well have done likewise.

Two further factors may have contributed to – or possibly even decided – the end of the Justinianic Pandemic. Both have been raised before as hypotheses, but molecular biology today offers the first real prospect of resolution. Now that the genome of *Y. pestis* has been identified and published, should not the modern DNA make increasingly clear where we should look in the aDNA to address this question? Microbiologists have cited the three plasmids as apparent factors in the virulence of modern *Y. pestis*.[82] And a proposed new biovar is reported to be avirulent in humans.[83] If those findings hold, it would be worthwhile to direct particular archaeobiological attention to the segments of early medieval aDNA that code for the virulence factor. Raoult and his colleagues may have identified one medieval mutation in the Pla gene, a probable virulence factor. If such mutations are confirmed and examples multiply, it would be possible to verify experimentally whether the mutations affect the virulence of *Y. pestis* in laboratory animals.

The question of diminished virulence shades into another possible contributor to the end of the Justinianic Pandemic. *Y. pestis* seems to be a fairly recent evolution from *Y. pseudotuberculosis*, and is a little more distantly related to *Y. enterocolitica*. *Y. pseudotuberculosis* and *Y. enterocolitica*

---

[80] John of Ephesus, *Historiae ecclesiasticae fragmenta*, fragmentum E, 229; Gregory of Tours, *Historia Francorum* 9.21–22, pp. 379–80. Procopius' description of the plague's penetration from the sea inland implies a similar understanding: *BP* 2.22.9, p. 251, 7–9.

[81] Desiderius of Cahors, *Epistolae* 2.20, pp. 74–75, dated c. 631–655 on the assumption that the "*Gallus peccator*" who wrote the letter was the bishop of Clermont of that name. If that assumption is correct, then the most likely known outbreak would be the one reported to have ravaged the Caliphate in 638–640; cf. Conrad, "Plague in the Early Medieval Near East," 167–246.

[82] Parkhill et al., "Genome Sequence of *Yersinia pestis*."

[83] Zhou et al., "Genetics of Metabolic Variations."

are also enzootic diseases that typically enter humans through the food chain and provoke gastrointestinal disorders from which healthy people usually recover. Belgian and French researchers' suspicion that the *Yersinia* ancestors do provide immunity to *Y. pestis* appears to find confirmation in recently published and preliminary epidemiological evidence. Chinese regions whose rodent and pig populations display the other *Yersinia* diseases are markedly resistant to *Y. pestis*; conversely, regions in which rodents show little sign of *Y. enterocolitica* or *Y. pseudotuberculosis* seem susceptible to plague.[84] If this medical research pans out, the question for historians of the ancient plague becomes obvious: Do ancient biomolecules attest the presence of these ancestral forms of non-deadly *Yersinia* infections in the regions from which the plague disappeared in the eighth century? If so, the molecular archaeology of such remains could perhaps finally unlock this great mystery, and shift the historical spotlight back to the enzootic, animal focuses of the plague.

Even so, it seems unlikely that any phenomenon as broad, deep, and complex as the Justinianic Pandemic will have ended for one sole cause. And this brings us back to our starting point, the great complexity of the phenomenon before us, and of the historical, archaeological, ecological, and molecular approaches needed to analyze, understand, and explain this most daunting historical question. Inventory of graves, data base of aDNA, phylogenetic characteristics of the putative pathogen that potentially illuminate dates and geographies of origin and contagion, the archaeology of rats and fleas: so many new approaches and techniques promise in coming years to produce new insights into the nature, course, and end of the Justinianic Pandemic. When we have them, it seems to me that the problem before us will take us closer than ever to answering the ancient question of the economic "fall" of the Roman Empire and the origins of the Middle Ages.

---

[84] Devignat, *La peste antique*, 33–34, hypothesized that *Y. pseudotuberculosis* (then believed to descend from *Y. pestis*, rather than vice versa), produced immunity to *Y. pestis* in Europe. Devignat; Audoin-Rouzeau, *Les chemins*, 279–83; Fukushima et al., "*Yersinia enterocolitica* O9;" cf. e.g., Alonso, "Interactions écologiques."

Bibliography

Abbreviations

AASS	*Acta sanctorum.* 3rd ed. Paris, Rome, Brussels, 1863–.
Bede, *EH*	*Bede's Ecclesiastical History of the English People.* Ed. B. Colgrave and R. A. B. Mynors. Oxford, 1969.
CCL	*Corpus christianorum, series latina.* Turnhout, 1953–.
CCCM	*Corpus christianorum, continuatio mediaevalis.* Turnhout, 1971–.
CFHB	*Corpus fontium historiae byzantinae.* Vienna, Washington, 1967–.
CIC	*Corpus Iuris Civilis.* Ed. P. Kreuger, T. Mommsen, R. Schoell, and G. Kroll. 3 vols. Berlin, 1880.
CMG	*Corpus medicorum Graecorum.* Berlin, Leipzig, 1908–.
CSCO	*Corpus scriptorum christianorum orientalium.* Ed. J.-B. Chabot et al. Paris, Louvain, 1903–.
CZ	*The Chronicle of Zūqnīn, Parts III and IV, A.D. 488–775.* Trans. A. Harrak. Medieval Sources in Translation 36. Toronto, 1999.
MGH	*Monumenta Germaniae Historica.* Hannover, Berlin, 1826–.
AA	*Auctores Antiquissimi*
Ep	*Epistolae*
LL	*Leges*
SRG	*Scriptores rerum Germanicarum*
SRL	*Scriptores rerum Langobardicarum*
SRM	*Scriptores rerum Merovingicarum*
SS	*Scriptores*
ODB	*Oxford Dictionary of Byzantium.* Ed. A. P. Kazhdan and A. M. Talbot. Oxford, 1991.
PG	*Patrologia cursus completus . . . series graeca.* Ed. J.-P. Migne. Paris, 1857–86.
PL	*Patrologia cursus completus . . . series latina.* Ed. J.-P. Migne. Paris, 1844–64.
PNAS	*Proceedings of the National Academy of Sciences*
PO	*Patrologia Orientalis*

Procopius Procopius of Caesaria
  BP   *De bello persico. Opera Omnia.* Ed. J. Haury, rev. G. Wirth, 4 vols.
          Leipzig, (1961–64), vol. 1.
  HA   *Historia arcana.* Ibid., vol. 3.
  PW   *The Persian War. Procopius, with an English Translation.* Ed. and trans.
          H. B. Dewing. The Loeb Classical Library. 7 vols. New York,
          1914–40. vol. 1.
  SH   *The Anecdota or Secret History.* Ibid., vol. 6.

Primary Sources

Abbon. *Libri duo bellorum Parisiacae urbis – Le Siège de Paris par les Normands.* Ed. and trans. H. Waquet. Les Classiques de l'histoire de France au Moyen Age 20. Paris, 1942.

Acta S. Sebastiani Martyris. PL 17:1113–50.

Adomnán. *Adomnán's Life of Columba.* Ed. and trans. A. O. and M. O. Anderson. Oxford, 1991.

Adomnán. *Life of St. Columba.* Trans. R. Sharpe. Harmondsworth, UK, 1995.

Æthelwulf. *De Abbatibus.* Ed. A. Campbell. Oxford, 1967.

Aetius of Amida. *Libri Medicinales V–VIII.* Ed. A. Olivieri. *CMG* VIII 2. Berlin, 1950.

Agapius. *Kitab al-Unvan.* Ed. A. Vasiliev. *PO* 8.

Agathias. *Agathiae Myrinei Historiarum Libri Quinque.* Ed. R. Keydell. *CFHB* 2. Berlin, 1967.

Agathias. *The Histories.* Trans. J. P. Frendo. Corpus Fontium Historiae Byzantinae II A. New York, 1975.

Agnellus. *Liber pontificalis ecclesiae Ravennatis. MGH, SRL.*

Ajbar Machmuâ, cronica anonima del siglo XI. Ed. and trans. E. Lafuente y Alcantara. 2 vols. Madrid, 1867.

Aldhelm: The Prose Works. Ed. M. Lapidge and M. Herren. Cambridge, 1979.

al-Masʿūdī. *Kitāb murūj al-dhahab.* Ed. Y. Daghir. Beirut, 1956.

al-Ṭabarī, 'A. *Ta'rīkh al-rusul wa 'l-mulūk.* Ed. M. J. de Goeje. 15 vols. Leiden, 1879.

Anastasius of Sinai. *Quaestiones. PG* 89:311–24.

Anecdota Syriaca. Ed. J. P. N. Land. 4 vols. Leiden, 1862–75.

The Annals of Clonmacnoise. Ed. D. Murphy. Dublin, 1896.

The Annals of Tigernach. Ed. W. Stokes. *Revue Celtique* 16–17 (1895–96). Reprint, 2 vols. Dyfed, 1993.

The Annals of Ulster (to A. D. 1131). Ed. S. MacAirt and G. MacNiocaill. 1. Dublin, 1983.

Anonymi auctoris Chronicon ad annum Christi 1234 pertinens, 1. *CSCO* 109/Syri 56.

Aretaeus. *The Extant Works of Aretaeus, the Cappodocian.* Ed. and trans. F. Adams. London, 1856.

Aretaeus. *Opera.* Ed. K. Hude. 2nd ed. *CMG* 2. Berlin, 1958.

Auctarium Marcellini in *MGH, AA* 11.

Audacht Morainn. Ed. F. Kelly. Dublin, 1976.

Basil of Caesaria. *Quod Deus non est auctor malorum. PG* 31:329–54.

Bede. *Bedae Venerabilis Opera,* pt1/1: *Opera Didascalia.* Ed. C. W. Jones. Corpus Christianorum. Turnhout, 1975.

Bede. *Opera historica.* Ed. C. Plummer. 2 vols. Oxford, 1896.

Beowulf. Ed. and trans. M. Swanton. Rev. ed. New York, 1997.

Beowulf: A New Verse Translation. Trans. R. M. Liuzza. Peterborough, Ont., 2000.

Boniface. *The Letters of Saint Boniface.* Trans. E. Emerton. New York, 1976.

Boniface. *S. Bonifatii et Lulli epistolae.* Ed. M. Tangl. *MGH, Epistolae selectae in usum scholarum.* Berlin, 1916. Reprint, 1989.

Cartularium Saxonicum. Ed. W. de Gray Birch. 3 vols. London, 1885–93.

Cassiodorus. *Variae.* Ed. T. Mommsen. *MGH, AA* 12.

The Chronicle of John Malalas. Trans. E. Jeffreys, M. Jeffreys, R. Scott. Melbourne, 1986.

Chronicon ad a. 846 in *CSCO* 4/Syri 4.

Chronicon ad annum Christi 1234 pertinens, 1. *CSCO* 81/Syri 36.

Chronicon ad a. 1234, 1. *CSCO*/Syri 14.

Chronicon anonymum ad A.D. 819 pertinens in *CSCO* 81/Syri 36.

Chronicon anonymum ad A.D. 819 pertinens in *CSCO* 109/Syri 56.

Chronicon anonymum ad annum 846, in *Chronica Minora. CSCO* 3/*CSCO* 4.

Chronicon Jacobi Edesseni, in *Chronica Minora,* 3. *CSCO* 5/Syri 5.

Chronicon miscellaneum ad annum p. Chr. 724 pertinens, in *Chronica Minora,* 2. *CSCO* 4/Syri 4.

Chronicon miscellaneum ad annum p. Chr. 724 pertinens, in *Chronica Minora,* 3. *CSCO* 3/Syri 3.

Chronicon Paschale. Trans. M. and M. Whitby. Liverpool, 1989.

Chronique de Michel le Syrien. Ed. J. B. Chabot. 4 vols. Paris, 1901. Repr. Bruxelles, 1963.

Claudii Galeni opera omnia. Ed. C. G. Kühn. 20 vols. Leipzig, 1821–33. Repr., Hildesheim, 1964–65.

Codex Justinianus, Novellae. Ed. R. Schöll and G. Kroll. 7th ed. Berlin, 1959.

Concilios visigóticos y hispano-romanos. Ed. J. Vives. Madrid, 1962.

Constantine VII Porphyrogenitus. *De thematibus.* Ed. Pertusi. Studi e testi 160. Vatican City, 1952.

Corippus. *Iohannidos seu de bellis libycis libri VIII.* Ed. J. Diggle and F. R. D. Goodyear. Cambridge, 1970.

Corpus Genealogiarum Sanctorum Hiberniae. Ed. P. Ó Riain. Dublin, 1985.

Corpus Inscriptionum Latinarum. New ed. Vol. 2, part 7. Berlin, 1995.

Crith Gablach. Ed. D. Binchy. Dublin, 1979.

Cronica Mozarabe de 754: Edicion critica y traduccion. Ed. and trans. J. E. Lopez Pereira. Zaragoza, 1989.

Cyprian of Carthage. *De mortalitate.* Ed. M. L. Hannan. The Catholic University of America. Patristic Series 36. Washington, 1933.

Delehaye, H. "Une vie inédite de Saint Jean l'Aumonier." *Analecta Bollandiana* 45(1927): 5–74.

Desiderius of Cahors. *Epistolae S. Desiderii Cadurcensis.* Ed. D. Norberg. Acta Universitatis Stockholmiensis, Studia latina Stockholmiensia 6. Stockholm, 1961.

Eddius Stephanus. *The Life of Bishop Wilfrid by Eddius Stephanus.* Ed. B. Colgrave. Cambridge, 1927.

Elias of Nisibis. *Opus Chronologicum* in *CSCO* 62/Syri 21.

English Historical Documents. Ed. D. C. Douglas. 12 vols. London, 1953–77.

Eulogium historiarum sive temporis: chronicon ab orbe condito usque ad annum domini M.CCC. LXVI. Ed. F. S. Haydon. 3 vols. Rolls Series 9. London, 1863.

Evagrius. *The Ecclesiastical History of Evagrius Scholasticus.* Trans. M. Whitby. Liverpool, 2000.

Evagrius. *The Ecclesiastical History of Evagrius, with the Scholia.* Ed. J. Bidez and L. Parmentier. London, 1898. Reprint New York, 1979.

Evagrius. "Evagre, *Histoire ecclésiastique.*" Trans. A. J. Festugière. *Byzantion* 45 (1975): 187–488.

Félire Óengusso Céli Dé: The Martyrology of Oengus the Culdee. Ed. W. Stokes. London, 1905.

Flodoard. *Annales.* Ed. P. Lauer. Collection de textes pour servir à l'étude et à l'énseignement de l'histoire 39. Paris, 1905.

Fredegar. *The Fourth Book of the Chronicle of Fredegar.* Ed. J. M. Wallace-Hadrill. London, 1960.

Gabriele de' Mussis. "Ystoria de morbo seu mortalitate qui fuit a 1348." Ed. H. Haeser. *Archive für die gesamte Medizin* 2 (1841): 26–59.

Gennadios Scholarios, *Oeuvres complètes.* Ed. L. Petit, X. A. Sidéridès, M. Jugie. 8 vols. Paris, 1928–36.

George Monachos. *Chronicon.* Ed. C. de Boor and P. Wirth. Vol 2. Stuttgart, 1978.

Gildas: the Ruin of Scotland and the Works. Ed. and trans. M. Winterbottom. Chicester, 1978.

Gregory of Tours. *Glory of the Confessors.* Trans. R. Van Dam. Liverpool, 1988.

Gregory of Tours. *Glory of the Martyrs.* Trans. R. Van Dam. Liverpool, 1988.

Gregory of Tours. *Historia Francorum.* Ed. B. Krusch and W. Arndt *MGH, SRM,* 1.

Gregory of Tours. *History of the Franks.* Trans. L. Thorpe. Harmondsworth, UK, 1974.

Gregory of Tours. *The History of the Franks.* Trans. O. M. Dalton. 2 vols. Oxford, 1927.

Gregory of Tours. *Liber de passionibus et virtutibis s. Iuliani. MGH, SRM,* 1.

Gregory of Tours. *Liber in gloria confessorum. MGH, SRM,* 1.

Gregory of Tours. *Liber in gloria martyrum. MGH, SRM,* 1.

Gregory of Tours. *Liber vitae patrum. MGH, SRM,* 1.

Gregory of Tours. *Life of the Fathers.* Trans. E. James. Liverpool, 1985.

Gregory the Great. *Dialogues.* Ed. A. de Vogüé. 3 vols. Sources chrétiennes 251, 260, 265. Paris, 1978–80.

Gregory the Great. *The Letters of Gregory the Great.* Trans. J. Martyn. Medieval Sources in Translation, 40. 3 vols. Toronto, 2004.

Gregory the Great. *S. Gregorii Magni Register epistularum.* Ed. D. Norberg. 2 vols. *CCL* 140–140A. Turnhout, 1982.

Guibert de Nogent. *De sanctis et eorum pigneribus.* Ed. R. B. C. Huygens. *CCCM* 127. Turnhout, 1993.

Guy de Chauliac. *Inventarium sive Chirurgia Magna.* Ed. M. R. McVaugh. *Guigonis de Caulhiaco (Guy de Chauliac) Inventarium sive Chirurgia Magna.* 2 vols. Leiden, 1997.

Hagios Nikolaos. Der heilige Nikolaos in der griechischen Kirche. Ed. G. Anrich. Berlin, 1913.

Helgaud de Fleury. *Epitoma Vitae regis Rotberti Pii – Vie de Robert le Pieux*. Ed. and trans. R.-H. Bautier and G. Labory. Sources d'histoire médiévale 1. Paris, 1965.

Hesychius Alexandrinus. *Lexicon*. Ed. K. Latte. 2 vols. Copenhagen, 1953, 1966.

Hippocrates. *De flatibus*. Ed. J. Jouanna. *Hippocrate*, V. 1. Paris, 1988.

Hippocrates. *Hippocratic Writings*. Trans. J. Chadwick and W. N. Mann. Harmondsworth, 1978.

Hippocrates. *De morbo sacro*. In *Hippocrates, with an English Translation*. Ed. and trans. W. H. S. Jones. 8 vols. Loeb Classical Library. Cambridge, Mass., 1984–95. Vol. 2:138–83.

Hippocrates. *De natura hominis*. Ed. J. Jouanna. *CMG*, I. 1.3. Berlin, 1975.

Hippocrates. *Oeuvres complètes d'Ippocrate*. Ed. E. Littré. 10 vols. Paris, 1839–61.

Histoire nestorienne inédite: (Chronique de Séert). Ed. and trans. A. Scher. 4 vols. *PO* 4,3; 5,2; 7,2; 13,4. Paris, 1908–50.

The History of Theophylact Simocatta. Ed. and trans. M. and M. Whitby. Oxford, 1986.

Homer. *The Iliad*. Trans. R. Fagles. Harmondsworth, UK, 1998.

Incerti auctoris chronicon pseudo-Dionysianum vulgo dictum, 2. *CSCO*, 104/Syri 53.

Inscriptiones Christianae Urbis Romae. Ed. G. B. De Rossi et al. Rome. 1922–.

Die irische Kanonensammlung. Ed. H. Wasserschleben. 2nd ed. Leipzig, 1885.

The Irish Liber Hymnorum. Henry Bradshaw Society 13. Ed. J. H. Bernard and R. Atkinson. London, 1898.

Irish Litanies. Ed. C. Plummer. London, 1925.

Itinerarium Antonini Placentini – un viaggio in terra Santa del 560–570 d.C. Ed. and trans. C. Milani. Rome, 1977.

Jahangir. *The Tūzūk-I-Jahāngīrī or Memoirs of Jahāngīr from the Thirteenth to the Beginning of the Nineteenth Year of his Reign*. Ed. A. Rogers and H. Beveridge. 2nd ed. 2 vols. London, 1914.

James of Voragine. *The Golden Legend*. Trans. W. G. Ryan. 2 vols. Princeton, 1993.

John Cantacuzenus. *Historiae. PG* 154.

John Malalas. *Chronographia*. Ed. I. Thurn. Berlin and New York, 2000.

John of Biclaro, *Chronica. MGH, AA* 9, 2.

John of Ephesus. *Lives of the Eastern Saints*. Ed. and trans. E. W. Brooks. *PO* 17.1, 18.4, 19.2. Paris, 1923–25.

John of Ephesus. *Historiae ecclesiasticae fragmenta*. Trans. W. J. Van Douwen and J. P. N. Land, "Joannis episcopi Ephesi Syri monophysitae . . . fragmenta," *Verhandelingen der koninklijke Akademie der wetenschappen, Afdeeling Letterkunde*, 18.2 (1889).

John of Naples. *Gesta episcoporum neapolitanorum. MGH, SRL*.

John of Worcester. *The Chronicle of John of Worcester*. Ed. R. R. Darlington and P. McGurk; trans. J. Bray and P. McGurk. 3 vols. Oxford, 1995.

John the Deacon. *Vita sancti Gregorii Magni. PL* 75:77–81.

Juan de Biclaro obispo de Gerona. Su vida y su obra. Ed. J. Campos. Madrid, 1960.

Kyrillos von Skythopolis. Ed. E. Schwartz. Leipzig, 1939.

Das Leben des heiligen Narren Symeon. Ed. L. Rydén. Acta Universitatis Upsaliensis. Studia Graeca Upsaliensia 4. Stockholm, Gothenburg, Uppsala, 1963.

Leges visigotorum. Ed. K. Zeumer. *MGH, LL* 1, sect. 1.

Lemerle, P. *Les plus anciens recueils des miracles de Saint Démétrius et la pénétration des Slavs dans les Balkans.* 2 vols. Paris, 1978–81.

Leontios. *Vie de Jean de Chypre.* Ed. A.-J. Festugière. Bibliothèque archéologique et historique 95. Paris, 1974.

Liber Historiae Francorum. MGH, SRM 2:215–328.

Liber pontificalis. Ed. T. Mommsen. *MGH, Gesta Pontificum Romanorum,* 1. Berlin, 1898.

Livy. *Ab urbe condita.* Trans. B. O. Foster. Loeb Classical Library. Rev. ed. 14 vols. Cambridge, Mass., 1988.

Marcellinus Comes. *Chronicon. MGH, AA* 9, 2.

Marius of Avenches, *Chronica. MGH, AA* 9, 2.

Mathias von Neuenburg. *Chronica. MGH, SRG,* new ser. 4.

Medieval Handbooks of Penance. Trans. J. T. McNeill and H. M. Gamer. New York, 1938.

Megas chronographos. Ed. P. Schreiner. *Die Byzantinischen Kleinchroniken,* 1. CFHB 12. Vienna, 1975.

Miracula sancti Artemii. Ed. A. Papadopoulos-Kerameus. Saint Petersburg, 1909.

Nicephorus. *Antirrhetikos III. PG* 100:205–850.

Nicephorus. *Breviarium.* Ed. C. Mango. CFHB 13. Washington, 1990.

Nicephorus Gregoras. *Historiae Byzantinae. PG* 74:61-962.

Opus chronologicum, 1. *CSCO* 62/Syri 21.

Oribasius. *Oribasii Collectionum Medicarum Reliquiae.* Ed. J. Raeder. Leipzig and Berlin, 1926; reprint *CMG* VI, 1–3.

De patriarchis nestorianorum commentaria. Ed. E. Grismondi. 2 vols. Rome, 1896–99.

The Patrician Texts in the Book of Armagh. Ed. L. Bieler. Dublin, 1979.

Paul the Deacon. *Historia Langobardorum.* Ed. L. Bethmann and G. Waitz. *MGH, SRL.*

Paul the Deacon. *History of the Lombards.* Ed. E. Peters, trans. W. D. Foulke. Philadelphia, 1974.

Paul of Aigina. *Epitomae medicae.* Ed. I. L. Heiberg. *CMG* IX 1 I. Berlin, 1921.

Peter of Blois. *Epistolae. PL* 207.

Philostratus. *The Life of Apollonius of Tyana.* Ed. F. C. Conybeare. The Loeb Classical Library 16 and 17. Cambridge (Mass.) and London, 1912. Reprint, 1950.

Pseudo-Dionysios of Tel-Mahrē. *Chronicle.* Trans. W. Witakowski. *Pseudo-Dionysios of Tel-Mahre, Chronicle (known also as the Chronicle of Zūqnīn), Part Three.* Liverpool, 1996.

Regesta pontificum Romanorum ab condita ecclesiae ad annum post Christum natum 1198. Ed. P. Jaffé, G. Wattenbach, P. Ewald, C. Loewenfeld, and F. Kaltenbrunner. 2 vols. Leipzig, 1885–88.

Romanos le Mélode. *Hymnes.* Ed. J. Grosdidier de Matons. Vol. 5. Paris, 1981.

Severus, *History of the Patriarchs. PO* 5.

Snorri Sturluson. "Ynglinga saga," in *Heimskringla. Sagas of the Norse Kings.* Trans. S. Laing. 3rd ed. rev. with introduction and notes by P. Foote. London, 1961.

Sources Syriaques. Ed. and trans. A. Mingana. Leipzig, 1907–8.

Suidae Lexicon. Ed. A. Adler. 5 vols. Leipzig, 1928–38.

Theodore Studites, *Laudatio Platonis. PG* 99.

Theophanes. *Chronographia.* Ed. C. de Boor. 2 vols. Leipzig, 1883–85; reprint Hildesheim, 1963, vol. 1.

Theophylactus Simocatta. *Historiae.* Ed. C. De Boor and P. Wirth. Stuttgart, 1972.

Theophylactus Simocatta. *The History of Theophylact Simocatta.* Ed. and trans. M. and M. Whitby. Oxford, 1986.

Thesaurus Palaeohibernicus. Vol. 2. Ed. W. Stokes and J. Strachan, Oxford, 1898.

Thomas Mallory. *The Book of Sir Launcelot and Queen Guinevere.* Ed. E. Vinaver. 2nd ed. Oxford, 1971.

Three Fragments of Irish Annals. Ed. Joan N. Radner. Dublin, 1978.

Thucydides. *History of the Peloponnesian War.* Ed. and trans. C. F. Smith. The Loeb Classical Library. Rev. ed. 4 vols. Cambridge, Mass., 1980.

La Topographie chrétienne de Cosmas Indicopleuste. Ed. and trans. W. Wolska-Conus. 3 vols. Sources chrétiennes, 141, 159, 197. Paris, 1968–73.

Two Lives of St. Cuthbert. Ed. B. Colgrave. Cambridge, 1940.

Victoris Tunnunensis Chronicon cum reliquiis ex consularibus Caesaraugustanis et Iohannis Biclarensis Chronicon. Ed. C. Cardelle de Hartmann. Corpus Christianorum, Series Latina 173A. Turnhout, 2001.

La vie ancienne de S. Syméon Stylite le jeune (521–592). Ed. P. Van den Ven. Subsidia Hagiographica 32. Brussels, 1962.

Vita of Andrew of Crete. Ed. A. Papadopoulos–Kerameus in Ἀνάλεκτα Ἱεροσολυμιτικῆς Σταχυολογίας V. St. Petersburg, 1898.

Vitae sanctorum Hiberniae. Ed. W. W. Heist. Subsidia hagiographica 28. Brussels, 1966.

Vittore da Tunnuna: Chronica. Chiesa e impero nell'età di Giustiniano. Ed. A. Placania. Florence, 1997.

Zacharias. *Historia ecclesiastica Zachariae rhetor vulgo adscripta,* 2. CSCO 84/Syri 39.

Zachariah, *Syriac Chronicle.* Trans. F. J. Hamilton and E. W. Brooks. London, 1899.

Zosimus. *Zosimus: New History.* Trans. R. T. Ridley. Byzantina Australiensia 2. Canberra, 1982.

Secondary Sources

Achtman, M., K. Zurth, G. Morelli, G. Torrea, A. Guiyoule, and E. Carniel. "*Yersinia pestis,* the Cause of Plague, is a Recently Emerged Clone of *Yersinia pseudotuberculosis.*" *PNAS* 96 (1999): 14043–48.

Ackerknecht, E. H. "Anticontagionism between 1821 and 1867." *Bulletin of the History of Medicine* 22 (1948): 562–93.

Adair, D. M., P. L. Worsham, K. K. Hill, A. M. Klevytska, P. J. Jackson, A. M. Friedlander, and P. Keim. "Diversity in a Variable-Number Tandem Repeat from *Yersinia pestis.*" *Journal of Clinical Microbiology* 38 (2000): 1516–19.

Adams, D. Q. and E. J. Barber. "Textile." *Encyclopedia of Indo-European Culture.* London and Chicago, 1997. pp. 569.

Adams, D. Q. and J. P. Mallory. "Medicine." *Encyclopedia of Indo-European Culture.* London and Chicago, 1997. pp. 375–77.

Aguilar Sáenz, A., P. Guichard, and S. Lefebvre. "La ciudad antigua de Lacimurga y su entorno rural." *Studia Historica, Historia Antigua* 10–11 (1992–1993): 109–30.

Agustí, B., L. E. Casellas, and J. Merino. "La necròpolis de les Goges (Sant Julià de Ramis, Girona)," in *IV Reunió d'arqueologia cristiana hispànica (Lisboa)*. Barcelona, 1995. pp. 107–13.

Albiach, R., A. Badía, M. Calvo, C. Marín, J. Piá, and A. Ribera. "Las últimas excavaciones (1992–1998) del solar de l'Almoina: Nuevos datos de la zona episcopal de *Valentia*," in *V Reunió d'arqueologia cristiana hispànica (Cartagena)*. Barcelona, 2000. pp. 63–86.

Alcock, L. *Bede, Eddius, and the Forts of the North Britons*. Jarrow Lecture. Jarrow, Tyne and Wear, 1988.

Alcock, L. *Neighbours of the Picts: Angles, Britons and Scots at War and at Home*. Rosemarkie, 1993.

Aleksova, B. and J. Wiseman. *Studies in the Antiquities of Stobi*. 3 vols. Belgrade, 1973–83.

Alexander, J. T. *Bubonic Plague in Early Modern Russia: Public Health and Urban Disaster*. Baltimore, 1980.

Alexander, P. *The Oracle of Baalbek*. Dumbarton Oaks Studies 10. Washington, D.C., 1967.

Allen, P. *Evagrius Scholasticus the Church Historian*. Leuven, 1981.

Allen, P. "The 'Justinianic' Plague." *Byzantion* 49 (1979): 5–20.

Allison, K., M. Beresford, and J. Hirst. *The Deserted Villages of Oxfordshire*. Leicester, 1965.

Alonso, J. M. "Interactions écologiques des Yersinia au sein de l'hôte réservoir commun, le rongeur." *Bulletin de la Société de pathologie exotique* 92 (1999): 414–17.

Altschuler, E. L. "Plague as HIV Vaccine Adjuvant." *Medical Hypotheses* 54 (2000): 1003–4.

Amiet, R. "Votive Masses." *Dictionary of the Middle Ages* 8:200–1.

Andersson, J. O. and S. G. E. Andersson. "Pseudogenes, Junk DNA, and the Dynamics of *Rickettsia* Genomes." *Molecular Biology and Evolution* 18 (2001): 829–39.

Anisimov, A. P., L. E. Lindler, and G. B. Pier. "Intraspecific Diversity of *Yersinia pestis*." *Clinical Microbiology Reviews* 17 (2004): 434–64.

Ansari, B. M. "An Account of Bubonic Plague in Seventeenth-Century India in an Autobiography of a Mughal Emperor." *Journal of Infection* 29 (1994): 351–52.

Antoniou, I. and A. K. Sinakos. "The Sixth-Century Plague, Its Repeated Appearances until 746 AD and the Explosion of the Rabaul Volcano." *Byzantinische Zeitschrift* 98 (2005): 1–4.

Appleby, A. B. "The Disappearance of Plague: A Continuing Puzzle." *Economic History Review* n.s. 33 (1980): 161–73.

Arbaji, A., S. Kharabsheh, S. Al-Azab, M. Al-Kayed, Z. S. Amr, M. Abu Baker, and M. C. Chu. "A 12-Case Outbreak of Pharyngeal Plague Following the Consumption of Camel Meat, in north-eastern Jordan." *Annals of Tropical Medicine and Parasitology* 99 (2005): 789–93.

Archi, A. "La peste presso gli Ittiti." *Parola del Passato* 33 (1978): 81–89.

Armitage, P. L. "Unwelcome Companions: Ancient Rats Reviewed." *Antiquity* 68 (1994): 231–40.

Armitage, P. L., B. West, and K. Steedman. "New Evidence of Black Rat in Roman London." *London Archaeologist* 4 (1984): 375–83.

Arnold, C. J. and P. Wardle. "Early Medieval Settlement Patterns in England." *Medieval Archaeology* 35 (1981): 145–49.

Arnold, D. *Colonizing the Body: State Medicine and Epidemic Disease in Nineteenth-Century India.* Berkeley, 1993.

Arrizabalaga, J. "Facing the Black Death: Perceptions and Reactions of University Medical Practitioners," in *Practical Medicine from Salerno to the Black Death.* Ed. L. García-Ballester, R. French, J. Arrizabalaga, and A. Cunningham. Cambridge, 1994. pp. 237–88.

Arrizabalaga, J., J. Henderson, and R. French. *The Great Pox: The French Disease in Renaissance Europe.* New Haven, 1997.

Arthur, P., ed. *Il complesso archeologico di Carminiello ai Mannesi, Napoli (Scavi 1983–1984).* Galatina, 1994.

Aston, M., D. Austin and C. Dyer, eds. *The Rural Settlements of Medieval England.* Oxford, 1989.

Audic, S. and E. Béraud-Colomb. "Ancient DNA is Thirteen Years Old." *Nature Biotechnology* 15 (1997): 855–58.

Audoin-Rouzeau, F. *Les chemins de la peste. Le rat, la puce et l'homme.* Rennes, 2003.

Audoin-Rouzeau, F. "La peste et les rats: les réponses de l'archéozoologie," in *Maladies et société (XIIᵉ–XVIIIᵉ siècles).* Actes du Colloque de Bielefeld. Ed. N. Bulst and R. Delort. Paris, 1989. pp. 65–71.

Audoin-Rouzeau, F. "Le rat noir (*Rattus rattus*) et la peste dans l'Occident antique et médiéval." *Bulletin de la Société de Pathologie Exotique* 92 (1999): 422–26.

Audoin-Rouzeau, F. and J. D. Vigne. "La colonisation de l'Europe par le rat noir (*Rattus rattus*)." *Revue de paléobiologie* 13 (1994): 124–45.

Backhouse, J. *The Lindisfarne Gospels.* London, 1981.

Backhouse, J. and L. Webster, eds. *The Making of England: Anglo-Saxon Art and Culture, A.D. 600–900.* London, 1991.

Bailey, G. A., P. M. Jones, F. Mormando, and T. W. Worcester. *Hope and Healing: Painting in Italy in a Time of Plague, 1500–1800.* Worcester, Mass., 2005.

Baillie, M. "Dendrochronology Raises Questions about the Nature of the AD 536 Dust-Veil Event." *The Holocene* 4 (1994): 212–17.

Baillie, M. *Exodus to Arthur. Catastrophic Encounters with Comets.* 2nd ed. London, 2000.

Baillie, M. "Marker Dates – Turning Prehistory into History." *Archaeology Ireland* 2 (1986): 154–55.

Baillie, M. "Patrick, Comets, and Christianity." *Emania* 13 (1995): 69–78.

Bakker, E. J. "Procopius en de pest van Justinian." *Hermeneus* 51 (1979): 147–52.

Ballard, R. D., F. T. Hiebert, D. F. Coleman, C. Ward, J. Smith, K. Willis, B. Foley, K. L. Croff, C. Major, and F. Torre. "Deepwater Archaeology of the Black Sea: The 2000 Season at Sinop, Turkey." *American Journal of Archaeology* 105 (2001): 607–23.

Baltazard, M., M. Bahmanyar, C. Mofidi, and B. Seydian. "Déclin et destin d'une maladie infectieuse: La peste." *Bulletin WHO* 23 (1960): 247–62.

Baltazard, M., M. Bahmanyar, C. Mofidi, and B. Seydian. "Le foyer de peste du Kurdistan." *Bulletin of the World Health Organisation* 5 (1952): 441–72.

Balty, J. "Apamée au VIe siècle," in *Apamée de Syrie. Bilan des recherches archéologiques, 1969–71*. Ed. J. Balty and J. C. Balty. Brussels, 1972. pp. 79–96.

Banaji, J. "Rural Communities in the Late Empire: Economic and Monetary Aspects." Ph. D. dissertation, Oxford University, 1992.

Barnes, D. S. *The Making of a Social Disease: Tuberculosis in Nineteenth-Century France.* Berkeley, 1995.

Barthélemy, D. *L'Ordre seigneurial, XIe–XIIe siècle.* Nouvelle histoire de la France médiévale 3. Paris, 1990.

Bartsocas, C. S. "Two Fourteenth-Century Greek Descriptions of the Black Death." *Journal of the History of Medicine and Allied Sciences* 21 (1966): 394–400.

Bassett, S., ed. *The Origins of the Anglo-Saxon Kingdoms.* Leicester, 1989.

Bauer, V. H. *Das Antonius-Feuer in Kunst und Medizin.* Berlin, Heidelberg, and New York, 1973.

Bazin-Tacchella, S. "Rupture et continuité du discours médical à travers les écrits sur la peste de 1348: Le '*Compendium de epidemia*' (1348) et ses adaptations françaises; La relation de peste contenue dans la '*Chirurgia Magna*' de Guy de Chauliac (1363)," in *Air, Miasmes et Contagion: Les épidémies dans l'Antiquité et au Moyen Âge.* Ed. S. Bazin-Tacchella, D. Quéruel, and E. Samana. Langres, 2001. pp. 105–56.

Beaucournu, J. C. "Diversité des puces vectrices en fonction des foyers pesteux." *Bulletin de la Société de pathologie exotique* 92 (1999): 419–21.

Beck, H. G. *Kirche und theologische Literatur im byzantinischen Reich.* Munich, 1959.

Becker, K. "*Rattus rattus*," in *Handbuch der Säugetiere Europas* 1. Ed. J. Niethammer and F. Krapp. Wiesbaden, 1978. pp. 382–400.

Bell, J. C., S. R. Palmer, and J. M. Payne. *Zoonoses: Infections Transmitted from Animals to Man.* London, 1988.

Benedict, C. "Bubonic Plague in Nineteenth-Century China." *Modern China* 14 (1988): 107–55.

Benedict, C. *Bubonic Plague in Nineteenth-Century China.* Stanford, 1996.

Benedictow, O. J. *The Black Death, 1346-1353: The Complete History.* Woodbridge, 2004.

Benedictow, O. J. "Morbidity in Historical Plague Epidemics." *Population Studies* 41 (1987): 401–31.

Benedictow, O. J. *Plague in the Late Medieval Nordic Countries.* Epidemiological Studies. Oslo, 1992.

Berrocal Caparrós, M. C. and M. D. Laiz Reverte. "Tipología de enterramientos en la necrópolis de San Antón, en Cartagena," in *IV Reunió d'arqueologia cristiana hispànica (Lisboa).* Barcelona, 1995. pp. 173–82.

Bertrand, J. B. *A Historical Relation of the Plague at Marseilles in the Year 1720.* Farnborough, 1805. Reprint, 1973 (original publication 1721).

Besnier, M. *L'Île Tibérine dans l'Antiquité.* Bibliothèque des Écoles Françaises d'Athènes et de Rome 87. Paris, 1902.

Biraben, J.-N. "Essai sur les réactions des sociétés éprouvées par de grands fléaux épidémiques," in *Maladie et société XIIe–XVIIIe siècles.* Ed. N. Bulst and R. Delort. Paris, 1989. pp. 367–74.

Biraben, J.-N. *Les Hommes et la peste en France et dans les pays européens et méditerranéens.* 2 vols. Paris, 1975.

Biraben, J.-N. "Rapport: la peste du VIe siècle dans l'Empire Byzantin," in *Hommes et richesses dans l'empire byzantin (IVe–VIIe siècles)*. Ed. V. Kraveri, C., Morrison, and J. Lefort. 2 vols. Paris, 1989–1991. pp. 121–25.

Biraben, J.-N. and J. Le Goff. "La Peste dans le Haut Moyen Age." *Annales: Economies, Sociétés, Civilisations* 24 (1969): 1484–510.

Biraben, J.-N. and J. Le Goff. "The Plague in the Early Middle Ages," in *Biology of Man in History*. Ed. R. Forster and O. Ranum, trans. E. Forster and P. M. Ranum. Baltimore, 1975. pp. 48–80.

Black, J. "Plague in East Suffolk 1906–1918." *Journal of the Royal Society of Medicine* 93 (2000): 540–43.

Blackburn, M. and P. Grierson. *Medieval European Coinage*. Vol. 1, *The Early Middle Ages*. Cambridge, 1986.

Blair, J. *Anglo-Saxon Oxfordshire*. Stroud, 1994.

Blair, J. "Debate: Ecclesiastical Organization and Pastoral Care in Anglo-Saxon England." *Early Medieval Europe* 4 (1995): 193–212.

Blair, J. "Minster Churches in the Landscape," in *Anglo-Saxon Settlements*. Ed. D. Hooker. Oxford, 1988.

Blanchard, R. "Notes historiques sur la peste." *Archives de parasitologie* 3 (1900): 589–648.

Blasco, J., V. Escrivà, A. Ribera, and R. Soriano. "Estat actual de la investigació arqueològica de l'antiguitat tardana a la ciutat de València," in *III Reunió d'arqueologia cristiana hispànica (Maó, Menorca)*. Barcelona, 1994. pp. 185–99.

Bleukx, K. "Was the Black Death (1348–49) a Real Plague Epidemic? England as a Case-Study," in *Serta devota in memoriam Guillelmi Lourdaux. Pars posterior: Cultura mediaevalis*. Mediaevalia Lovaniensia series I, studia XXI. Ed. W. Verbeke, M. Haverals, R. De Keyser, and J. Goossens. Leuven, 1995. pp. 65–113.

Bloch, M. *Les Rois thaumaturges*. New ed. Paris, 1983.

Blondheim, S. H. "The First Recorded Epidemic of Pneumonic Plague: The Bible, I. Sam. VI." *Bulletin of the History of Medicine* 29 (1955): 337–45.

Blum, C. "The Meaning of *stoicheion* and its Derivatives in the Byzantine Age." *Eranos* 44 (1946): 315–25.

Blum, J. "The Rise of Serfdom in Eastern Europe." *American Historical Review* 62 (1957): 807–36.

Bobrov, A. G. and A. A. Filippov. "Prevalence of IS285 and IS100 in *Yersinia pestis* and *Yersinia pseudotuberculosis* Genomes." *Mol. Gen. Mikrobiol. Virusol.* 2 (1997): 36–40 (article in Russian).

Bodson, L. "Le vocabulaire latin des maladies pestilentielles et épizootiques," in *Le Latin médical: La constitution d'une langage scientifique*. Centre Jean Palerne, Mémoires 10. Saint-Etienne, 1991. pp. 215–41.

Boisier, P., L. Rahalison, M. Rasolomaharo, M. Ratsitorahina, M. Mahafaly, M. Razafimahefa, J.-M. Duplantier, L. Ratsifasoamanana, and S. Chanteau. "Epidemiologic Features of Four Successive Annual Outbreaks of Bubonic Plague in Mahajanga, Madagascar." *Emerging Infectious Diseases* 8 (2002): 311–16.

Boll, F., C. Bezold, and W. Gundel. *Sternglaube und Sterndeutung*. Ed. H. G. Gundel. 5th ed. Stuttgart, 1966.

Bonnassie, P. *From Slavery to Feudalism in South-Western Europe.* Trans. J. Birrell. Cambridge, 1991.

Bonner, C. *Studies in Magical Amulets.* Ann Arbor, 1950.

Bonser, W. "Epidemics During the Anglo-Saxon Period." *Journal of the British Archaeological Association,* 3rd. ser. 9 (1944): 48–71.

Bonser, W. *The Medical Background of Anglo-Saxon England.* London, 1963.

Bornmann, F. "Motivi Tucididei in Procopio." *Atene e Roma* 19 (1974): 138–50.

Bowen, E. G. *Saints, Seaways and Settlements in Celtic Lands.* Cardiff, 1977.

Bowsky, W. M. "The Impact of the Black Death upon Sienese Government and Society." *Speculum* 39 (1964): 1–34.

Brandes, W. "Anastasios ho dikoros: Endzeiterwartung und Kaiserkritik in Byzanz um 500 n. Chr." *Byzantinische Zeitschrift* 90 (1997): 24–63.

Brandes, W. "Byzantine Cities in the Seventh and Eighth Centuries – Different Sources, Different Histories?" in *The Idea and the Ideal of the Town Between Late Antiquity and the Early Middle Ages.* Ed. C. P. Brogiolo and B. Ward-Perkins. Leiden, 1999. pp. 25–58.

Brandes, W. "Die Entwicklung des byzantinischen Städtewesens von der Spätantike bis ins 9. Jahrhundert," in *Die byzantinische Stadt im Rahmen der allgemeinen Stadtentwicklung.* Ed. K. P. Matschke. Leipzig, 1995.

Brandt, A. M. *No Magic Bullet: A Social History of Venereal Disease in the United States since 1880.* New York, 1987.

Bratton, T. L. "The Identity of the Plague of Justinian. Parts I & II." *Transactions and Studies of the College of Physicians of Philadelphia* ser. 5, 3 (1981): 113–24 and 174–80.

Bray, R. S. *Armies of Pestilence: The Effects of Pandemics on History.* Cambridge, 1996.

Breatnach, L. "Canon Law and Secular Law in Early Ireland: The Significance of 'Bretha Nemed.'" *Peritia* 3 (1984): 39–59.

Brenner, R. "Agrarian Class Structure and Economic Development in Pre-Industrial Europe." *Past and Present* 70 (1976): 30–75.

Briggs, G., J. Cook, and T. Rowley, eds. *The Archaeology of the Oxford Region.* Oxford, 1986.

Brock, S. P. "North Mesopotamia in the Late Seventh Century. Book XV of John Bar Penkāyē's *Rīš Mellē.*" *Jerusalem Studies in Arabic and Islam* 9 (1987): 51–75.

Brocke, T. D. *Robert Koch: A Life in Medicine and Microbiology.* Washington, D. C., 1999.

Brooks, N. *The Early History of the Church of Canterbury.* Leicester, 1984.

Brothen, J. A. "Population Decline and Plague in Late Medieval Norway." *Annales de Démographie Historique* (1996): 137–49.

Brothwell, D. and A. T. Sandison, eds. *Diseases in Antiquity: A Survey of the Diseases, Injuries and Surgery of Early Populations.* Springfield, Illinois, 1967.

Brown, P. R. L. *The Rise of Western Christendom.* Oxford, 1996.

Brown, P. R. L. *Society and the Holy in Late Antiquity.* Berkeley and Los Angeles, 1982.

Brown, P. R. L. *The World of Late Antiquity.* London, 1971.

Brubaker, R. R. "The Recent Emergence of Plague: A Story of Felonious Evolution." *Microbial Ecology* 47 (2004): 293–99.

Bryer, A. "The Means of Agricultural Production: Muscle and Tools," in *The Economic History of Byzantium From the Seventh through the Fifteenth Century.* Ed. A. E. Laiou. 3 vols. Washington, D. C, 2002. 1:101–13.

Bryder, L. *Below the Magic Mountain: A Social History of Tuberculosis in Twentieth-Century Britain.* Oxford, 1988.

Buckland, P. C., P. I. Buckland, and P. Skidmore. "Insect Remains from GUS: An Interim Report," in *Man, Culture and Environment in Ancient Greenland.* Ed. J. Arneborg and H. C. Gulløv. Copenhagen, 1998. pp. 74–79.

Buckland, P. C. and J. P. Sadler. "A Biogeography of the Human Flea, *Pulex irritans* L. (Siphonaptera: Pulicidae)." *Journal of Biogeography* 16 (1989): 115–20.

Burgess, C. "Population, Climate and Upland Settlement," in *Upland Settlement in Britain: The Second Millennium B.C. and After.* BAR British Series 143. Eds. D. Spratt and C. Burgess. Oxford, 1985. pp. 195–229.

Burroughs, A. L. "Sylvatic Plague Studies. The Vector Efficiency of Nine Species of Fleas Compared with *Xenopsylla cheopis*." *Journal of Hygiene* 45 (1947): 371–96.

Butler, T. *Plague and other Yersinia Infections.* New York, 1983.

Byrne, F. J. *Irish Kings and High-Kings.* London, 1973.

Byrne, F. J. "Tribes and Tribalism in Early Ireland." *Ériu* 22 (1971): 149–53.

Cabrol, F. "Litanies." *Dictionnaire d'Archéologie chrétienne et de liturgie* 9.2, 1540–71.

Calvi, G. *Histories of a Plague Year: The Social and the Imaginary in Baroque Florence.* Berkeley, 1989.

Cameron, A. "Images of Authority: Elites and Icons in Late Sixth-Century Byzantium," in *Byzantium and the Classical Tradition.* Ed. M. Mullett and R. Scott. Birmingham, 1981.

Campbell, J. "Elements in the Background to the Life of St. Cuthbert," in *St. Cuthbert, His Cult and His Community to AD 1200.* Ed. G. Bonner, D. Rollason, and C. Stancliffe. Woodbridge, UK, 2002. pp. 3–19.

Campbell, J. *Essays in Anglo-Saxon History.* London, 1986.

Campbell, J. "The Impact of the Sutton Hoo Discovery on the Study of Anglo-Saxon History," in *Voyage to the Other World: The Legacy of Sutton Hoo.* Ed. C. B. Kendall and P. Wells. Minneapolis, 1992. pp. 79–101.

Canivet, P. and J.-P. Rey-Coquais, eds. *La Syrie de Byzance à l'Islam: VIIe–VIIIe siècles.* Damascus, 1992.

Cantlie, J. "The Signs and Symptoms of Bubonic, Pneumonic, and Septicaemic Plague." *British Medical Journal* 2 (1900): 1229–32.

Cantor, N. F. *In the Wake of the Plague: The Black Death and the World it Made.* London, 2001.

Carmichael, A. G. "Contagion Theory and Contagion Practice in Fifteenth-Century Milan." *Renaissance Quarterly* 44 (1991): 213–56.

Carmichael, A. G. "Infection, Hidden Hunger, and History," in *Hunger and History: The Impact of Changing Food and Consumption Patterns on Society.* Ed. R. I. Rotberg and T. K. Rabb. Cambridge, 1985. pp. 51–66.

Carmichael, A. G. *Plague and the Poor in Renaissance Florence.* Cambridge, 1986.

Carpentier, E. "Autour de la peste noire: Famines et épidémies dans l'histoire du XIVe siècle." *Annales: Economies Sociétés Civilisations* 17 (1962): 1062–92.

Carpentier, E. *Une ville devant la peste: Orvieto et la peste noire de 1348.* 2nd ed. Brussels, 1993.

Carreté, J.-M., S. J. Keay, and M. Millett. *A Roman Provincial Capital and Its Hinterland: The Survey of the Territory of Tarragona, Spain, 1985–1990. Journal of Roman Archaeology*, Supplementary Series 15. Ann Arbor, 1995.

Casson, L. *Ships and Seamanship in the Ancient World.* Princeton, 1971.

Cassano, W. F. "Cystic Fibrosis and the Plague." *Medical Hypotheses* 18 (1985): 51–52.

Castel Sant'Angelo. Ed. N. Giustozzi. Milan, 2003.

Cavanaugh, D. C. and J. E. Williams. "Plague: Some Ecological Interrelationships," in *Fleas: Proceedings of the International Conference on Fleas, Ashton Wold, Peterborough, UK, 21–25 June 1977.* Ed. R. Traub and H. Starcke. Rotterdam, 1980. pp. 245–56.

Chambers, M., D. Herlihy, T. K. Rabb, I. Woloch, and R. Grew. *The Western Experience.* 5th ed. New York, 1991.

Champion, J. A. I., ed. *Epidemic Disease in London.* London, 1993.

Champion, T. "Chalton." *Current Archaeology* 59 (1977): 364–69.

Chanteau, S., M. Ratsitorahina, L. Rahalison, B. Rasoamanana, F. Chan, P. Boisier, D. Rabeson, and J. Roux. "Current Epidemiology of Human Plague in Madagascar." *Microbes and Infection* 2 (2000): 25–31.

Charles-Edwards, T. M. *Early Christian Ireland.* Cambridge, 2000.

Charles-Edwards, T. M. *Early Irish and Welsh Kinship.* Oxford, 1993.

Cipolla, C. M. *Christofano and the Plague: A Study in the History of Public Health in the Age of Galileo.* Berkeley, 1973.

Cipolla, C. M. *Faith, Reason, and the Plague in Seventeenth-Century Tuscany.* Ithaca, 1979.

Cipolla, C. M. *Fighting the Plague in Seventeenth-Century Italy.* Madison, 1981.

Cipolla, C. M. "The Plague and Pre-Malthus Malthusians." *Journal of European Economic History* 3 (1974): 277–84.

Cipolla, C. M. *Public Health and the Medical Profession in the Renaissance.* Cambridge, 1976.

Claude, D. "Remarks About Relations Between Visigoths and Hispano-Romans in the Seventh-Century," in *Strategies of Distinction. The Construction of Ethnic Communities, 300–800.* Ed. W. Pohl and H. Reimitz. Leiden, 1998. pp. 117–30.

Cliff, A. D. and P. Haggett. "Epidemic Control and Critical Community Size: Spatial Aspects of Eliminating Communicable Diseases in Human Populations," in *Spatial Epidemiology.* Ed. R. W. Thomas. London, 1990. pp. 93–110.

Cliff, A. D. and P. Haggett. *The Spread of Measles in Fiji and the Pacific: Spatial Components in the Transmission of Epidemic Waves through Island Communities.* Canberra, 1985.

Cockburn, T. A. "Infectious Diseases in Ancient Populations." *Current Anthropology* 12 (1971): 45–54.

Cohn, S. K. "The Black Death: End of a Paradigm." *American Historical Review* 107 (2002): 703–38.

Cohn, S. K. *The Black Death Transformed: Disease and Culture in Early Renaissance Europe.* London, 2002.

Cole, S. T., K. Eiglmeier, J. Parkhill, K. D. James, N. R. Thompson, P. R. Wheeler, N. Honoré, et al. "Massive Gene Decay in the Leprosy Bacillus." *Nature* 409 (2001): 1007–11.

Collins, R. "Isidore, Maximus and the *Historia Gothorum*," in *Historiographie im frühen Mittelalter*. Ed. A. Scharer and G. Scheibelreiter. Munich, 1994. pp. 345–58.

Congourdeau, M.-H. "La peste noire à Constantinople de 1348 à 1466." *Medicina nei Secoli* 11 (1999): 377–89.

Congourdeau, M.-H. "La société byzantine face aux grandes pandémies," in *Maladie et société à Byzance*. Ed. E. Patlagean. Spoleto, 1993. pp. 22–41.

Congourdeau, M.-H. and M. Melhaoui. "La perception de la peste en pays chrétien byzantin et musulman." *Revue des Études Byzantines* 59 (2001): 95–124.

Conrad, L. I. "Arabic Plague Chronologies and Treatises: Social and Historical Factors in the Formation of a Literary Genre." *Studia Islamica* 54 (1981): 51–93.

Conrad, L. I. "The Biblical Tradition for the Plague of the Philistines." *Journal of the American Oriental Society* 104 (1984): 281–87.

Conrad, L. I. "Epidemic Disease in Central Syria in the Late Sixth Century: Some New Insights from the Verse of Hassan ibn Thābit." *Byzantine and Modern Greek Studies* 18 (1994): 12–58.

Conrad, L. I. "Epidemic Disease in Formal and Popular Thought in Early Islamic Society," in *Epidemics and Ideas: Essays on the Historical Perception of Pestilence*. Ed. T. Ranger and P. Slack. Cambridge, 1992. pp. 77–99.

Conrad, L. I. "Historical Evidence and the Archaeology of Early Islam," in *Quest for Understanding: Arabic and Islamic Studies in Memory of Malcolm H. Kerr*. Ed. S. Seikaly, R., Baalbaki, and P. Dodd. Beirut, 1991. pp. 263–82.

Conrad, L. I. "Die Pest und ihr soziales Umfeld im Nahen Osten des frühen Mittelalters." *Der Islam* 73 (1996): 81–112.

Conrad, L. I. "The Plague in Bilād al-Shām in Pre-Islamic Times," in *Proceedings of the Symposium on Bilād al-Shām during the Byzantine Period*. Ed. M. A. al-Bakhīt and M. Asfur. 2 vols. Amman, 1986. 2: 143–63.

Conrad, L. I. "Plague in the Early Medieval Near East." Ph. D. dissertation, Princeton University, 1981.

Conrad, L. I. "*Ṭā' ūn* and *Wabā*: Conceptions of Plague and Pestilence in Early Islam." *Journal of the Economic and Social History of the Orient* 25 (1982): 268–307.

Conrad, L. and D. Wujastyk, eds. *Contagion: Perspectives from Pre-Modern Societies*. Aldershot, 2000.

Contis, G. "The Impact of the Plague Pandemics on the Byzantine Empire," in *Acts of the XVIIIth International Congress of Byzantine Studies: Summaries of Communications*. Moscow, 1991. 1:241–42.

Cooper, A. and H. N. Polinnar. "Ancient DNA: Do it Right or Not at All." *Science* 289 (2000): 1139.

Coram-Mekkey, S. "Peste et rat: Un couple indissociable?" *Moyen Age* 103 (1997): 139–52.

Cornelis, G. R. "Molecular and Cell Biology Aspects of Plague." *PNAS* 97 (2000): 8778–83.

Cramp, R. "Monkwearmouth and Jarrow: The Archaeological Evidence," in *Famulus Christi: Essays in Commemoration of the Thirteenth Centenary of the Venerable Bede*. Ed. G. Bonner. London, 1976.

Cramp, R. "Northumberland and Ireland," in *Sources of Anglo-Saxon Culture.* Ed. P. E. Szarmach. Kalamazoo, 1986.

Crawfurd, R. H. P. *Plague and Pestilence in Literature and Art.* Oxford, 1914.

Creighton, C. *A History of Epidemics in Britain.* London, 1894. Repr., New York, 1965.

Cróinín, D. Ó. *Early Medieval Ireland, 400–1200.* London, 1995.

Crone, P. *Meccan Trade and the Rise of Islam.* Oxford, 1987.

Cronje, G. "Tuberculosis and Mortality Decline in England and Wales, 1851–1910," in *Urban Disease and Mortality in Nineteenth-Century England.* Ed. R. Woods and J. Woodward. New York, 1984. pp. 79–101.

Crosby, A. W. *America's Forgotten Pandemic: The Influenza of 1918.* Cambridge, 1989.

Crosby, A. W. *Ecological Imperialism: The Biological Expansion of Europe, 900–1900.* Cambridge, 1986.

Crosby, A. W. "Hawaiian Depopulation as a Model for the Amerindian Experience," in *Epidemics and Ideas: Essays on the Historical Perception of Pestilence.* Ed. T. Ranger and P. Slack. Cambridge, 1992. pp. 175–201.

Culte et pèlerinage à saint Michel en occident: Les trois monts dédiés à l'archange. Ed. P. Bouet, G. Otranto, and A. Vauchez. Collection de l'Ecole française de Rome 316. Rome, 2003.

Cumont, F., F. Boll, W. Kroll, F. Skutsch, and K. Ziegler, eds. *Catalogus Codicum Astrologorum Graecorum.* 12 vols, in 20 parts. Brussels, 1898–1936.

Cunliffe, B. "Saxon and Medieval Settlement-Pattern in the Region of Chalton, Hampshire." *Medieval Archaeology* 16 (1972): 1–12.

Cunningham, A. "Transforming Plague: The Laboratory and the Identification of Infectious Disease," in *The Laboratory Revolution in Medicine.* Ed. A. Cunningham and P. Williams. Cambridge, 1992. pp. 209–44.

Curson, P. and K. McCracken. *Plague in Sydney: The Anatomy of an Epidemic.* Kensington, 1986.

Curtin, P. D. *Death by Migration: Europe's Encounter with the Tropical World in the Nineteenth Century.* Cambridge, 1989.

Dagron, G. *Constantinople imaginaire. Études sur le recueil des "Patria."* Bibliothèque byzantine 8. Paris, 1984.

Dagron, G. *Hommes et richesse dans l'Empire Byzantin.* Paris, 1989.

Dagron, G. "Quand la terre tremble," in *Hommage à M. Paul Lemerle.* Paris, 1981. pp. 87–103.

Dagron, G. "Le saint, le savant, l'astrologue: Etudes de thèmes hagiographiques à travers quelques recueils de 'Questions et réponses' des Ve–VIIe siècles," in *Hagiographie, cultures et sociétés (IVe–VII siècles).* Paris, 1981. pp. 143–56.

Daley, B. *The Hope of the Early Church: A Handbook of Patristic Eschatology.* Cambridge, 1991.

Daniels, R. "The Anglo-Saxon Monastery at Church Close, Hartlepool, Cleveland." *Archaeological Journal* 145 (1988): 158–210.

Daniels, R. "Hartlepool," *Current Archaeology* 104 (1987): 273–83.

Dar, L., R. Thakur, and V. S. Dar. "India: Is it Plague?" *Lancet* 344 (1994): 1359.

Darby, C., J. W. Hsu, N. Ghori, and S. Falkow. "Plague Bacteria Biofilm Blocks Food Intake." *Nature* 417 (2002): 243–44.

D'Arrigo, R., D. Frank, G. Jacoby, and N. Pederson. "Spatial Response to Major Volcanic Events in or about AD 536, 934, and 1258: Frost Rings and Other Dendrochronological Evidence from Mongolia and Northern Siberia: Comment on R. B. Stothers 'Volcanic Dry Fogs, Climate Cooling, and Plague Pandemics in Europe and the Middle East' [*Climatic Change* 42 (1999)]." *Climatic Change* 49 (2001): 239–46.

Dauphin, C. *La Palestine byzantine. Peuplement et populations.* BAR International Series 726. Oxford, 1998.

Davis, D. E. "The Scarcity of Rats and the Black Death: An Ecological History." *Journal of Interdisciplinary History* 16 (1986): 455–70.

Davis, E. M. "Palaeoecological Studies at Stobi," in *Studies in the Antiquities of Stobi.* Ed. B. Aleksova and J. Wiseman. Belgrade, 1983. 3: 87–94.

Davis, S., M. Begon, L. De Bruyn, V. S. Ageyev, N. L. Klassovskiy, S. B. Pole, H. Viljugrein, N. C. Stenseth, and H. Leirs. "Predictive Thresholds for Plague in Kazakhstan." *Science* 304 (2004): 736–39.

Dawes, H. "*Yersinia pestis*: Sequence Sheds Light on the Plague's Past." *Current Biology* 27 (2001): R949–51.

Debré, P. *Louis Pasteur.* Trans. E. Forster. Baltimore, 1998.

del Amo, M. D. *Estudio crítico de la necrópolis paleocristiana de Tarragona.* 3 vols. Tarragona, 1979–1989.

Delefosse, T. and A. D. Yoder. "Ancient DNA," in *McGraw-Hill Yearbook of Science and Technology, 2002.* New York, 2001. pp. 9–14.

Del Panta, L. *Le epidemie nella storia demografica italiana (secoli XIV–XIX).* Turin, 1980.

Deng, W., V. Burland, G. Plunkett, A. Boutin, G. F. Mayhew, P. Liss, N. T. Perna, et al. "Genome Sequence of *Yersinia pestis* KIM." *Journal of Bacteriology* 184 (2002): 4601–11.

Dennis, D. T., K. L. Gage, N. Gratz, J. D. Poland, and E. Tikhomirovcan, eds. *Plague Manual: Epidemiology, Distribution, Surveillance and Control.* Geneva, 1999.

Derbes V. J. "De Mussis and the Great Plague of 1348: A Forgotten Episode of Bacteriological Warfare." *Journal of the American Medical Association* 196.1 (1966): 179–82.

Detorakes, T. E. "Ἀνέκδοτον ἐγκώμιον εἰς Ἀνδρέαν Κρήτης." *Epeteris Etairias Byzantinon Spoudon* 37 (1969–70).

Devignat, R. "Comportement biologique et biochimique de *Pasteurella pestis* et de *P. pseudotuberculosis.*" *Bulletin of the World Health Organization* 10 (1954): 463–94.

Devignat, R. *La peste antique du Congo belge dans le cadre de l'histoire et de la géographie.* Institut royal colonial belge, Section des sciences naturelles et médicinales, Mémoires, Collection 23, fasc. 4. Brussels, 1953.

Devignat, R. "Variétés de l'espèce *Pasteurella pestis*: Nouvelle hypothèse." *Bulletin of the World Health Organization* 4 (1951): 247–63.

De Vries, J. *Altgermanische Religionsgeschichte.* Grundriss der germanischen Philologie 12. 3rd ed. Berlin, 1970.

Devroey, J.-P. *Economie rurale et société dans l'Europe franque (VIe–IXe siècles).* Paris, 2003.

Dictionary of the Irish Language and Contributions to a Dictionary of the Irish Language. Dublin, 1913–76.

Digby, A. *Pauper Palaces.* London, 1978.

Doll, J. M., P. S. Zeitz, P. Ettestad, A. L. Bucholtz, T. Davis, and K. Gage. "Cat-Transmitted Fatal Pneumonic Plague in a Person Who Travelled from Colorado to Arizona." *American Journal of Tropical Medicine and Hygiene* 51 (1994): 109–14.

Dols, M. W. *The Black Death in the Middle East.* Princeton, 1977.

Dols, M. W. "The Comparative Communal Responses to the Black Death in Muslim and Christian Societies." *Viator* 5 (1974): 169–87.

Dols, M. W. "Geographical Origin of the Black Death: Comment." *Bulletin of the History of Medicine* 52 (1978): 112–20.

Dols, M. W. "Plague in Early Islamic History." *Journal of the American Oriental Society* 94 (1974): 371–83.

Dols, M. W. "The Second Plague Pandemic and its Recurrences in the Middle East: 1347–1394." *Journal of the Economic and Social History of the Orient* 22 (1979): 162–89.

Dong, L., M. Xi, and F. Thann. *Les maux épidémiques dans l'empire chinois.* Paris 1995.

D'Onofrio, C. *Castel S. Angelo e Borgo tra Roma e Papato.* Rome, 1978.

Downey, G. *A History of Antioch in Syria.* Princeton, 1961.

Drancourt, M. and D. Raoult. "Molecular Detection of *Yersinia pestis* in Dental Pulp." *Microbiology* 150 (2004): 263–4.

Drancourt, M. and D. Raoult. "Molecular Insights into the History of Plague." *Microbes and Infection* 4 (2002): 105–9.

Drancourt, M., G. Aboudharam, M. Signoli, O. Dutour, and D. Raoult. "Detection of 400-year-old *Yersinia pestis* DNA in Human Dental Pulp: An Approach to the Diagnosis of Ancient Septicemia." *PNAS* 95 (1998): 12637–40.

Driesch, A. von den and J. Boessneck. "A Roman Cat Skeleton from Quseir on the Red Sea Coast." *Journal of Archaeological Science* 10 (1983): 205–11.

Dubos, R. and J. Dubos. *The White Plague: Tuberculosis, Man, and Society.* New Brunswick, 1952. Rep., 1987.

Duby, G. *The Early Growth of the European Economy.* Trans. H. B. Clarke. Ithaca, 1974.

Ducos, J. "L'air corrompu dans les traités de peste," in *Air, Miasmes et Contagion: Les épidémies dans l'Antiquité et au Moyen Âge.* Ed. S. Bazin-Tachella, D. Quéruel, and E. Samana. Langres, 2001. pp. 87–104.

Dumville, D. "Gildas and Melgwn: Problems of Dating," in *Gildas: New Approaches.* Ed. M. Lapidge and D. Dumville. Woodbridge, 1984.

Duncan, K. "The Possible Influence of Climate on the Plague in Scotland." *Scottish Geographical Magazine* 108 (1992): 29–34.

Duncan-Jones, R. "The Impact of the Antonine Plague." *Journal of Roman Archaeology* 9 (1996): 108–36.

Durey, M. *The Return of the Plague: British Society and the Cholera, 1831–1832.* Dublin, 1979.

Durliat, J. "La peste du VIe siècle: Pour un nouvel examen des sources byzantines," in *Hommes et richesses dans l'empire byzantin.* Eds. V. Kravari, C. Morrison, and J. Lefort. 2 vols. Paris, 1989–91. pp. 107–119.

Duval, N., P. Périn, and J.-C. Picard. "Nouvelles recherches d'archéologie et d'épigraphie chrétienne à Sufetula (Byzacène)." *Mélanges d'archéologie de l'école française de Rome* 68 (1956): 277–80.

Duval, N., P. Périn and J.-C. Picard. "Paris," in *Topographie chrétienne des cités de la Gaule, des origines au milieu du VIIIe siècle.* Paris, 1992. 8: 97–129.

Dyer, A. D. "The Influence of Bubonic Plague in England, 1500–1667." *Medical History* 22 (1978): 308–26.

Dykhuizen, D. E. "*Yersinia pestis* – an Instant Species?" *Trends in Microbiology* 8 (2000): 297–98.

Ebied, R. Y. and M. L. J. Young. "A Treatise in Arabic on the Nestorian Patriarchs." *Le Museón* 87 (1974): 87–113.

Eckert, E. A. "The Retreat of Plague from Central Europe, 1640–1720: A Geomedical Approach." *Bulletin of the Institute of the History of Medicine* 74 (2000): 1–28.

Eckert, E. A. *The Structure of Plagues and Pestilences in Early Modern Europe: Central Europe, 1560–1640.* Basle, 1996.

Eckstein, F. and J. H. Waszink. "Amulett." *Reallexicon für Antike und Christentum* 1: 397–411.

Edis, R. "The Byzantine Era in Tunisia: A Forgotten Footnote?" *The Journal of North African Studies* 4 (1999): 45–61.

Edmunds, L. *Oedipus. The Ancient Legend and Its Later Analogues.* Baltimore and London, 1985.

Ell, S. R. "Immunity as a Factor in the Epidemiology of Medieval Plague." *Reviews of Infectious Diseases* 6.6 (1984): 866–79.

Ell, S. R. "Interhuman Transmission of Medieval Plague." *Bulletin of the History of Medicine* 54 (1980): 497–510.

Ell, S. R. "Iron in Two Seventeenth-Century Plague Epidemics." *Journal of Interdisciplinary History* 15 (1985): 445–57.

Elton, C. S. "Plague and the Regulation of Numbers in Wild Mammals." *Journal of Hygiene* 24 (1925): 138–63.

Elvin, S. J., D. E. Williamson, J. C. Scott, J. N. Smith, G. Pérez de Lema, S. Chilla, P. Clapham, K. Pfeffer, D. Schlöndorff, and B. Luckow. "Ambiguous Role of CCR5 in *Y. pestis* Infection." *Nature* 430 (2004): 418.

Engemann, J. "Zur Verbreitung magischer Übelabwehr in der nichtschristlichen und christlichen Spätantike." *Jahrbuch für Antike und Christentum* 18 (1975): 22–48.

Enright, M. *Lady with a Mead Cup. Ritual, Prophecy and Lordship in the European Warband from La Tène to the Viking Age.* Dublin, 1996.

Enscore, R. E., B. J. Biggerstaff, T. L. Brown, R. E. Fulgham, P. J. Reynolds, D. M. Engelthaler, C. E. Levy, et al. "Modeling Relationships Between Climate and the Frequency of Human Plague Cases in the Southwestern United States, 1960–97." *American Journal of Tropical Medicine and Hygiene* 66 (2002): 186–96.

Ervynck, A. "Sedentism or Urbanism: On the Quest for the Oldest Commensal Rodent," in *Bones and the Man: Studies in Honour of Don Brothwell.* Ed. K. Dobney and T. O'Connor. Oxford, 2002. pp. 95–110.

Escrivá Torres, V. and R. Soriano Sánchez. "El área cementerial asociada a la Basílica de la Almoina." *III Congreso de Arqueología Medieval* 2 (1994): 103–109.

Escrivá Torres, V. and R. Soriano Sánchez. "El área episcopal de Valentia." *Archivo Español de Arqueología* 63 (1990): 347–54.

Etchingham, C. "Early Medieval Irish History," in *Progress in Early Medieval Irish Studies.* Maynooth Monographs 7. Ed. K. McCone and K. Simms. Maynooth, 1996.

Evans, J. A. S. *The Age of Justinian: The Circumstances of Imperial Power.* London and New York, 1996.

Evin, J., A. Ferdière, and G.-N. Lambert, eds. *Les méthodes de datation en laboratoire.* Collection "Archéologiques." Paris, 1990.

Farley, J. *Bilharzia: A History of Imperial Tropical Medicine.* Cambridge, 1991.

Farris, W. W. *Population, Disease, and Land in Early Japan, 645–690.* Cambridge, Mass., 1985.

Fee, E. and D. M. Fox, eds. *AIDS: The Burdens of History.* Berkeley, 1988.

Fee, E. and D. M. Fox, eds. *AIDS: The Making of a Chronic Disease.* Berkeley, 1992.

Feldberg, G. D. *Disease and Class: Tuberculosis and the Shaping of Modern North American Society.* New Brunswick, 1995.

Fenner, F., D. A. Henderson, I. Arita, Z. Ježek, and I. D. Ladnyi. *Smallpox and Its Eradication.* WHO. Geneva, 1988.

Fernández Corrales, J. M. *El asentamiento romano en Extremadura y su analisis espacial.* Cáceres, 1988.

Festugière, A. J., ed. *Vie de Jean de Chypre.* Institut Français d'archéologie de Beyrouth. Bibliothéque archéologique et historique 95. Paris, 1974.

Festugière, A. J., ed. *Vie de Théodore de Sykéon.* Subsidia Hagiographica 48. Brussels, 1970.

Findlay, R. and M. Lundahl. "Demographic Shocks and the Factor Proportions Model: From the plague of Justinian to the Black Death," a paper given at Barnard College in 2003; see at http://www.econ.barnard.columbia. edu/~econhist/papers/Findlay%20Justinian.pdf.

Flinn, M. "Plague in Europe and the Mediterranean Countries." *Journal of European Economic History* 8 (1979): 131–48.

Ford, J. *The Role of Trypanosomiases in African Ecology: A Study of the Tsetse Fly Problem.* Oxford, 1971.

Foss, C. "Syria in Transition, A.D. 550–750." *Dumbarton Oaks Papers* 51 (1997): 189–270.

Fossier, R. *The Cambridge Illustrated History of the Middle Ages.* Trans. S. H. Tension. 3 vols. New York, 1986.

Fotiou, A. "Recruitment Shortages in Sixth-Century Byzantium." *Byzantion* 58 (1988): 65–77.

Franz, L. "Zur Bevölkerungsgeschichte des frühen Mittelalters." *Deutsches Archiv für Landes- und Volksforschung* 2 (1938): 404–16.

Freedman, P. *Images of the Medieval Peasant.* Stanford, 1999.

Frieden, N. M. "The Russian Cholera Epidemic of 1892–93 and Medical Professionalization." *Journal of Social History* 10 (1977): 538–59.

Fukushima, H., Q. Hao, K. Wu, X. Hu, J. Chen, Z. Guo, H. Dai, C. Qin, S. Lu, and M. Gomyoda. "*Yersinia enterocolitica* O9 as a Possible Barrier against *Y. pestis* in Natural Plague Foci in Ningxia." *Current Microbiology* 42 (2001): 1–7.

Fyodorov, V. N. "The Question of the Existence of Natural Foci of Plague in Europe in the Past." *Journal of Hygiene, Epidemiology, Microbiology and Immunology* 4 (1960): 135–41.

Gage, K. L., D. T. Dennis, K. A. Orloski, P. Ettestad, T. L. Brown, P. J. Reynolds, W. J. Pape, C. L. Fritz, L. G. Carter, and J. D. Stein. "Cases of Cat-Associated Human Plague in the Western US, 1977–1998." *Clinical Infectious Diseases* 30 (2000): 893–900.

Galimand, J., A. Guiyoule, G. Gerbaud, B. Rasoamanana, S. Chanteau, E. Carniel, and P. Courvalin. "Multidrug Resistance in *Yersinia pestis* Mediated by a Transferable Plasmid." *New England Journal of Medicine* 337 (1997): 677–80.

Galvani, A. P. and M. Slatkin. "Evaluating Plague and Smallpox as Historical Selective Pressures for the CCR5-Δ32 HIV-resistance Allele." *PNAS*, 100 (2003): 15276–79.

García Moreno, L. A. *El fin del reino visigodo de Toledo. Decadencia y catastrofe, una contribución a su crítica.* Madrid, 1975.

Garrelt, C. and I. Wiechmann. "Detection of *Yersinia pestis* in early and late medieval bavarian burials," in *Decyphering Ancient Bones. The Research Potential of Bioarchaeological Collections.* Ed. G. Grupe and J. Peters. Rahden, 2003. pp. 247–54.

Garrett, L. *Betrayal of Trust: The Collapse of Global Public Health.* New York, 2000.

Gates, T. and C. O'Brien. "Cropmarks at Milfield and New Bewick and the Recognition of Grubenhaüser in Northumberland." *Archaoelogia Aeliana.* 5th ser. 16 (1988): 1–9.

Gelpi, A. P. "Saint Sebastian and the Black Death." *Vesalius*, 4 (1998): 23–30.

Gerberding, R. *The Rise of the Carolingians and the Liber Historiae Francorum.* Oxford Historical Monographs. Oxford, 1987.

Getz, F. M. "Black Death and the Silver Lining: Meaning, Continuity, and Revolutionary Change in Histories of Medieval Plague." *Journal of the History of Biology* 24 (1991): 265–89.

Ghosh, N. C. and K. Ismael. "Two Foreign Gold Coins from Excavations at Kudvalli, District Mhabubnagar, Andhra Pradesh." *Journal of the Numismatic Society of India* 42 (1980): 11–17.

Gilbert, M. T. P., J. Cuccui, W. White, N. Lynnerup, R. W. Titball, A. Cooper, and M. B. Prentice. "Absence of *Yersinia pestis*-Specific DNA in Human Teeth from Five European Excavations of Putative Plague Victims." *Microbiology* 150 (2004): 341–54.

Gilbert, M. T. P., J. Cuccui, W. White, N. Lynnerup, R. W. Titball, A. Cooper, and M. B. Prentice. "Response to Drancourt and Raoult." *Microbiology* 150 (2004): 264–5.

Gill, C. A. *The Genesis of Epidemics and the Natural History of Disease: An Introduction to the Science of Epidemiology Based upon the Study of Epidemics of Malaria, Influenza, and Plague.* London, 1928.

Gilliam, J. F. "The Plague under Marcus Aurelius." *American Journal of Philology* 82 (1961): 225–51.

Girard, G. "Les ectoparasites de l'homme dans l'épidémiologie de la peste." *Bulletin de la Société de Pathologie Exotique* 36 (1943): 4–43.

Girard, G. "A quelle époque remonte la présence du rat (*Rattus rattus*) en Europe?" *Bulletin de la Société de Pathologie Exotique* 67 (1974): 601–6.

Girard, J. M., D. M. Wagner, A. J. Vogler, C. Keys, C. J. Allender, L. C. Drickamer, and P. Keim. "Differential Plague-Transmission Dynamics Determine *Yersinia pestis* Population Genetic Structure on Local, Regional, and Global Scales." *PNAS* 101 (2004): 8408–13.

Glucker, C. A. M. *The City of Gaza in the Roman and Byzantine Periods*. BAR International Series 325. Oxford, 1987.

Goar, J. *Euchologion sive rituale graecorum*. Venice, 1730. Repr. Graz, 1960.

Goffart, W. *The Narrators of Barbarian History: Jordanes, Gregory of Tours, Bede and Paul the Deacon*. Princeton, 1988.

Gómez Santa Cruz, J. "Aproximación al poblamiento rural hispano-romano en la provincia de Soria," in *Actas Sorianas II* (1989): 937–56.

Gonzalez, M. D., C. A. Lichtensteiger, R. Caughlan, and E. R. Vimr. "Conserved Filamentous Prophage in *Escherichia coli* O18:K1:H7 and *Yersinia pestis* Biovar *orientalis*." *Journal of Bacteriology* 184 (2002): 6050–55.

González-Conde, M. P. *Romanidad e indigenismo en Carpetania*. Alicante, 1987.

Gordh, G. and D. Headrick, eds. *A Dictionary of Entomology*. Wallingford, 2001.

Gorges, J.-G. *Les villas hispano-romaines*. Paris, 1979.

Gottfried, R. S. *The Black Death: Natural and Human Disaster in Mediaeval Europe*. London, 1983.

Gottfried, R. S. "Review of Twigg, *Black Death: A Biological Reappraisal*." *Speculum* 61 (1986): 217–19.

Grattan, J. P. and F. B. Pyatt. "Volcanic Eruptions, Dry Fogs and the European Palaeoenvironmental Record: Localised Phenomena or Hemispheric Impacts?" *Global and Planetary Change* 21 (1999): 173–79.

Gratz, N. "Rodent Reservoirs and Flea Vectors of Natural Foci of Plague," in Dennis et al., *Plague Manual*, 63–96.

Greatrex, G. *Rome and Persia at War 502–532*. Leeds, 1996.

Gregg, C. T. *Plague: An Ancient Disease in the Twentieth Century*. Albuquerque, 1985.

Gregg, C. T. *Plague! The Shocking Story of a Dread Disease in America Today*. New York, 1978.

Gregoire, H., R. Goossens, and M. Mathieu. *Asklèpios, Apollon Smintheus et Rudra. Études sur le dieu à la taupe et le dieu au rat dans la Grèce et dans l'Inde*. Académie royale de Belgique, Classe des Lettres et des Sciences morales et politiques. Mémoires 45. Brussels, 1949.

Grégoire, R. *Les homéliaires du Moyen Âge: Inventaire et analyse des manuscrits*. Rome, 1966.

Griffin, J. P. "Bubonic Plague in Biblical Times." *Journal of the Royal Society of Medicine* 93 (2000): 449.

Grmek, M. "Les conséquences de la peste de Justinien dans l'Illyricum," in *Radovi XIII. međunarodnog kongresa za starokršćansku arheologiju*. Ed. N. Cambi and E. Marin. Split, 1998. 2: 787–94.

Grosjean, P. "La Date du Colloque de Whitby." *Analecta Bollandiana*. 78 (1960): 233–74.

Guidoboni, E., A. Comastri, and G. Traina. *Catalogue of Ancient Earthquakes in the Mediterranean Area up to the 10th Century*. Rome, 1994.

Guirand, F. ed. *New Larousse Encyclopedia of Mythology.* Trans. R. Aldington and D. Ames. London, 1987.

Guiyoule, A., F. Grimont, F. Iteman, P. A. Grimont, M. Lefevre, and F. Carniel. "Plague Pandemics Investigated by Ribotyping of *Yersinia pestis* Strains." *Journal of Clinical Microbiology* 32 (1994): 634–41.

Guiyoule, A., B. Rasoamanana, C. Buchrieser, P. Michel, S. Chanteau, and E. Carniel. "Recent Emergence of New Variants of *Yersinia pestis* in Madagascar." *Journal of Clinical Microbiology* 35 (1997): 2826–33.

Gunn, J. D., ed. *The Years Without Summer: Tracing A.D. 536 and its Aftermath.* BAR International Series 872. Oxford, 2000.

Gutiérrez Lloret, S. "Eastern Spain in the Sixth Century in the Light of Archaeology," in *The Sixth Century: Production, Distribution, and Demand.* Ed. R. Hodges and W. Bowden. Leiden, 1998. pp. 161–84.

Gutsmiedl, D. "Die justinianische Pest nördlich der Alpen? Zum Doppelgrab 166/167 aus dem frühmittelalterlichen Reihengräberfeld von Aschheim-Bajuwarenring." *Cum grano salis. Beiträge zur europäischen Vor- und Frühgeschichte. Festschrift für Volker Bierbrauer zum 65. Geburtstag.* Ed. B. Päffgen, E., Pohl, and M. Schmauder. Friedberg, 2005. pp. 199–208.

Haldon, J. *Byzantium in the Seventh Century: The Transformation of a Culture.* Revised ed. Cambridge, 1997.

Haldon, J. "Production, Distribution and Demand in the Byzantine World, c. 660–840," in *The Transformation of the Roman World.* Ed. I. L. Hansen and C. Wickham. Leiden, 2000. 2: 225–64.

Haldon, J. "The Works of Anastasius of Sinai: A Key Source for the History of Seventh-Century East Mediterranean Society and Belief," in *The Byzantine and Early Islamic Near East I: Problems in the Literary Source Material.* Ed. A. Cameron and L. I. Conrad. Princeton, 1992. pp. 107–48.

Hall, R. A. "York, 700–1050," in *The Rebirth of Towns in the West.* Council for British Archaeology, Research Report 68. Ed. R. Hodges and B. Hobley. London, 1988. pp. 125–32.

Hall, R. A. and H. K. Kenward. "Environmental Evidence from the Colonia: General Accident and Rougier Street," in *The Archaeology of York.* Ed. P. V. Addyman and V. E. Black. Dorchester, 1990. 14:289–434.

Hamerow, H. *Excavations at Mucking.* 2 vols. London, 1993.

Hamerow, H. "Settlement Mobility and the 'Middle Saxon Shift': Rural Settlements and Settlement Patterns in Anglo-Saxon England." *Anglo-Saxon England* 20 (1991): 1–18.

Hamilton, F. J. and E. W. Brooks. *The Syriac Chronicle Known as That of Zachariah of Mitylene.* London, 1899.

Han, Y. W. and V. L. Miller. "Reevaluation of the Virulence Phenotype of the *inv yadA* Double Mutants of *Yersinia pseudotuberculosis.*" *Infection and Immunity* 65 (1997): 327–30.

Hankin, E. H. "On the Epidemiology of Plague." *Journal of Hygiene* 5 (1905): 48–83.

Hardy, A. "Urban Famine or Urban Crisis? Typhus in the Victorian City." *Medical History* 32 (1988): 401–25.

Harrison, D. "Plague, Settlement and Structural Change at the Dawn of the Middle Ages." *Scandia* 59 (1993): 15–48.

Harrison, P. M. and M. Gerstein. "Studying Genomes through the Aeons: Protein Families, Pseudogenes and Proteome Evolution." *Journal of Molecular Biology* 318 (2002): 1155–74.

Hart, C. R. *The Early Charters of Eastern England.* Leicester, 1966.

Hasday, J. D., K. D. Fairchild, and D. Shanholtz. "The Role of Fever in the Infected Host." *Microbes and Infection* 2 (2002): 1891–904.

Hatcher, J. "England in the Aftermath of the Black Death." *Past and Present* 144 (1994): 3–35.

Hatcher, J. *Plague, Population and the English Economy, 1348–1530.* London, 1977.

Hecker, J. F. C. *The Black Death.* London, 1844. Repr., Lawrence, 1972.

Heinzelmann, M. *Gregory of Tours: History and Society in the Sixth Century.* Trans. C. Carroll. Cambridge, 2001.

Helleiner, K. F. "The Population of Europe from the Black Death to the Vital Revolution," in *The Cambridge Economic History of Europe.* Ed. E. E. Rich and C. H. Wilson. Cambridge, 1967. 4: 1–95.

Hendy, M. F. "Light Weight Solidi, Tetartera, and the Book of the Prefect." *Byzantinische Zeitschrift* 65 (1972): 57–80.

Herlihy, D. *The Black Death and the Transformation of the West.* Ed. S. K. Cohn. Cambridge, Mass., 1997.

Herlihy, D. *Opera Muliebria. Women and Work in Medieval Europe.* New York, 1990.

Hershleifer, J. *Disaster and Recovery.* Santa Monica, 1966.

Hertzberg, H. *Die Historien und die Chroniken des Isidorus. Eine Quellenuntersuchung. Erster Theil: Die Historien.* Göttingen, 1874.

Hill, D. and D. M. Metcalf, eds. *Sceattas in England and on the Continent.* British Archaeological Report. Brit. Ser. 128. Oxford, 1984.

Hinnebusch, B. J. "Bubonic Plague: A Molecular Genetic Case History of the Emergence of an Infectious Disease." *Journal of Molecular Medicine* 75 (1997): 645–52.

Hinnebusch, B. J., A. E. Rudolph, P. Cherepanov, J. E. Dixon, T. G. Schwan, and A. Forsberg. "Role of Yersinia Murine Toxin in Survival of *Yersinia pestis* in the Midgut of the Flea Vector." *Science* 296 (2002): 733–35.

Hinton, D. A. *Archaeology, Economy and Society: England from the Fifth to the Fifteenth Century.* London, 1990.

Hirst, L., F. *The Conquest of Plague: A Study of the Evolution of Epidemiology.* Oxford, 1953.

Hocart, A. M. *Kings and Councillors. An Essay in the Comparative Anatomy of Human Society.* Ed. R. Needham. Chicago and London, 1970.

Hodges, R. and D. Whitehouse. *Mohammed, Charlemagne and the Origins of Europe: Archaeology and the Pirenne Thesis.* Thesis Ithaca, 1983.

Hofreiter, M., D. Serre, H. N. Poinar, M. Kuch, and S. Pääbo. "Ancient DNA." *Nature Reviews. Genetics* 2 (2001): 353–9.

Holdsworth, P. *Excavations at Melbourne Street, Southampton, 1971–76.* London, 1980.

Holladay, A. J. and J. C. F. Poole. "Thucydides and the Plague of Athens." *Classical Quarterly* 29 (1979): 282–300.

Hollingsworth, M. F. and T. H. Hollingsworth. "Plague Mortality Rates by Age and Sex in the Parish of St. Botolph's Without Bishopsgate, London, 1603." *Population Studies* 25 (1971): 131–46.

Hollingsworth, T. H. *Historical Demography*. London, 1969.

Hooker, E. M. "Buboes in Thucydides?" *Journal of Hellenic Studies* 78 (1958): 78–83.

Hope-Taylor, B. *Yeavering: An Anglo-British Centre of Early Northumbria*. London, 1977.

Hopkins, G. H. E. and M. Rothschild. *An Illustrated Catalogue of the Rothschild Collection of Fleas (Siphonaptera) in the British Museum*, 1. London, 1953.

Horden, P. "Mediterranean Plague in the Age of Justinian," in *The Cambridge Companion to the Age of Justinian*. Ed. M. Maas. Cambridge, 2005. pp. 134–60.

Horrox, R., ed. and trans. *The Black Death*. Manchester Medieval Sources. Manchester, 1994.

Höss, M., P. Jaruga, T. H. Zastawny, M. Dizdaroglu, and S. Pääbo. "DNA Damage and DNA Sequence Retrieval from Ancient Tissues." *Nucleic Acids Research* 24 (1996): 1304–7.

Howard-Johnston, J. D. "'Heraclius' Persian Campaigns and the Revival of the East Roman Empire." *War and History*. 6.1 (1999): 1–44.

Howard-Johnston, J. D. "The Two Great Powers in Late Antiquity: A Comparison," in *The Byzantine and Early Islamic Near East, III: States, Resources and Armies*. Ed. A. Cameron. Princeton, 1995.

Hudson, G. F. "The Medieval Trade of China," in *Islam and the Trade of Asia*. Ed. D. S. Richards. Oxford, 1970. pp. 159–67.

Hughes, K. and A. Hamlin. *Celtic Monasticism: The Modern Traveler to the Early Irish Church*. New York, 1981.

Hummel, S. *Ancient DNA Typing: Methods, Strategies, and Applications*. Berlin, 2003.

Hummel, S., G. Nordsiek, J. Rameckers, C. Lassen, H. Zierdt, H. Baron and B. Herrmann. "aDNA-Ein neuer Zugang zu alten Fragen." *Zeitschrift für Morphologie und Anthropologie* 81 (1995): 41–65.

Inglesby, T. V., D. T. Dennis, D. A. Henderson, J. G. Bartlett, M. S. Ascher, E. Eitzen, A. D. Fine, et al. "Plague as a Biological Weapon: Medical and Public Health Management." *Journal of the American Medical Association* 283 (2000): 2281–90.

Jacoby, A. "La population de Constantinople à l'époque byzantine: Un problème de démographie urbaine." *Byzantion* 31 (1961): 81–109.

James, E. "Ireland and Western Gaul in the Merovingian Period," in *Ireland in Early Medieval Europe: Studies in Memory of Kathleen Hughes*. Ed. D. Whitelock, R. McKitterick, and D. Dumville. Cambridge, 1982. pp. 362–86.

James, S. and M. Millett. "Excavations at Cowdery's Down, Basingstoke, Hampshire, 1978–81." *Archaeology Journal* 140 (1983): 151–279.

James, T. "Procopius and the Great Plague of 542 AD." *Adler Museum Bulletin* 5.3 (1979): 5–9.

Jaski, B. *Early Irish Kingship and Succession*. Dublin, 2000.

Jennings, W. E. *A Manual of Plague*. London, 1903.

John, T. J. "India: Is it Plague?" *Lancet* 344 (1994): 1359–60.

Jones, A. H. M. *The Later Roman Empire, 284–602: A Social, Economic and Administrative Survey.* 2 vols. Baltimore, 1964.

Jones, A. H. M., Martindale, J. R., and J. Morris. *The Prosopography of the Later Roman Empire.* 3 vols. Cambridge, 1971–92.

Kalabukhov, N. I. "The Structure and Natural Dynamics of Natural Foci of Plague." *Journal of Hygiene, Epidemiology, Microbiology and Immunology* 9 (1965): 147–59.

Kaplan, M. *Les hommes et la terre à Byzance du VIe au XIe siècle: propriété et exploitation du sol.* Byzantina Sorbonensia 10. Paris, 1992.

Karimi, Y., M. Eftekhari, and C. R. Almeida. "Sur l'écologie des puces impliquées dans l'épidémiologie de la peste et le rôle éventuel de certains insectes hématophages dans son processus au Nord-est du Brésil." *Bulletin de la Société de Pathologie Exotique* 67 (1974): 583–91.

Karlsson, G. "Plague without Rats: The Case of Fifteenth-Century Iceland." *Journal of Medieval History* 22 (1996): 263–84.

Kearns, G. "Zivilis or Hygaeia: Urban Public Health and the Epidemiologic Transition," in *The Rise and Fall of Great Cities: Aspects of Urbanization in the Western World.* Ed. R. Lawton. London, 1989. pp. 96–124.

Keeling, M. J. and C. A. Gilligan. "Bubonic Plague: A Metapopulation Model of a Zoonosis." *Proceedings of the Royal Society of London, series B, Biological sciences* 267 (2000): 2219–30.

Keeling, M. J. and C. A. Gilligan. "Metapopulation Dynamics of Bubonic Plague." *Nature* 407 (2000): 903–6.

Keen, M. H. *English Society in the Later Middle Ages.* London, 1990.

Kennedy, H. "Antioch: From Byzantium to Islam," in *The City in Late Antiquity.* Ed. J. Rich. London, 1992. pp. 181–98.

Kerenyi, K. *Der göttliche Arzt. Studien über Asklepios und seine Kultstätter.* Darmstadt, 1956.

Keys, D. *Catastrophe. An Investigation into the Origins of the Modern World.* London, 1999.

King, P. D. *Law and Society in the Visigothic Kingdom.* Cambridge, 1972.

Kirby, D. P. "Bede, Eddius Stephanus and the 'Life of Wilfrid.'" *English History Review* 98 (1983): 106–08.

Kirby, D. P. "Bede's Native Sources for the *Historia Ecclesiastica*." *Bulletin of the John Rylands Library* 48 (1966): 341–71.

Kirk, G. E. and C. B. Welles. "The Inscriptions," in *Excavations at Nessana I.* Ed. H. D. Colt. London, 1962. pp. 131–97.

Kislinger, E. "Ein Angriff zu viel. Zur Verteidigung der Thermopylen in justinianischer Zeit." *Byzantinische Zeitschrift* 91 (1998): 49–58.

Kislinger, E. and D. Stathakopoulos. "Pest und Perserkrieg bei Prokop. Chronologische Überlegungen zum Geschehen 540–545." *Byzantion* 69 (1999): 76–98.

Knowles, D. *The Religious Orders in England.* 3 vols. Cambridge, 1948–59.

Kobischanov, Y. M. *Axum.* Trans. L. T. Kapitanoff. London, 1979.

Koder, J. "Ein inschriftlicher Beleg zur 'justinianischen' Pest in Zora (Azra'a)." *Byzantinoslavica* 56 (1995): 13–18.

Koder, J. "Climatic Change in the Fifth and Sixth Centuries?" in *The Sixth Century: End or Beginning?* Byzantina Australiensia 10. Ed. P. Allen and E. Jeffreys. Brisbane, 1996. pp. 270–85.

Köhler, W. "Pest, Pestheilige, Blutwunder und andere Begebenheiten aus der Geschichte der Bakteriologie." *Leopoldina* 37 (1992): 211–38.

Kötting, B. "Endzeitprognosen zwischen Lactantius und Augustinus." *Historisches Jahrbuch* 77 (1958): 125–39.

Kolman, C. J. and N. Tuross. "Ancient DNA Analysis of Human Populations." *American Journal of Physical Anthropology* 111 (2000): 5–23.

Kondoleon, C. *Antioch: The Lost Ancient City.* Princeton, 2000.

Krappe, A. H. "Apollon Σμίνθεύς and the Teutonic Mysing." *Archiv für Religionswissenschaft* 33 (1936): 40–56.

Krautheimer, R. *Rome, Profile of a City, 312–1308.* Princeton, 1980.

Kudlick, C. *Cholera in Post-Revolutionary Paris: A Cultural History.* Berkeley, 1996.

Kudlien, F. "Poseidonios und die Ärzteschule der Pneumatiker." *Hermes* 90 (1962): 419–29.

Kulikowski, M. "The Interdependence of Town and Country in Late Antique Spain," in *Urban Centers and Rural Contexts in Late Antiquity.* Ed. T. S. Burns and J. W. Eadie. East Lansing, 2001. pp. 147–61.

Kulikowski, M. *Late Roman Spain and Its Cities.* Baltimore, 2004.

Laforce, F. M., I. L. Acharya, G. Stott, P. S. Brachman, A. F. Kaufman, R. F. Clap, and N. K. Shah. "Clinical and Epidemiological Observations on an Outbreak of Plague in Nepal." *Bulletin WHO* 45 (1971): 693–706.

Lagerlöf, N.-P. "Diseases and Growth." 2002. Available from World Wide Web: ⟨http://www.alcor.concordia.ca/~nippe/scandjournmalthus3.pdf⟩.

Lamb, H. H. *Climate, History and the Modern World.* London, 1982.

Lapidge, M. "The Archetype of Beowulf." *Anglo-Saxon England* 29 (2000): 5–41.

Lastufka K. "Bohemia during the Medieval Black Death: A Pocket of Immunity." *East European Quarterly* 19 (1985): 275–80.

Leach, P. E. *Archaeology in Kent to AD 1500.* London, 1982.

Leclercq, H. "Rogations." *Dictionnaire d'Archéologie chrétienne et de liturgie* 14.2:2459.

Lemerle, P. *Les plus anciens recueils des Miracles de Saint Démétrius et la pénétration des Slaves dans les Balkans.* Vol I. Paris, 1979.

Lenski, R. E. "Evolution of Plague Virulence." *Nature* 334 (1988): 473–74.

Lerner, R. E. "The Black Death and Western European Eschatological Mentalities," in *The Black Death: The Impact of the Fourteenth-Century Plague.* Ed. D. Williman. Binghamton, New York, 1982. pp. 77–105.

Le Roy Ladurie, E. "Un concept: L'unification microbienne du monde (XIVe– XVIIe siècles)." *Schweizerische Zeitschrift für Geschichte* 23 (1973): 627–96.

Leven, K. H. "*Athumia* and *Philanthropia*: Social Reactions to Plagues in Late Antiquity and Early Byzantine Society." *Clio Medica* 28 (1995): 393–407.

Leven, K. H. "Die 'Justinianische' Pest." *Jahrbuch des Instituts für Geschichte der Medizin der Robert Bosch Stiftung* 6 (1987): 137–61.

Leven, K. H. "Krankheiten – historische Deutung versus retrospective Diagnose," in *Medizingeschichte: Aufgaben, Probleme, Perspektiven.* Ed. N. Paul and T. Schlich. New York, 1998. pp. 153–85.

Levison, W. "Bede as Historian," in *Bede: His Life, Times and Writings.* Ed. A. H. Thompson. Oxford, 1935. pp. 111–51.

Lewinstein, K. "The Revaluation of Martyrdom in Early Islam," in *Sacrificing the Self: Perspectives on Martyrdom and Religion.* Ed. M. Cormack. New York, 2001. pp. 78–91.

Liebeschuetz, J. *Decline and Fall of the Roman City.* Oxford, 2001.

Lilie, R. J. *Die byzantinische Reaktion auf die Ausbreitung der Araber.* Miscellenea Byzantina Monascensia 22. Munich, 1976.

Limberis, V. *Divine Heiress. The Virgin Mary and the Creation of Christian Constantinople.* London and New York, 1994.

Lindley, P. and M. Ormrod, eds. *The Black Death in England.* Stamford, 1996.

Link, V. *A History of Plague in the United States.* U.S.P.H.S. Public Health Monograph 26. Washington, D.C., 1953.

Lloyd, A. and O. Springer. *Etymologisches Wörterbuch des Althochdeutschen.* Vol. 1. Göttingen and Zurich, 1988.

Lloyd, J. E. *A History of Wales from the Earliest Times to the Edwardian Conquest.* 3rd ed. 2 vols. London, 1939.

Lobel, M. D., ed. *The City of London from Prehistoric Times to c.1520.* The British Atlas of Historic Towns. Vol. 3. Oxford, 1989.

Loosjes, F. E. "Is the Brown Rat (Rattus norvegicus Berkenhout) Responsible for the Disappearance of Plague from Western Europe?" *Documents in Medicine and Geography of the Tropics* 8 (1956): 175–78.

López i Vilar, J. "Un nuevo conjunto paleocristiano en las afueras de Tarraco." *Revista de Arquelogía* 197 (1997): 58–64.

Lounghis, T. Επισκόπιση βυζαντινής ιστορίας. 2nd ed. Vol. 1. Athens, 1998.

Loyn, H. R. *Anglo-Saxon England and the Norman Conquest.* 2nd ed. London, 1991.

Lucier, T. S. and R. R. Brubaker. "Determination of Genome Size, Macrorestriction Pattern Polymorphism, and Non-Pigmentation-Specific Deletion in *Yersinia pestis* by Pulsed-Field Gel Electrophoresis." *Journal of Bacteriology* 174 (1992): 2078–86.

Lucotte, G. "Distribution of the CCR5 Gene 32-Basepair Deletion in West Europe: A Hypothesis about the Possible Dispersion of the Mutation by the Vikings in Historical Times." *Human Immunology* 62 (2001): 933–36.

MacArthur, W. "The Identification of Some Pestilences Recorded in the Irish Annals." *Irish Historical Studies* 6 (1949): 169–88.

MacArthur, W. "The Medical Identification of Some Pestilences of the Past." *Transactions of the Royal Society of Tropical Medicine and Hygiene* 53 (1959): 423–39.

Macchiarelli, R. and L. Salvadei. "Early Medieval Human Skeletons from the Thermae of Venosa, Italy. Skeletal Biology and Life Stresses in a Group Presumably Inhumed Following an Epidemic." *Rivista di antropologia* 67 (1989): 105–28.

MacLagan, T. J. "The Early Cases of a Typhus Outbreak." *Edinburgh Medical Journal* 19 (1873/74): 965–87.

MacLean, D. "Scribe as Artist not Monk: The 'Canon Tables of Ailerán the Wise' and the Book of Kells." *Peritia* 17–18 (2003–4): 433–68.

MacNeill, M. *Festival of Lughnasa.* Oxford, 1962.

Maddicott, J. R. "Plague in Seventh-Century England." *Past and Present* 156 (1997): 7–54.

Magdalino, P. "The History of the Future and its Uses: Prophecy, Policy and Propaganda," in *The Making of Byzantine History. Studies Dedicated to Donald M. Nicol on his Seventieth Birthday.* Ed. R. Beaton and C. Roueché. Aldershot, 1993. pp. 3–34.

Manganaro, G. "Byzantina Siciliae." *Minima Epigraphica et Papyrologica* 4 (2001): 133.

Mar, R., J. López i Vilar, O. Tobías, I. Peña, and L. Palahí. "El conjunto pale-ocristiano del Francolí en Tarragona. Nuevas aportaciones." *Antiquité Tardive* 4 (1996): 320–24.

Marasco, G. "Cléopâtre et les sciences de son temps," in *Sciences exactes et sciences appliquées à Alexandrie (IIIe siècle av. J.-C.-Ier siècle ap. J.-C.).* Ed. G. Argoud and J.-Y. Guillaumin. Saint-Étienne, 1998. pp. 39–53.

Margerison, B. J. and C. J. Knusel. "Paleodemographic Comparison of a Catastrophic and an Attritional Death Assemblage." *American Journal of Physical Anthropology* 119 (2002): 134–43.

Marienlexikon. Ed. R. Baümer and L. Scheffczyk. 8 vols. St. Ottilien, 1988–94.

Marín Jordá, C., J. Piá Brisa, and M. Rosselló i Mesquida. *El foro romano de Valentia.* Quaderns de Difusió Arqueològica 4. Valencia, 1999.

Marín Jordá, C., A. Ribera i Lacomba, and M. Rossello i Mesquida. *L'Almoina: De la fundació de València als orígens del cristianisme.* Valencia, 1999.

Márquez Villora, J. C. *El comercio romano en el Portus Ilicitanus.* Alicante, 1999.

Marshall, A. and G. Marshall. "Differentiation, Change and Continuity in Anglo-Saxon Buildings." *Archaeology Journal* 150 (1993): 366–402.

Marshall, L. "Manipulating the Sacred: Image and Plague in Renaissance Italy." *Renaissance Quarterly* 45 (1992): 485–532.

Mateos Cruz, P. *La basílica de Santa Eulalia de Mérida. Arqueología y urbanismo.* Anejos del Archivo Español de Arqueología 19. Madrid, 1999.

Matthews, C. and S. Hawkes. "Early Anglo-Saxon Settlements and Burials on Puddlehill, Near Dunstable, Bedfordshire." *Anglo-Saxon Studies in Archaeology and History* 4 (1985): 59–115.

Mavalankar, D. V. "Indian 'Plague' Epidemic: Unanswered Questions and Key Lessons." *Journal of the Royal Society of Medicine* 88 (1995): 547–51.

Mayr-Harting, H. *The Coming of Christianity to Anglo-Saxon England.* London, 1972.

McArthur, N. *Island Populations of the Pacific.* Canberra, 1968.

McCarthy, D. "The Chronology of Saint Colum Cille," papers given at the School of Celtic Studies. Dublin, 2001. Consult http://www.celt.dias.ie/english/tionol/tionolo1.html.

McCormick, M. "Bateaux de vie, bateaux de mort: Maladie, commerce, transports annonaires et le passage économique du Bas-Empire au Moyen Âge," in *Morfologie sociali e culturali in Europa fra tarda antichità e alto Medioevo.* Settimane di studio del Centro italiano di studi sull'alto Medioevo 45. Spoleto, 1998. pp. 35–118.

McCormick, M. *Origins of the European Economy. Communications and Commerce, A. D. 300–900.* Cambridge, 2001.

McCormick, M. "Rats, Communications, and Plague: Toward an Ecological History." _Journal of Interdisciplinary History_ 34 (2003): 1–25.

McKeough, A. "Ring-A-Ring-A-Rosy: Can DNA Analysis Identify the Presence of the Plague Bacillus in Archaeological Remains?" B.A. Thesis, University of Queensland, 2001.

McKeough, A. and T. Loy. "Ring-A-Ring-A-Rosy: DNA Analysis of the Plague Bacillus from Late Mediaeval London," in Abstracts of the 6th International Ancient DNA Conference. Tel Aviv, 2002, in _Ancient Biomolecules_ 4 (2002): 145.

McNeill, W. H. _Plagues and Peoples_. New York, 1976. Rep. with new preface, New York, 1998.

McVaugh, M. R. "Review of Cohn, _Black Death Transformed._" _Bulletin of the History of Medicine_ 78 (2004): 212–13.

Meaney, A. _A Gazeteer of Early Anglo-Saxon Burial Sites_. London, 1964.

Meaney, A. and S. Hawkes. _Two Anglo-Saxon Cemeteries at Winnall_. London, 1970.

Mecsas, J., G. Franklin, W. A. Kuziel, R. R. Brubaker, S. Falkow, and D. E. Mosier. "CCR5 Mutation and Plague Protection." _Nature_ 427 (2004): 606.

Meier, M. "Beobachtungen zu den sogenannten Pestschilderungen bei Thukydides II 47–54 und bei Prokop, Bell. Pers. II 22–23." _Tyche_ 14 (1999): 177–210.

Mendenhall, G. E. _The Tenth Generation: The Origins of the Biblical Tradition_. Baltimore, 1973.

Metcalf, D. M. "The Metrology of Justinian's Follis." _Numismatic Chronicle_ 20 (1960): 210–19.

Metcalf, D. M. "Sceattas Found at the Iron-Age Hill Fort of Walbury Camp, Berkshire." _British Numismatic Journal_ 44 (1974): 1–12.

Meyer, K. "The Laud Genealogies and Tribal Histories." _Zeitschrift für celtische Philologie_ 8 (1912): 292–338.

Meyvaert, P. "Church Paintings at Wearmouth Jarrow." _Anglo-Saxon England_ 8 (1979): 63–77.

Migliani, R., M. Ratsitorahina, L. Rahalison, I. Rakotoarivony, J. B. Duchemin, J. M. Duplantier, J. Rakotonomenjanahary, and S. Chanteau. "Résurgence de la peste dans le district d'Ikongo B Madagascar en 1998. 1. Aspects épidémiologiques dans la population humaine." _Bulletin de la Société de pathologie exotique_ 94 (2001): 115–18.

Miket, R. and C. O'Brien. "The Early Medieval Settlement of Thirlings, Northumberland." _Durham Archaeology Journal_ 7 (1991): 57–91.

Miller, T. S. _The Birth of the Hospital in the Byzantine Empire_. 2nd ed. Baltimore and London, 1997.

Miller, T. S. "The Plague in John VI Cantacuzenus." _Greek, Roman and Byzantine Studies_ 17 (1976): 385–95.

Mills, I. D. "The 1918–1919 Influenza Pandemic – The Indian Experience." _Indian Economic and Social History Review_ 23 (1986): 17–32.

Miskimin, H. A. _The Economy of Early Renaissance Europe, 1300–1460_. Cambridge, 1975.

Mollaret, H. and J. Brossollet. _Alexandre Yersin, 1863–1943: Un pasteurien en Indochine_. Paris, 1993.

Morin, G., ed. _Liber comicus sive lectionarius missae quo Toletana Ecclesia ante annos mille et ducentos utebatur_. Anecdota Maredsolana 1. Mardesous, 1893.

Morony, M. G. "Michael the Syrian as a Source for Economic History." *Hugoye: Journal of Syriac Studies* (electronic) 3.2 (2000). See http://syrcom.cua.edu/ Hugoye/.

Morpurgo, P. "La peste: Dinamiche di interpretazione storiografica," in *The Regulation of Evil: Social and Cultural Attitudes to Epidemics in the Late Middle Ages.* Ed. A. P. Bagliani and F. Santi. Florence, 1998. pp. 41–61.

Morris, C. "Plague in Britain," in *The Plague Reconsidered: A New Look at its Origins and Effects in 16th and 17th Century England.* Matlock, 1977.

Morris, C. "Review of Shrewsbury, *History of Bubonic Plague.*" *The Historical Journal* 14 (1971): 205–15.

Morris, J. *The Age of Arthur.* London, 1973.

Morris, R. J. *Cholera 1832: The Social Response to an Epidemic.* New York, 1976.

Morton, R. D., ed. *Excavations at Hamwic.* Council for British Archaeology, Research Report 84, London, 1992.

Motin, V. L., A. M. Georgescu, J. M. Elliott, P. Hu, P. L. Worsham, L. L. Ott, T. R. Slezak, et al. "Genetic Variability of *Yersinia pestis* Isolates as Predicted by PCR-Based IS*100* Genotyping and Analysis of Structural Genes Encoding Glycerol-3-Phosphate Dehydrogenase (*glpD*)." *Journal of Bacteriology* 184 (2002): 1019–27.

Müller, A. E. "Getreide für Konstantinopel. Überlegungen zu Justinians Edikt XIII als Grundlage für Aussagen zur Einwohnerzahl Konstantinopels im 6. Jahrhundert." *Jahrbuch der Österreichischen Byzantinistik* 43 (1993): 1–20.

Munro-Hay, S. *Aksum. An African Civilisation of Late Antiquity.* Edinburgh, 1991.

Muratori, L. A. *Del governo della peste.* Rome, 1743.

Narasmahmurthy, A. V. "Numismatic Studies in Karnataka." *Journal of the Numismatic Society of India* 47 (1985): 1–10.

Nau, F. "Analyse de la seconde partie inédite de l'Histoire ecclésiastique de Jean d'Asie, patriarche jacobite de Constantinople († 585)." *Revue de l'Orient chrétien* 2 (1897): 455–493.

Nau, F. "Un colloque du patriarch Jean avec l'émir des Agaréens et faits divers des années 712 à 716 d'après le ms. British Museum Add. 17193." *Journal Asiatique* 11, 5 (1915): 225–79.

Navarre, O. *"Ludi Publici,"* in *Dictionnaire des antiquités grecques et romaines.* Ed. Charles Daremberg and Edmond Saglio. Vol. 3, part 2. Paris, 1904. pp. 1362–79.

Negev, A. *The Greek Inscriptions from the Negev.* Studium Biblicum Franziscanum, Collectio Minor 25. Jerusalem, 1981.

Noddle, B. A. *Animal Bones from Jarrow.* Unpublished Ancient Monuments Laboratory Report 80/87. London, n.d.

Noethlichs, L. "Heidenverfolgung." *Reallexicon für Antike und Christentum* 13: 1169–71.

Norris J. "East or West? The Geographic Origin of the Black Death." *Bulletin of the History of Medicine* 51 (1977): 1–24.

Oakley, S. P. *A Commentary on Livy, Books VI–X.* 2 vols. Oxford, 1998,

Oberhelman, S. M. "On the Chronology and Pneumatism of Aretaios of Cappadocia," in *Aufstieg und Niedergang der römischen Welt* 37.2 (1994): 941–66.

O'Connor, T. P. *Animal Bones from Flaxengate, Lincoln, c.870–1500.* Archaeology of Lincoln, 18, pt 1. London, 1982.

O'Connor, T. P. *Bones from Anglo-Scandinavian Levels at 16–22 Coppergate.* The Archaeology of York 15, fasc. 3. London, 1989.

O'Connor, T. P. *Bones from 46–54 Fishergate.* The Archaeology of York 15, fasc. 4. London, 1991.

O'Connor, T. P. *Bones from the General Accident Site, Tanner Row.* The Archaeology of York 15, fasc. 2. London, 1988.

O'Connor, T. P. "On the Lack of Bones of the Ship Rat *Rattus rattus* from Dark Age York." *Journal of Zoology, London* 224 (1991): 318–20.

Ó Cróinín, D. *Early Medieval Ireland, 400–1200.* London, 1995.

Orchard, A. *A Critical Companion to Beowulf.* Cambridge, 2003.

Orlandis, J. *Hispania y Zaragoza en la antigüedad tardia: Estudios varios.* Zaragoza, 1984.

Orlandis, J. *Historia del reino visigodo español.* Madrid, 1988.

Orlandis, J. "Homilías visigóticas de Clade," in *Hispania y Zaragoza en la antigüedad tardía.* Zaragoza, 1984. pp. 115–22.

Orssaud, D. "Le passage de la céramique byzantine à la céramique islamique," in *La Syrie de Byzance à l'Islam.* Ed. P. Canivet and J.-P. Rey-Coquais. Damascus, 1992, pp. 219–28.

Otten, L. "The Problem of the Seasonal Prevalence of Plague." *Journal of Hygiene* 32 (1932): 396–405.

Ovitt, G. "Manual Labor and Early Medieval Monasticism." *Viator* 17 (1986): 1–18.

Oyston, P. "Plague Virulence." *Journal of Medical Microbiology* 50 (2001): 1015–17.

Paine, R. R. "If a Population Crashes in Prehistory, and There is No Paleodemographer There to Hear It, Does It Make a Sound?" *American Journal of Physical Anthropology* 112 (2000): 181–190.

Palmer, A. *The Seventh-Century in the West-Syrian Chronicles.* Liverpool, 1993.

Panagiotakopulu, E. *Archaeology and Entomology in the Eastern Mediterranean: Research into the History of Insect Synanthropy in Greece and Egypt.* British Archaeological Reports, International Series 836. Oxford, 2000.

Panzac, D. *La peste dans l'Empire ottoman, 1700–1850.* Leuven, 1985.

Papastratos, D. Χάρτινες Εικόνες. Ορθόδοξα θρησκευτικά χαρακετικά 1665–1899. Vol. 1. Athens, 1986.

Parker, R. *Miasma: Pollution and Purification in Early Greek Religion.* Oxford, 1983.

Parkes. M. *The Scriptorium of Wearmouth-Jarrow.* Jarrow Lecture, 1982.

Parkhill, J., B. W. N. Wren, R. Thomson, R. W. M. Titball, T. G. Holden, M. B. Prentice, M. Sebaihia, et al. "Genome Sequence of *Yersinia pestis*, the Causative Agent of Plague." *Nature* 413 (2001): 523–27.

Parmenter, R. R., E. P. Yadav, C. A. Parmenter, P. Ettestad, and K. L. Gage. "Incidence of Plague Associated with Increased Winter-Spring Precipitation in New Mexico." *American Journal of Tropical Medicine and Hygiene* 61 (1999): 814–21.

Patlagean, E. *Pauvreté économique et pauvreté sociale à Byzance 4e-7e siècles.* Civilisations et sociétés 48. Paris, 1977.

Paul, J. R. *A History of Poliomyelitis.* New Haven, 1971.

Payne-Smith, J. *A Compendious Syriac Dictionary.* Oxford, 1903.

Penhallurick, R. D. *Tin in Antiquity.* London, 1986.

Périn, P. *Catalogues d'art et d'histoire du Musée Carnavalet.* Vol. 2. *Collections mérovingiennes.* Paris, 1985.

Perry, R. D. and J. D. Fetherston. "*Yersinia pestis* – Etiologic Agent of Plague." *Clinical Microbiology Reviews* 10 (1997): 35–66.

Pesci, B. "Il culto di San Sebastiano a Roma nell' Antichità e nel medioevo." *Antonianum* 20 (1945): 177–200.

La peste nera: Dati di una realtà ed elementi di una interpretazione. Atti del XXX Convegno storico internazionale, Todi, 10–13 ottobre 1993. Spoleto, 1994.

Petrie, G. F. and R. E. Todd. "A Report on Plague Investigations in Egypt." *Journal of Hygiene* 23 (1924): 117–50.

Peters, W. and H. M. Gilles. *A Colour Atlas of Tropical Medicine and Parasitology.* London, 1977.

Phillimore, E. "The Annales Cambriae and Old-Welsh Genealogies from Harlein MS 3859." *Y Cymmrodor* 9 (1888): 141–83.

Phillips, J. "Punt and Aksum: Egypt and the Horn of Africa." *Journal of African History* 38 (1997): 423–57.

Picard, J. M. "Adomnán's *Vita Columbae* and the Cult of Colum Cille in Continental Europe." *Proceedings of the Royal Irish Academy* 98C (1998): 1–23.

Piganiol, A. *Recherches sur les jeux romains. Notes d'archéologie et d'histoire religieuse.* Publications de la Faculté des Lettres de l'Université de Strasbourg 13. Paris, 1923.

Piotrovski, M. B. "L'économie de l'Arabie préislamique," in *L'Arabie avant l'Islam.* Ed. B. Chiesa, V. Colomba, G. Crespi, G. Garbini, S., Noja, and M. Piotrovski. Aix-en-Provence, 1994.

Pitsakes, K., "Η θέση των ομοφυλοφίλων στη βυζαντινή κοινωνία," in *Οι Πριθωριακοί στο Βυζάντιο.* Ed. C. Maltezou. Athens, 1993. pp. 207–18.

Poirier, S. *Chicago's War on Syphilis, 1937–1940: The Times, the 'Trib,' and the Clap Doctor.* Urbana, 1995.

Pollitzer, R. *Plague.* Geneva, 1954.

Potts, D. T. *Mesopotamian Civilization: The Material Foundations.* London, 1997.

Pounds, N. J. G. *An Economic History of Medieval Europe.* 2nd ed. London, 1994.

Pourcel, C., F. André-Mazeaud, H. Neubauer, F. Ramisse, and G. Vergnaud. "Tandem Repeats Analysis for the High Resolution Phylogenetic Analysis of *Yersinia pestis.*" *BMC Microbiology* (electronic) 4 (2004): article no. 22.

Powell, J. H. *Bring Out Your Dead: The Great Plague of Yellow Fever in Philadelphia in 1793.* Philadelphia, 1949.

Power, E. *Medieval English Nunneries, c. 1275–1535.* Cambridge, 1922.

Prentice, M. B., K. D. James, J. Parkhill, S. G. Baker, K. Stevens, M. N. Simmonds, K. L. Mungall, et al. "*Yersinia pestis* pFra Shows Biovar-Specific Differences and Recent Common Ancestry with a Salmonella Enterica Serovar Typhi Plasmid." *Journal of Bacteriology* 183 (2001): 2586–94.

Prins, G. "But What Was the Disease? The Present State of Health and Healing in African Studies." *Past and Present* 124 (1989): 159–79.

Pullan, B. "Plague and Perceptions of the Poor in Early Modern Italy," in *Epidemics and Ideas: Essays on the Historical Perception of Pestilence.* Ed. T. Ranger and P. Slack. Cambridge, 1992. pp. 101–23.

Pusch, C. M., L. Rahalison, N. Blin, G. J. Nicholson, and A. Czarnetzki. "Yersinial F1 Antigen and the Cause of Black Death." *Lancet: Infectious Diseases* 4 (2004): 484–85.

Quétel, C. *History of Syphilis*. Baltimore, 1990.

Rackham, J. *Environment and Economy in Anglo-Saxon England*. Council for British Archaeology Research Report 89, London, 1994.

Rackham, J. "*Rattus Rattus*: the Introduction of the Black Rat into Britain." *Antiquity* 53 (1979): 112–20.

Radnedge, L., P. G. Agron, P. L. Worsham, and G. L. Andersen. "Genome Plasticity in *Yersinia pestis*." *Microbiology* 148 (2002): 1687–98.

Ramaley, P. A., N. French, P. Kaleebu, C. Gilks, J. Whitworth, and A. V. S. Hill. "Chemokine Receptor Genes and AIDS Risk." *Nature* 417 (2002): 140.

Ramírez Sádaba, J. L. "Panorámica religiosa de *Augusta Emerita*," in *Religio Deorum: Actas del Coloquio Internacional de Epigrafía: Culto y Sociedad en Occidente*. Ed. M. Mayer. Barcelona, 1988. pp. 389–98.

Ramsay, J. H. *Genesis of Lancaster*. 2 vols. Oxford, 1913.

Raoult, D., G. Aboudharam, E. Crubé, G. Larrouy, B. Ludes, and M. Drancourt. "Molecular Identification by 'Suicide PCR' of *Yersinia pestis* as the Agent of Medieval Black Death." *PNAS* 97 (2000): 12880–83.

Ratsitorahina, M. "Seroepidemiology of Human Plague in the Madagascar Highlands." *Tropical Medicine and International Health* 5.2 (2000): 94–98.

Ratsitorahina, M., S. Chanteau, L. Rahalison, L. Ratsifasoamanana, and P. Boisier. "Epidemiological and Diagnostic Aspects of the Outbreak of Pneumonic Plague in Madagascar." *Lancet* 355 (2000): 111–13.

Razi, Z. *Life, Marriage and Death in a Medieval Parish: Economy, Society, and Demography in Halesowen, 1270–1400*. Cambridge, 1980.

Reimann, D., K. Düwel, and A. Bartel. "Vereint in den Tod – Doppelgrab 166/167 aus Aschheim." *Das archäologische Jahr in Bayern, 1999*. Stuttgart, 2000. pp. 83–85.

Renardy, C. "Un témoin de la grande peste: Maître Simon de Couvin, chanoine de Saint-Jean L'Évangéliste à Liège (†1367)." *Revue Belge de Philologie et d'Histoire* (1974): 273–92.

Renouard, Y. "Conséquences et intérêt démographiques de la peste noir de 1348." *Population* 2 (1948): 459–66.

Reports of the Advisory Committee on Plague Investigations in India. XXI. "Digest of Recent Observations on the Epidemiology of Plague." *Journal of Hygiene* 7 (1907): 694–723.

Reports of the Advisory Committee on Plague Investigations in India. XXIII. "Epidemiological Observations in the Villages of Sion, Wadhala, Parel and Worli in Bombay Village." *Journal of Hygiene* 7 (1907): 799–873.

Reports of the Advisory Committee on Plague Investigations in India. XXII. "The Epidemiological Observations Made by the Commission in Bombay City." *Journal of Hygiene* 7 (1907): 724–98.

Reports of the Advisory Committee on Plague Investigations in India. XX. "A Note on Man as a Host of the Indian Rat Flea (*P. cheopis*)." *Journal of Hygiene* 7 (1907): 472–76.

Reports of the Advisory Committee on Plague Investigations in India. XLVI. "Observations on Plague in Eastern Bengal and Assam." *Journal of Hygiene* 13 (1912): 157–92.

Reports of the Advisory Committee on Plague Investigations in India. II. "On the Existence of Chronic Plague in Rats in Localities Where Plague is Endemic." *Journal of Hygiene* 6 (1906): 530–36.

Reports of the Advisory Committee on Plague Investigations in India. XIX. "On the Natural Occurrence of Chronic Plague in Rats." *Journal of Hygiene* 7 (1907): 457–71.

Reports of the Advisory Committee on Plague Investigations in India. XXXIV. "Resolving (Chronic) Plague in Rats." *Journal of Hygiene* 10 (1910): 335–48.

Reynolds, P. *Settlement and Pottery in the Vinalopó Valley (Alicante, Spain) A.D. 400–700*. British Archaeological Reports International Series 588. Oxford, 1993.

Ribera, A. and R. Soriano. "Enterramientos de la Antigüedad tardía en Valentia." *Lucentum* 6 (1987): 139–64.

Ribera i Lacomba, A. and M. Rosselló i Mesquida. *L'Almoina: El nacimiento de la Valentia cristiana*. Quaderns de Difusió Arqueològica 5. Valencia, 1999.

Ribera i Lacomba, A., and R. Soriano Sánchez. "Los cementerios de época visigoda." *Saitabi* 46 (1996): 195–230.

Riché, P. "Problèmes de démographie historique du Haut Moyen Age (V^e–VIIIe) siècles." *Annales de démographie historique* (1966): 37–55.

Riedinger, U. *Die Heilige Schrift im Kampf der griechischen Kirche gegen die Astrologie*. Innsbruck, 1956.

Rijkels, D. F. *Agnosis en Diagnosis, Over Pestilentiën in het Romeinse Keizerrijk*. Leiden, 2005.

Roberts, C. A. and A. Grauer. "Commentary: Bones, Bodies and Representativity in the Archaeological Record." *International Journal of Epidemiology* 30 (2001): 109–10.

Rochow, I. *Kaiser Konstantin V. (741–775)*. Berliner Byzantinistische Studien 1. Frankfurt, 1994.

Röhser, G. *Metaphorik und Personifikation der Sünde. Antike Sündenvorstellungen und paulinische Hamartia*. Wissenschaftliche Untersuchungen zum Neuen Testament II/25. Tübingen, 1987.

Rojas Rodríguez-Malo, J. M. and J. R. Villa González. "Consejería de Obras Públicas," in *Toledo: Arqueología en la ciudad*. Ed. F. J. Sánchez-Palencia. Toledo, 1996. pp. 225–37.

Rollason, D. W. "Why was St. Cuthbert so Popular?" in *Cuthbert, Saint and Patron*. Ed. D. W. Rollason. Durham, 1987.

Rose, L. J., R. Donlan, S. N. Banerjee, and M. J. Arduino. "Survival of *Yersinia pestis* on Environmental Surfaces." *Applied and Environmental Microbiology*, 69 (2003): 2166–71.

Rosenberg, C. E. *The Cholera Years: The United States in 1832, 1849, and 1866*. Chicago, 1962.

Rosenberg, C. E. *Explaining Epidemics and Other Studies in the History of Medicine*. Cambridge, 1992.

Rosqvist, R., M. Skurnik, and H. Wolf-Watz. "Increased Virulence of *Yersinia pseu-dotuberculosis* by Two Independent Mutations." *Nature* 334 (1988): 522–25.

Rothschild, N. C. "Note on the Species of Fleas Found upon Rats, *Mus rattus* and *Mus decumanus*, in Different Parts of the World, and on Some Variations in the Proportion of Each Species in Different Localities." *Journal of Hygiene* 6 (1906): 483–85.

Rouche, M. "Europe Accumulates its First Gains," in Fossier, *History of the Middle Ages*, 1:474–80.

Rouche, M. "Une révolution mentale du Haut Moyen Age: Loisir et travail," in *Horizons marins et itinéraires spirituels (Ve-XVIIIe siècles)*. Ed. H. Dubois, J.-C. Hocquet, and A. Vauchez. 2 vols. Paris, 1987. 1:233–37.

Rougé, J. "La navigation hivernale sous l'Empire romain." *Revue des études anciennes* 54 (1952): 316–25.

Rubin, B. *Das Zeitalter Justinians.* 2 vols. Berlin, 1960, 1995.

Ruddiman, W. F. "The Anthropogenic Greenhouse Era Began Thousands of Years Ago." *Climatic Change* 61 (2003): 261–93.

Russel, J. "The Archaeological Context of Magic in the Early Byzantine Period," in *Byzantine Magic.* Ed. H. Maguire. Washington, D.C., 1995. pp. 35–50.

Russell, J. C. *The Control of Late Ancient and Medieval Population.* Philadelphia, 1985.

Russell, J. C. "That Earlier Plague." *Demography* 5 (1968): 174–84.

Russell, J. C. "The Earlier Medieval Plague in the British Isles." *Viator* 7 (1976): 65–78.

Saint-Denis, E. de. "Mare clausum." *Revue des études latines* 25 (1947): 196–214.

Salinas de Frías, M. "El poblamiento rural antiguo de la provincia de Salamanca: Modelos e implicaciones históricas." *Studia Historica, Historia Antigua* 10–11 (1992–1993): 177–88.

Sallares, R. *The Ecology of the Ancient Greek World.* London, 1991.

Sallares, R. *Malaria and Rome: A History of Malaria in Ancient Italy.* Oxford, 2002.

Sallares, R. "Pathocoenoses Ancient and Modern." *History and Philosophy of the Life Sciences* 27.2 (2005): 221–40.

Sallares, R. and S. Gomzi. "Biomolecular Archaeology of Malaria." *Ancient Biomolecules* 3 (2001): 195–213.

Samama, E. "Thucydide et Procope: Le regard des historiens sur les épidémies," in *Air, Miasmes et Contagion: Les épidémies dans l'Antiquité et au Moyen Âge.* Ed. S. Bazin-Tacchella, D., Quéruel, and E. Samana. Langres, 2001. pp. 55–74.

Sarris, P., "Economy and Society in the Age of Justinian." Ph. D. dissertation, Oxford University, 1999.

Sarris, P. "The Justinianic Plague: Origins and Effects." *Continuity and Change* 17 (2002): 169–82.

Sawyer, P. H. *From Roman Britain to Norman England.* London, 1978.

Saxena, V. K. and T. Verghese. "Ecology of Flea-Transmitted Zoonotic Infection in Village Mamla, District Beed." *Current Science* 71 (1996): 800–2.

Scarborough, J. and A. Kazhdan. "Plague." *ODB* 3: 1681.

Scheidel, W. *Death on the Nile: Disease and the Demography of Roman Egypt.* Leiden, 2001.

Schliekelman, P., C. Garner, and M. Slatkin. "Natural Selection and Resistance to HIV." *Nature* 411 (2001): 545–46.

Schoten, E. J. "Joannes VI Cantacuzenus over de pest in Constantinopel." *Hermeneus* 51 (1979): 153–57.

Schubert, S., B. Picard, S., Gouriou, J. Heesemann, and E. Denamur. "*Yersinia* High-Pathogenicity Island Contributes to Virulence in *Escherichia coli* Causing Extraintestinal Infections." *Infection and Immunity* 70 (2002): 5335–37.

Scott, S. and C. J. Duncan. *Biology of Plagues. Evidence from Historical Populations.* Cambridge, 2001.

Seger, T. "The Plague of Justinian and Other Scourges: An Analysis of the Anomalies in the Development of the Iron Age Population in Finland." *Fornvännen* 77 (1982): 191–97.

Seibel, V. *Die grosse Pest zur Zeit Justinians I. und die ihr voraus und zur Seite gehenden ungewöhnlichen Natur-Ereignisse.* Dillingen, 1857.

Sendrail, M. *Histoire culturelle de la maladie.* Toulouse, 1980.

Serrano Ramos, E. and F. Alijo Hidalgo. "Una necrópolis de época hispano-visigoda en las eras de Peñarrubia (Málaga)," in *Actas del III congreso de arqueología medieval española, Oviedo, 1989.* Oviedo, 1992. 2: 110–20.

Seyberlich, R. "Die Judenpolitik Kaiser Justinians I," in *Byzantinistische Beiträge.* Ed. J. Irmscher. Berlin, 1964. pp. 73–80.

Sfikas, G. *Birds and Mammals of Crete.* Athens, 1994.

Shivaji, S., N. Vijaya Bhanu, and R. K. Aggarwal. "Identification of *Yersinia pestis* as the Causative Organism of Plague in India as Determined by 16S rDNA Sequencing and RAPD-Based Genomic Fingerprinting." *FEMS Microbiology Letters* 189 (2000): 247–52.

Shrewsbury, J. F. D. *A History of Bubonic Plague in the British Isles.* Cambridge, 1970.

Shrewsbury, J. F. D. "The Plague of the Philistines." *Journal of Hygiene* 47 (1949): 244–52.

Shrewsbury, J. F. D. *The Plague of the Philistines and Other Medical-Historical Essays.* London, 1964.

Shrewsbury, J. F. D. "The Yellow Plague." *Journal of the History of Medicine* 4 (1949): 5–47.

Sigerist, H. E. *Civilization and Disease.* Ithaca, 1943. Repr., Chicago, 1962.

Sigerist, H. E. "Sebastian – Apollo." *Archiv für Geschichte der Medizin* 29 (1927): 301–17.

Signoli, M. and O. Dutour. "Etude anthropologique d'un charnier de la grande peste de Marseille (1720–1722). Premiers résultats." *Anthropologie et préhistoire* 108 (1997): 147–58.

Signori, G. *Maria zwischen Kathedrale, Kloster und Welt. Hagiographische und historiographische Annäherung an eine hochmittelalterliche Wunderpredigt.* Sigmaringen, 1995.

Skurnik, M., A. Peippo, and E. Ervelä. "Characterization of the O-Antigen Gene Clusters of *Yersinia pseudotuberculosis* and the Cryptic O-Antigen Gene Cluster of *Yersinia pestis* Shows that the Plague Bacillus is Most Closely Related to and has Evolved from *Y. pseudotuberculosis* Serotype O:1b." *Molecular Microbiology* 37 (2000): 316–30.

Slack, P. "The Disappearance of Plague: An Alternative View." *Economic History Review*, n.s. 34 (1981): 469–76.

Slack, P. *The Impact of Plague in Tudor and Stuart England.* London, 1985.

Smith, F. B. *The Retreat of Tuberculosis, 1850–1950*. London, 1988.

Snowden, F. M. *Naples in the Time of Cholera, 1884–1911*. Cambridge, 1995.

Sodini, J.-P., G. Tate, B. Bavant, D. Orssaud, and J.-L. Biscop. "Déhes (Syrie du Nord): Recherches sur l'Habitat Rural." *Syria* 57 (1980): 1–305.

Sodini, J.-P. and E. Villeneuve. "Le passage de la céramique byzantine à la céramique omeyyade en Syrie du nord, en Palestine et en Transjordanie," in *La Syrie de Byzance à l'Islam*. Ed. P. Canivet and J.-P. Rey-Coquais. Damascus, 1992, 195–218.

Sontag, S. *AIDS and its Metaphors*. New York, 1989.

Soriano Sánchez, R., ed. *La arqueología cristiana en la ciudad de Valencia: De la leyenda a la realidad*. Quaderns de Difusió Arqueològica 1. Valencia, 1990.

Soriano Sánchez, R., ed. *Cripta arqueológica de la Cárcel de San Vicente*. Valencia, 1998.

Soriano Sánchez, R., ed. "Las excavaciones arqueológicas de la Cárcel de San Vicente (Valencia)." *Saguntum: Papeles del Laboratorio de Arqueología de Valencia* 27 (1994): 173–86.

Soriano Sánchez, R., ed. "Los restos arqueológicos de la sede episcopal valentina: Avance preliminar," in *IV Reunió d'arqueologia cristiana hispànica (Lisboa)*. Barcelona, 1995. pp. 133–40.

Sreevatsan, S., X. Pan, K. E. Stockbauer, N. D. Connell, B. N. Kreiswirth, T. S. Whittam, and J. M. Musser. "Restricted Structural Gene Polymorphism in the *Mycobacterium tuberculosis* Complex Indicates Evolutionarily Recent Global Dissemination." *PNAS* 94 (1997): 9869–74.

Stancliffe, C. "Cuthbert and the Polarity between Pastor and Solitary," in *St. Cuthbert, His Cult and His Community to AD 1200*. Ed. G. Bonner, D. Rollason, and C. Stancliffe. Woodbridge, UK, 1989. pp. 21–44.

Stannard, D. E. *Before the Horror: The Population of Hawai'i on the Eve of Western Contact*. Honolulu, 1989.

Stathakopoulos, D. *Famine and Pestilence in the Late Roman and Early Byzantine Empire: A Systematic Survey of Subsistence Crises and Epidemics*. Birmingham Byzantine and Ottoman Monographs. Aldershot, UK, 2004.

Stathakopoulos, D. "The Justinianic Plague Revisited." *Byzantine and Modern Greek Studies* 24 (2000): 256–76.

Stathakopoulos, D. "Die Terminologie der Pest in byzantinischen Quellen." *Jahrbuch der österreichischen Gesellschaft für Byzantinistik* 48 (1998): 1–7.

Stathakopoulos, D. "Travelling with the Plague," in *Travel in the Byzantine World*. Society for the Promotion of Byzantine Studies 10. Ed. R. Macrides. Aldershot, 2002. pp. 99–102.

Steel, D. "Plague Writing: From Boccaccio to Camus." *Journal of European Studies* 11 (1981): 88–110.

Stein, E. *Histoire du Bas-Empire*. 2 vols. Paris, 1949–59.

Stenton, F. M. *Anglo-Saxon England*. 3rd ed. Oxford, 1971.

Stephens, J. C., D. E. Reich, D. B. Goldstein, H. D. Shin, M. W. Smith, M. Carrington, C. Winkler et al. "Dating the Origin of the CCR5-D32 AIDS-Resistance Allele by the Coalescence of Haplotypes." *American Journal of Human Genetics* 62 (1998): 1507–15.

Sticker, G. *Abhandlungen aus der Seuchengeschichte und Seuchenlehre.* 1 *Die Pest.* Giessen, 1908.

Stoclet, A. J. "Entre Esculape et Marie: Paris, la peste et le pouvoir aux premiers temps du Moyen Age." *Revue Historique* 301 (1998): 691–746.

Stoclet, A. J. "From Baghdad to *Beowulf.* Eulogizing 'Imperial' Capitals East and West in the Mid-Eighth Century." Proceedings of the Royal Irish Academy 105C (2005): 151–95.

Stothers, R. B. "Mystery Cloud of AD 536." *Nature* 307 (1984): 344–45.

Stothers, R. B. "Volcanic Dry Fogs, Climate Cooling, and Plague Pandemics in Europe and the Middle East." *Climatic Change* 42 (1999): 713–23.

Sublet, J. "La peste prise aux rêts de la jurisprudence." *Studia Islamica* 33 (1971): 141–49.

Sudhoff, K. "Johanns von Tornamira '*Praeservatio et cura apostematum antrosorum pestilentialium*'." *Archiv für Geschichte der Medizin* 5 (1912): 46–53.

Sudhoff, K. "Ein Pestkonsilium Magister Bernhards von Frankfurt, 1381." *Archiv für Geschichte der Medizin* 9 (1915): 244–52.

Sudhoff, K. "Pestschriften aus den ersten 150 Jahren nach der Epidemie des 'Schwarzen Todes' 1348." *Archiv Für Geschichte der Medizin* 4–16 (1910–1925).

Tate, G. *Les Campagnes de la Syrie du Nord.* Paris, 1992.

Taylor, A. *William Cooper's Town. Power and Persuasion on the Frontier of the Early American Republic.* New York, 1996.

Taylor, C. *Village and Farmstead.* London, 1983.

Tchalenko, G. *Villages antiques de la Syrie du Nord: Le massif du Bélus à l'époque romaine.* 3 vols. Paris, 1953–58.

Teall, J. "The Barbarians in Justinian's Armies." *Speculum* 40 (1965): 294–322.

TED'A. *Els enterraments del Parc de la Ciutat i la problemàtica funerària de Tàrraco.* Tarragona, 1987.

Teh, W. L. "Plague in the Orient with Special Reference to the Manchurian Outbreaks." *Journal of Hygiene* 21 (1922/23): 62–76.

Teh, W. L. *A Treatise on Pneumonic Plague.* Geneva, 1926.

Teh, W. L., J. W. H. Chun, and R. Pollitzer. "Clinical Observations upon the Manchurian Plague Epidemic, 1920–21." *Journal of Hygiene* 21 (1922/23): 289–306.

Teh, W. L., J. W. H. Chun, and R. Pollitzer. "Observations Made during and after the Second Manchurian Plague Epidemic of 1920–21." *Journal of Hygiene* 21 (1922/23): 307–28.

Thacker, A. "Lindisfarne and the Origins of the Cult of St. Cuthbert," in *St Cuthbert, His Cult and His Community to AD 1200.* Ed. G. Bonner, D. Rollason, and C. Stancliffe. Woodbridge, 1989. pp. 103–22.

Thacker, A. "Monks, Preaching and Pastoral Care in Early Anglo-Saxon England," in *Pastoral Care before the Parish.* Ed. J. Blair and R. Sharpe. Leicester, 1992.

Thomas, C. *A Provisional List of Imported Pottery in Post-Roman Western Britain and Ireland.* Redruth, 1981.

Thomas, M., P. Gilbert, J. Cuccui, W. White, N. Lynnerup, R. W. Titball, A. Cooper, and M. B. Prentice. "Absence of *Yersinia pestis*-specific DNA in Human Teeth from Five European Excavations of Putative Plague Victims." *Microbiology* 150 (2004): 341–54.

Thompson, J. A. "On the Epidemiology of Plague." *Journal of Hygiene* 6 (1906): 537–69.

Thüry, G. E. *Müll und Marmorsäulen. Siedlungshygiene in der römischen Antike.* Mainz, 2001.

Thüry, G. E. "Zur Infektkette der Pest in hellenistisch-römischer Zeit," in *Festschrift 75 Jahre Anthropologische Staatssammlung München 1902–1977.* Munich, 1977. pp. 275–83.

Tomkins, S. "The Failure of Expertise: Public Health Policy in Britain during the 1918–19 Influenza Epidemic." *Social History of Medicine* 5 (1992): 435–54.

Treadgold, W. *A History of the Byzantine State and Society.* Stanford, 1997.

Tsafrir, Y. "The Greek Inscriptions," in *Excavations at Rehovot-in-the-Negev.* 1 *The Northern Church.* Qedem Monographs of the Institute of Archaeology 25. Jerusalem, 1988.

Tuchman, B. W. *A Distant Mirror: The Calamitous 14th Century.* New York, 1978.

Tucker, W. F. "Natural Disasters and the Peasantry in Mamluk Egypt." *Journal of the Economic and Social History of the Orient* 24 (1981): 215–24.

Turner, D. "The Politics of Despair: The Plague of 746–747 and Iconoclasm in the Byzantine Empire." *Annual of the British School at Athens* 85 (1990): 419–34.

Twigg, G. *The Black Death: A Biological Reappraisal.* London, 1984.

Twigg, G. "The Black Death in England: An Epidemiological Dilemma," in *Maladies et société (XIIᵉ–XVIIIᵉ siècles).* Actes du Colloque de Bielefeld. Ed. N. Bulst and R. Delort. Paris, 1989. pp. 75–98.

Twigg, G. "Bubonic Plague: Doubts and Diagnoses." *Journal of Medical Microbiology* 42 (1995): 383–85.

Twitchett, D. "Population and Pestilence in T'ang China," in *Studia Sino-Mongolica.* Ed. W. Bauer. Wiesbaden, 1979. pp. 35–68.

U.S. Food and Drug Administration. Center for Food Safety & Applied Nutrition. *Foodborne Pathogenic Microorganisms and Natural Toxins Handbook*, s.v. "*Yersinia enterocolitica*," online at http://vm.cfsan.fda.gov/~mow/chap5.html&isbol–0.

van Loghem, J. J. "The Plague of the 17th Century Compared with the Plague of Our Days." *Janus* 23 (1918): 95–107.

van Zwanenberg, D. "The Last Epidemic of Plague in England? Suffolk 1906–1918." *Medical History* 14 (1970): 63–74.

Vasiliev, A. "Medieval Ideas of the End of the World: West and East." *Byzantion* 16 (1942/43): 462–502.

Victoria County History. Oxfordshire 6. Oxford, 1956.

Villeneuve, F. "L'économie rurale et la vie des campagnes," in *Hauran I.* Ed. J.-M. Dentzer. Paris, 1985: pp. 63–136.

von Hagen, B. *Die Pest im Altertum.* Jena, 1939.

von Kremer, A. "Über die grossen Seuchen des Orients nach arabischen Quellen." *Sitzungsberichte der kaiserlichen Akademie der Wissenschaften, Philosophisch-historische Classe* 96 (1880): 69–156.

von Siebenthal, W. *Krankheit als Folge der Sünde.* Heilkunde und Geisteswelt 2. Hannover, 1950.

Waldron, H. A. "Are Plague Pits of Particular Use to Palaeoepidemiologists?" *International Journal of Epidemiology* 30 (2001): 104–8.

Walløe, L. "Was the Disruption of the Mycenaean World Caused by Repeated Epidemics of Bubonic Plague?" *Opuscula Atheniensia* 24 (1999): 121–26.

Walmsley, A. "Production, Exchange and Regional Trade in the Islamic East Mediterranean: Old Structures, New Systems?" in *The Long Eighth Century.* Ed. I. L. Hansen and C. Wickham. The Transformation of the Roman World 2. Leiden, 2000. pp. 264–343.

Ward-Perkins, B. "Land, Labour and Settlement," in *The Cambridge Ancient History.* Ed. Averil Cameron, B. Ward Perkins, and M. Whitby. Cambridge, 2000. 14: 315–45.

Watson, P. "Change in Foreign and Regional Economic Links with Pella in the seventh century AD: the Ceramic Evidence," in *La Syrie de Byzance à l'Islam.* Ed. P. Canivet and J.-P. Rey-Coquais. Damascus, 1992. pp. 233–47.

Watts, J. "Victims of Japan's Notorious Unit 731 Sue." *The Lancet* 360 (2002): 628.

Watts, S. *Epidemics and History: Disease, Power and Imperialism.* New Haven, 1997.

Watts, S. Review of J. N. Hays, *The Burdens of Disease: Epidemics and Human Response in Western History. Bulletin of the History of Medicine* 73 (1999): 491.

Weale, M. E., D. A. Weiss, R. F. Jager, N. Bradman, and M. G. Thomas. "Y Chromosome Evidence for Anglo-Saxon Mass Migration." *Molecular Biology and Evolution* 19 (2002): 1008–21.

Weekly Epidemiological Record, no. 33. August 13, 2004, p. 302.

Welch, M. *Anglo-Saxon England.* London, 1992.

West, S. *West Stow: The Anglo-Saxon Village.* East Anglian Archaeology Report 24. 2 vols. Ipswich, 1985.

Whitby, M. "John of Ephesus and the Pagans: Pagan Survivals in the Sixth Century," in *Paganism in the Late Roman Empire and in Byzantium.* Byzantina et Slavica Cracoviensia 1. Ed. M. Salamon. Cracow, 1991. pp. 111–31.

Whitby, M. "Recruitment in Roman Armies from Justinian to Heraclius," in *The Byzantine and Early Islamic Near East, III: States, Resources And Armies.* Ed. A. Cameron. Princeton, 1995. pp. 61–124.

White, K. A. "Pittsburgh in the Great Epidemic of 1918." *Western Pennsylvania Historical Magazine* 68 (1985): 221–42.

Whitehouse, D. See Hodges, R. and D. Whitehouse.

Whittow, M. *The Making of Orthodox Byzantium 600–1025.* London, 1996.

Whittow, M. "Ruling the Late Roman and Early Byzantine City: A Continuous History." *Past and Present* 129 (1990): 2–29.

Wickham, C. *Land and Power: Studies in Italian and European Social History, 400–1200.* London, 1994.

Wiechmann, I. and G. Grupe. "Detection of *Yersinia pestis* DNA in Two Early Medieval Skeletal Finds From Aschheim (Upper Bavaria, 6th Century A.D.)." *American Journal of Physical Anthropology* 126 (2005): 48–55.

Wilcocks, C. and P. E. C. Manson-Bahr. *Manson's Tropical Diseases.* 17th ed. London, 1972.

Williams, E. W. "The End of an Epoch." *Greece and Rome.* 2nd s. 9 (1962): 109–25.

Williams, E. W. "The Sickness at Athens." *Greece and Rome.* 2nd s. (1957): 98–103.

Wills, C. *Yellow Fever Black Goddess: The Coevolution of People and Plagues.* Reading, Mass., 1996.

Witakowski, W. *The Syriac Chronicle of Pseudo-Dionysius of Tel-Mahrē: A Study in the History of Historiography.* Uppsala, 1987.

Wood, I. *The Most Holy Abbot Ceolfrid.* Jarrow Lecture. 1995.

Wooding, J. M. *Communication and Commerce Along the Western Sea Lanes, AD 400–800.* British Archaeological Reports International Series 654. Oxford, 1996.

Woods, D. "Acorns, the Plague and the 'Iona Chronicle.'" *Peritia* 17–18 (2003–4): 495–502.

Wu, Lien-Teh. *A Treatise on Pneumonic Plague.* Paris, 1926.

Yvinec, J. H., P. Ponel, and J. C. Beaucournu. "Premiers apports archéoentomologiques de l'étude des Puces: Aspects historiques et anthropologiques (Siphonaptera)." *Bulletin de la Société entomologique de France* 105 (2000): 419–25.

Zeller, M. *Rochus: Die Pest und ihr Patron.* Nürnberg, 1989.

Zhou, D., Y. Han, Y. Song, Z. Tong, J. Wang, and Z. Guo. "DNA Microarray Analysis of Genome Dynamics in *Yersinia pestis*: Insights into Bacterial Genome Microevolution and Niche Adaptation." *Journal of Bacteriology* 186 (2004): 5138–46.

Zhou, D., Z. Tong, Y. Song, Y. Han, D. Pei, and X. Pang. "Genetics of Metabolic Variations between *Yersinia pestis* Biovars and the Proposal of a New Biovar, Microtus." *Journal of Bacteriology* 186 (2004): 5147–52.

Zhou, S., W. Deng, T. S. Anantharaman, A. Lim, E. T. Dimalanta, J. Wang, J. Wu et al. "A Whole-Genome Shotgun Optical Map of Yersinia pestis Strain KIM." *Applied and Environmental Microbiology* 68 (2002): 6321–31.

Ziegler, P. *The Black Death.* London, 1969.

Zimmermann, V. "Krankheit und Gesellschaft: Die Pest." *Sudhof's Archiv für Geschichte der Medizin* 72 (1988): pp. 1–13.

Zink, A. R., U. Reischl, H. Wolf, and A. G. Nerlich. "Molecular Analysis of Ancient Microbial Infections." *FEMS* [Federation of European Microbiological Societies] *Microbiology Letters* 213 (2002): 141–47.

Zupko, R. E. and R. A. Laures. *Straws in the Wind: Medieval Urban Environmental Law – the Case of Northern Italy.* Boulder, CO, 1996.

Index